2013
YEAR BOOK OF
VASCULAR SURGERY®

The 2013 Year Book Series

Year Book of Critical Care Medicine®: Drs Dries, Zanotti-Cavazzoni, Latenser, Martinez, Rincon, and Zwank

Year Book of Emergency Medicine®: Drs Hamilton, Bruno, Handly, Minczak, Quintana, and Ramoska

Year Book of Endocrinology®: Drs Schott, Apovian, Clarke, Eugster, Meikle, Oetgen, Ovalle, Schteingart, and Toth

Year Book of Hand and Upper Limb Surgery®: Drs Yao, Adams, Isaacs, and Rizzo

Year Book of Medicine®: Drs Barker, Garrick, Gersh, Khardori, LeRoith, Panush, Talley, and Thigpen

Year Book of Neonatal and Perinatal Medicine®: Drs Fanaroff, Benitz, Donn, Neu, Papile, and Van Marter

Year Book of Neurology and Neurosurgery®: Drs Klimo, Minagar, Gandhi, Liu, Panagariya, Rezania, Riel-Romero, Riesenburger, Robottom, Schwendimann, Shafazand, and Yang

Year Book of Obstetrics, Gynecology, and Women's Health®: Drs Dungan and Shulman

Year Book of Oncology®: Drs Arceci, Bauer, Chiorean, Gordon, Lawton, Murphy, Thigpen, and Tsao

Year Book of Ophthalmology®: Drs Rapuano, Cohen, Flanders, Hammersmith, Milman, Myers, Nagra, Nelson, Penne, Pyfer, Sergott, Shields, Talekar, and Vander

Year Book of Orthopedics®: Drs Morrey, Huddleston, Rose, Swiontkowski, and Trigg

Year Book of Otolaryngology-Head and Neck Surgery®: Drs Sindwani, Balough, Franco, Gapany, and Mitchell

Year Book of Pathology and Laboratory Medicine®: Drs Raab and Bissell

Year Book of Pediatrics®: Dr Stockman

Year Book of Plastic and Aesthetic Surgery™: Drs Miller, Boehmler, Gosman, Gutowski, Ruberg, Salisbury, and Smith

Year Book of Psychiatry and Applied Mental Health®: Drs Talbott, Ballenger, Buckley, Frances, Krupnick, and Mack

Year Book of Pulmonary Disease®: Drs Barker, Jones, Maurer, Spradley, Tanoue, and Willsie

Year Book of Sports Medicine®: Drs Shephard, Cantu, Feldman, Galea, Jankowski, Janssen, Lebrun, and Nieman

Year Book of Surgery®: Drs Behrns, Daly, Fahey, Hines, Howe, Huber, Klodell, Mozingo, and Pruett

Year Book of Urology®: Drs Andriole and Coplen

Year Book of Vascular Surgery®: Drs Gillespie, Bush, Passman, Starnes, and Watkins

2013

The Year Book of VASCULAR SURGERY®

Editor-in-Chief

David L. Gillespie, MD, RVT, FACS

*Professor of Surgery, Division of Vascular Surgery,
University of Rochester School of Medicine and Dentistry,
Rochester, New York*

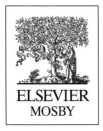

ELSEVIER
MOSBY

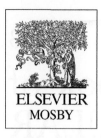

ELSEVIER
MOSBY

Senior Vice President, Content: Linda Belfus
Editor: Jessica McCool
Production Supervisor, Electronic Year Books: Donna M. Skelton
Electronic Article Manager: Mike Rainey
Illustrations and Permissions Coordinator: Dawn Vohsen

2013 EDITION

Composition by TNQ Books and Journals Pvt Ltd, India

Printed and bound by CPI Group (UK) Ltd, Croydon, CR0 4YY

Transferred to digital print 2012

Editorial Office:
Elsevier
Suite 1800
1600 John F. Kennedy Blvd.
Philadelphia, PA 19103-2899

International Standard Serial Number: 0749-4041
International Standard Book Number: 978-1-4557-7293-3

Associate Editors

Ruth L. Bush, MD, MPH
Professor of Surgery and Interim Vice Dean, Bryan/College Station Campus, Texas A&M Health Science Center College of Medicine, Bryan, Texas

Marc A. Passman, MD
Professor of Surgery, Section of Vascular Surgery and Endovascular Therapy, University of Alabama at Birmingham, Birmingham, Alabama

Benjamin W. Starnes, MD
Professor of Surgery and Chief, Division of Vascular Surgery; University of Washington, Seattle, Washington

Michael T. Watkins, MD
Associate Professor of Surgery, Harvard Medical School; Director, Vascular Surgery Research Laboratory, Massachusetts General Hospital, Boston, Massachusetts

Contributors

James H. Black, III, MD, FACS
Bertram M. Bernheim, MD Associate Professor of Surgery, Division of Vascular Surgery and Endovascular Therapy, Johns Hopkins Hospital, Baltimore, Maryland

Matthew A. Corriere, MD, MS
Assistant Professor, Department of Vascular and Endovascular Surgery, Wake Forest University School of Medicine, Winston-Salem, North Carolina

John P. Cullen, PhD
Research Associate Professor of Surgery, Division of Vascular Surgery, University of Rochester School of Medicine and Dentistry, Rochester, New York

Kakra Hughes, MD
Director of Endovascular Surgery, Howard University Hospital, Assistant Professor of Surgery, Howard University School of Medicine, Washington, DC

Brian G. Peterson, MD, FACS
Associate Professor of Surgery, Division of Vascular Surgery, Saint Louis University Health Sciences Center; Chief, Vascular Surgery Division, St. Anthony's Medical Center, St Louis, Missouri

Joseph D. Raffetto, MD, FACS, FSVM
Assistant Professor of Surgery, Harvard Medical School, Brigham and Women's Hospital; Chief, Vascular Surgery Division, VA Boston Healthcare System, West Roxbury, Massachusetts

Table of Contents

Journals Represented

Journals represented in this YEAR BOOK are listed below.

AJR American Journal of Roentgenology
American Journal of Cardiology
American Journal of Pathology
American Surgeon
Annals of Surgery
Annals of Vascular Surgery
Archives of Surgery
British Journal of Surgery
Cardiovascular and Interventional Radiological
Circulation
European Journal of Radiology
European Journal of Vascular and Endovascular Surgery
Eye
Journal of Cardiothoracic and Vascular Anesthesia
Journal of Stroke and Cerebrovascular Diseases
Journal of Surgical Research
Journal of the American College of Cardiology
Journal of the American College of Surgeons
Journal of the American Medical Association
Journal of Thoracic and Cardiovascular Surgery
Journal of Vascular and Interventional Radiology
Journal of Vascular Surgery
Nephrology Dialysis Transplantation
Seminars In Interventional Radiology
Stroke
Surgery

STANDARD ABBREVIATIONS

The following terms are abbreviated in this edition: acquired immunodeficiency syndrome (AIDS), cardiopulmonary resuscitation (CPR), central nervous system (CNS), cerebrospinal fluid (CSF), computed tomography (CT), deoxyribonucleic acid (DNA), electrocardiography (ECG), health maintenance organization (HMO), human immunodeficiency virus (HIV), intensive care unit (ICU), intramuscular (IM), intravenous (IV), magnetic resonance (MR) imaging (MRI), ribonucleic acid (RNA), and ultrasound (US).

NOTE

The YEAR BOOK OF VASCULAR SURGERY® is a literature survey service providing abstracts of articles published in the professional literature. Every effort is made to assure the accuracy of the information presented in these pages. Neither the editors nor the publisher of the YEAR BOOK OF VASCULAR SURGERY® can be responsible for errors in the original materials. The editors' comments are their own opinions. Mention of specific products within this publication does not constitute endorsement.

To facilitate the use of the YEAR BOOK OF VASCULAR SURGERY® as a reference tool, all illustrations and tables included in this publication are now identified as they appear in the original article. This change is meant to help the reader recognize that any illustration or table appearing in the YEAR BOOK OF VASCULAR SURGERY® may be only one of many in the original article. For this reason, figure and table numbers will often appear to be out of sequence within the YEAR BOOK OF VASCULAR SURGERY®.

1 Basic Considerations

Skeletal Muscle Adaptation in Response to Supervised Exercise Training for Intermittent Claudication
Beckitt TA, Day J, Morgan M, et al (Bristol Royal Infirmary, UK)
Eur J Vasc Endovasc Surg 44:313-317, 2012

Objectives.—There is evidence that the improvement following supervised exercise for claudication results from skeletal muscle adaptation. The myosin heavy chain (MHC) determines muscle fibre type and therefore efficiency. Immunohistochemical analysis has failed to take account of hybrid MHC expression within myofibres. This study sought evidence of differential MHC protein expression following supervised exercise for claudication.

Design.—38 claudicants were recruited. Subjects undertook a three-month supervised exercise programme. Controls were patients awaiting angioplasty for claudication.

Materials and Methods.—Subjects underwent paired gastrocnemius biopsy. Relative expression of MHC proteins was determined by SDS-PAGE electrophoresis. Non-parametric data is presented as median with the inter-quartile range and parametric as the mean ± standard deviation.

Results.—Upon completion of the exercise programme there was a 94% increase (124 (106−145) to 241 (193−265) metres, $p = 0.002$) in maximum walking distance, which was not evident in the control group. An 11.1% ($p = 0.02$) increase in MHC I expression was observed in the exercise but not the control group (34.3% ± 6.8 to 45.4% ± 4.4). There was a positive correlation between the change in MHC I expression and the improvement in claudication distance ($r = 0.69$, $p < 0.05$).

Conclusions.—Supervised exercise training for claudication results in an increase in the proportion of MHC type I expression within the symptomatic gastrocnemius muscle.

▶ As vascular surgeons, we advocate for structured exercise programs before moving forward with arterial intervention. The mechanism for walking distance improvement has been postulated as more efficient oxygen extraction or hypertrophy or angiogenesis (or really any combination thereof). The authors elegantly show solid evidence for the increased expression of myosin-heavy chain I protein (MHC I) in the patients' gastrocnemius muscles. The authors further propose that exercise may be a potent stimulator for local skeletal muscle adaptation, and the local muscle event may be the key event in symptomatic improvement in claudicants. What is most interesting to contemplate in the article is what occurs in the control group—those who were awaiting angioplasty and had no discernible change in MHC I protein. In such patients, improvement in circulation if an angioplasty was to be done would not be expected to deliver an improvement in walking distance if the skeletal muscle adaptation had not occurred. Indeed, could this be the explanation of the failure of iliac revascularization in the CLEVER trial to show a difference in walking distance?

J. Black, MD

The Relative Position of Paired Valves at Venous Junctions Suggests Their Role in Modulating Three-dimensional Flow Pattern in Veins
Lurie F, Kistner RL (Univ of Hawaii, Honolulu)
Eur J Vasc Endovasc Surg 44:337-340, 2012

Purpose.—The aim of the study is to investigate the relative position of orifices of two valves within the most proximal segments of the great saphenous vein (GSV), and the femoral vein (FV).

Methods.—A total of 15 volunteers with no signs or symptoms of venous disease and 13 unaffected limbs of patients with unilateral primary chronic venous disease (CVD) were included. Two most proximal valves of the GSV and the FV were identified. The angle between the two valves, and the distance between the valves were measured.

Results.—The mean distance between the two valves in the GSV was 3.8 ± 0.4 cm, and in the FV was 4.6 ± 0.3 cm. In one limb, the distance between the FV valves was 1 cm less than GSV valves, and in two limbs the distances were equal. In the remaining 12 limbs available for comparison, the valves in the FV were 1-2 cm further apart compared to the GSV ($P = 0.002$, paired t-test). All studied pairs of valves were positioned at a minimum 60° angle to each other. The mean angle between the two valves was 84.3 ± 8.4° in the GSV, and 88.3 ± 6.7° in the FV ($P = 0.24$). The angle between the two valves correlated with the distance between the valves ($r = 0.68$, $P = 0.000005$). No significant relations were found between the diameter of the studied vein, and the angle between the two valves. There was no difference in valve orientation between volunteers and unaffected limbs of the patients with CVD.

Conclusion.—When two valves are present in the areas of venous junctions, they consistently positioned at a significant angle to each other. A hypothesis that venous valves at the junctions increase efficiency of venous return by creating a helical flow pattern can be postulated and deserves further investigation.

▶ Although a 3-dimensional helical or spiral flow pattern has been identified in normal arteries, its existence in veins has not been previously described. In this interesting anatomic study, a pattern related to angle and distance between paired valves in the proximal great saphenous and femoral vein segments is described. Although the significance of this pattern is unknown, the authors postulate that a natural 3-dimensional helical or spiral flow pattern could be created by this anatomic orientation, thereby augmenting venous flow. While additional confirmatory work is still needed to better define the physiologic significance, this study also raises the possible question of what happens when this 3-dimensional flow pattern is dysfunctional. There may also be future implications in how to better restore this flow pattern with operations directed at valve reconstruction or potential technology related to artificial venous valves.

M. A. Passman, MD

Dietary Nitrate Supplementation Improves Revascularization in Chronic Ischemia
Hendgen-Cotta UB, Luedike P, Totzeck M, et al (Univ Hosp Düsseldorf, Germany; et al)
Circulation 126:1983-1992, 2012

Background.—Revascularization is an adaptive repair mechanism that restores blood flow to undersupplied ischemic tissue. Nitric oxide plays an important role in this process. Whether dietary nitrate, serially reduced to nitrite by commensal bacteria in the oral cavity and subsequently to nitric oxide and other nitrogen oxides, enhances ischemia-induced remodeling of the vascular network is not known.

Methods and Results.—Mice were treated with either nitrate (1 g/L sodium nitrate in drinking water) or sodium chloride (control) for 14 days. At day 7, unilateral hind-limb surgery with excision of the left femoral artery was conducted. Blood flow was determined by laser Doppler. Capillary density, myoblast apoptosis, mobilization of CD34$^+$/Flk-1$^+$, migration of bone marrow—derived CD31$^+$/CD45$^-$, plasma S-nitrosothiols, nitrite, and skeletal tissue cGMP levels were assessed. Enhanced green fluorescence protein transgenic mice were used for bone marrow transplantation. Dietary nitrate increased plasma S-nitrosothiols and nitrite, enhanced revascularization, increased mobilization of CD34$^+$/Flk-1$^+$ and migration of bone marrow—derived CD31$^+$/CD45$^-$ cells to the site of ischemia, and attenuated apoptosis of potentially regenerative myoblasts in chronically ischemic tissue. The regenerative effects of nitrate treatment were abolished by eradication of the nitrate-reducing bacteria in the oral cavity through the use of an antiseptic mouthwash.

Conclusions.—Long-term dietary nitrate supplementation may represent a novel nutrition-based strategy to enhance ischemia-induced revascularization (Figs 1, 4-6).

▶ This study uses an animal model to provide detailed insight into mechanistic relationships between dietary nitrate supplementation and extremity perfusion, apoptosis, and mobilization and migration of endothelium-regenerating CD34$^+$/Flk-1$^+$ cells (Figs 1, 4-6). The use of control animals treated with antibacterial mouthwash also generated valuable pharmacokinetic information with potential to inform development of in-human therapeutic interventions. It is interesting to note that an equivalent level of nitrate supplementation to that used in

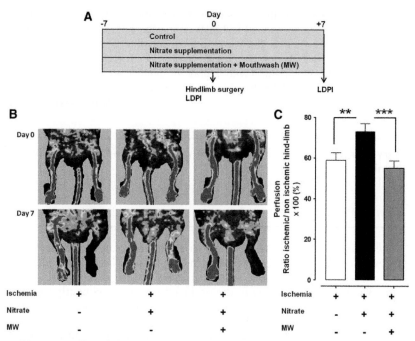

FIGURE 1.—Effect of dietary nitrate supplementation on perfusion recovery. **A,** Experimental protocol. **B,** Original laser Doppler perfusion images (LDPIs) display hind-limb perfusion before and 7 days after excision of the femoral artery. Mice receiving nitrate (middle row) show increased perfusion compared with control animals (left row). Mice receiving antiseptic mouthwash (MW) did not exhibit the nitrate-induced gain of perfusion (right row). **C,** Nitrate-supplemented mice showed increased perfusion recovery in chronic hind-limb ischemia (black bars; $P < 0.02$); this effect was not observed in mice receiving antiseptic mouthwash (gray bars; $P < 0.02$). Data are expressed as mean $\pm$ SEM (n = 21−23). (Reprinted from Hendgen-Cotta UB, Luedike P, Totzeck M, et al. Dietary nitrate supplementation improves revascularization in chronic ischemia. *Circulation.* 2012;126:1983-1992, © 2012, American Heart Association, Inc.)

these experiments is attainable through dietary intake in humans (described by the authors as consistent with rich vegetable intake). Because the observed beneficial effects appeared to be dependent on oral nitrate-reducing bacteria, nitrate supplementation may be most beneficial in the setting of chronic ischemia. Because the experimental model utilized involved a period of ischemia lasting one week, it remains to be seen whether this model is consistent with chronic (as described in the title) or acute ischemia in humans. Further investigation will also be necessary to determine whether the observed effects on secondary endpoints are accompanied by significant impact on limb salvage or functional outcomes.

M. A. Corriere, MD, MS

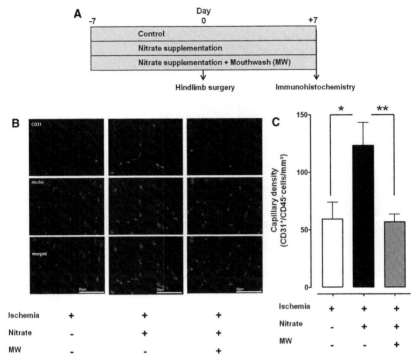

FIGURE 4.—Effect of dietary nitrate on revascularization. **A,** Experimental protocol. **B,** Representative original micrographs of hind-limb sections show amounts of endothelial cells per 1 mm^2. Dietary nitrate—treated mice show higher numbers of CD31$^+$/CD45$^-$ cells 7 days after hind-limb surgery, whereas the mice receiving mouthwash (MW) did not exhibit this effect. Top row micrographs show CD31$^+$/CD45$^-$-stained cells (red); middle row, DAPI-stained nuclei (blue); bottom row, double-stained (merged) cells indicating endothelial cells. **C,** Quantitative analysis of capillary density displayed as CD31$^+$/CD45$^-$-stained cells per 1 mm^2 hind limb. Bars show higher capillary density in dietary nitrate—supplemented mice at day 7 (black bars; $P = 0.045$). Treatment with an antiseptic mouthwash did not exhibit the nitrate-mediated increase in capillary density (gray bars; $P < 0.02$). Data are expressed as mean ± SEM (n=6). For Interpretation of the references to color in this figure legend, the reader is referred to web version of this article. (Reprinted from Hendgen-Cotta UB, Luedike P, Totzeck M, et al. Dietary nitrate supplementation improves revascularization in chronic ischemia. *Circulation.* 2012;126:1983-1992, © 2012, American Heart Association, Inc.)

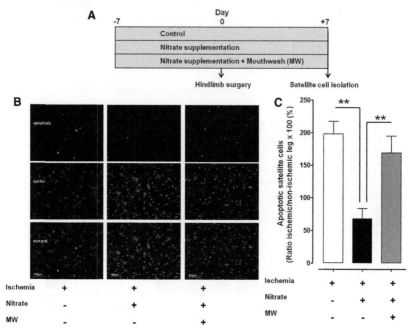

FIGURE 5.—Effect of dietary nitrate on apoptosis in myoblasts. A, Experimental protocol. B, Terminal deoxynucleotidyl transferase dUTP nick-end labeling (TUNEL) staining of isolated myoblasts demonstrating lower amounts of apoptotic cells in mice receiving dietary nitrate supplementation (middle) compared with those receiving control treatment (left) or antiseptic mouthwash (MW; right). Top row micrographs show TUNEL-positive nuclei indicating apoptotic cells (green); middle row, DAPI-positive cells indicating nuclei (blue); bottom, double-stained cells (merged) indicating apoptotic cells. C, Quantitative analysis of TUNEL-stained myoblasts per hind limb displayed as the ratio between ischemic and nonischemic hind limb and expressed as percent. Bars show significantly decreased apoptosis in mice supplemented with dietary nitrate (black bar). Mice without dietary nitrate supplementation (white bar; $P < 0.001$) or with antiseptic mouthwash (gray bar; $P < 0.02$) did not show nitrate-mediated regenerative effects. Data are expressed as mean ± SEM (n=9–11). For Interpretation of the references to color in this figure legend, the reader is referred to web version of this article. (Reprinted from Hendgen-Cotta UB, Luedike P, Totzeck M, et al. Dietary nitrate supplementation improves revascularization in chronic ischemia. *Circulation.* 2012;126:1983-1992, © 2012, American Heart Association, Inc.)

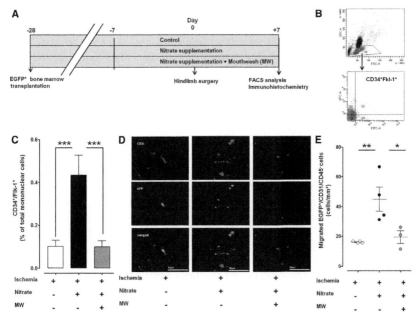

FIGURE 6.—Impact of dietary nitrate on mobilization and migration of endothelium-regenerating cells. **A,** Experimental protocol. **B,** Exemplary flow cytometric analysis shows the total mononuclear cells in peripheral blood analyzed at day 7 after the onset of hind-limb ischemia. The gated population displays isolated blood cells, stained with FITC rat anti-mouse CD34 and APC rat anti-mouse Flk-1. **B** and **C,** The amount of CD34⁺/Flk-1⁺ cells was higher in the nitrate-treated group compared with those receiving standard drinking water ($P < 0.001$). Antiseptic mouthwash (MW) did not show this effect and distinctly prevented accumulation of CD34⁺/Flk-1⁺ cells despite nitrate supplementation ($P < 0.01$; n=7–10). **D,** Representative original micrographs of hind-limb sections show amounts of enhanced green fluorescence protein–positive (EGFP⁺)/CD31⁺/CD45⁻ cells per 1 mm². Mice receiving dietary nitrate showed an increased migration of EGFP⁺/CD31⁺/CD45⁻ cells 7 days after hind-limb surgery (middle) compared with mice receiving the mouthwash procedure (right). **E,** Bars show significantly increased EGFP⁺/CD31⁺/CD45⁻ cell migration in mice supplemented with dietary nitrate at day 7 (black bars; $P = 0.029$), whereas antiseptic mouthwash–treated mice displayed a markedly attenuated nitrate-mediated increase in EGFP⁺/CD31⁺/CD45⁻ cell migration in chronic hind-limb ischemia (gray bars; $P = 0.034$; n=3–4). Data are expressed as mean ± SEM. FACS indicates fluorescence-activated cell sorting. (Reprinted from Hendgen-Cotta UB, Luedike P, Totzeck M, et al. Dietary nitrate supplementation improves revascularization in chronic ischemia. *Circulation.* 2012;126:1983-1992, © 2012, American Heart Association, Inc.)

Carotid Endarterectomy in Asymptomatic Patients With Limited Life Expectancy

Wallaert JB, De Martino RR, Finlayson SRG, et al (Dartmouth-Hitchcock Med Ctr, Lebanon NH; et al)
Stroke 43:1781-1787, 2012

Background and Purpose.—Data from randomized trials assert that asymptomatic patients undergoing carotid endarterectomy (CEA) must live 3 to 5 years to realize the benefit of surgery. We examined how commonly CEA is performed among asymptomatic patients with limited life expectancy.

Methods.—Within the American College of Surgeons National Quality Improvement Project we identified 8 conditions associated with limited life expectancy based on survival estimates using external sources. We then compared rates of 30-day stroke, death, and myocardial infarction after CEA between asymptomatic patients with and without life-limiting conditions.

Results.—Of 12 631 CEAs performed in asymptomatic patients, 2525 (20.0%) were in patients with life-limiting conditions or diagnoses. The most common conditions were severe chronic obstructive pulmonary disease and American Society of Anesthesiologists Class IV designation. Patients with life-limiting conditions had significantly higher rates of perioperative complications, including stroke (1.8% versus 0.9%, $P < 0.001$), death (1.4% versus 0.3%, $P < 0.001$), and stroke/death (2.9% versus 1.1%, $P < 0.001$). Even after adjustment for other comorbidities, patients with life-limiting conditions were nearly 3 times more likely to experience perioperative stroke or death than those without these conditions (OR, 2.8; 95% CI, 2.1–3.8; $P < 0.001$).

Conclusion.—CEA is performed commonly in asymptomatic patients with life-limiting conditions. Given the high rates of postoperative stroke/death in these patients as well as their limited life expectancy, the net benefit of CEA in this population remains uncertain. Health policy research examining the role of CEA in asymptomatic patients with life-limiting conditions is necessary and may serve as a potential source for significant healthcare savings in the future.

▶ This article addresses important and controversial issues in the treatment of patients with carotid artery occlusive disease. The article's title reflects both issues: 1, Whether to offer carotid revascularization in the form of endarterectomy (CEA) to patients with asymptomatic disease and, whether to offer CEA to patients with a limited life expectancy. Both of these issues are important in the decision-making process for patients with carotid disease. This study addresses these issues by looking at a large validated national dataset—the American College of Surgeons National Surgical Quality Improvement Project. I do disagree with the first statement of the introduction: that evidence supporting CEA on asymptomatic patients is well-established. Many recent articles question or flat-out refute this previously held dogma in this era of modern and improved medical management. Studies are being designed or are underway to reevaluate CEA versus medical management in the asymptomatic patient. Even more disturbing is that 20% of the patients treated in the American College of Surgeons National Surgical Quality Improvement Program had documentation of limited life expectancy. However, this percentage is difficult to interpret given some of the conditions labeled as indicative of shortened life expectancy, such as chronic obstructive pulmonary disease, may vary in actual severity among individuals.

The patients in this dataset who underwent CEA with a life-threatening condition or diagnosis had a 1.4% stroke and death rate and for the patients older than 80 years of age, 2.2%. Because these patients have a limited life expectancy as determined by congestive heart failure, disseminated cancer, or the like, why subject them to an unnecessary risk of stroke or death from a CEA? As the authors stated in their discussion, these patients need to live long enough to realize the benefits of a prophylactic CEA. Surgeons need to examine their personal biases concerning CEA in the asymptomatic patient, take a critical look at current literature, peruse the patient's chart and history, and then individualize treatment for their patient.

R. L. Bush, MD, MPH

2 Epidemiology

Regional Disparities in Incidence, Handling and Outcomes of Patients with Symptomatic and Ruptured Abdominal Aortic Aneurysms in Norway
Brattheim BJ, Eikemo TA, Altreuther M, et al (Sør-Trøndelag Univ College (HiST), Trondheim, Norway; Norwegian Univ of Science and Technology (NTNU), Trondheim, Norway; Univ Hosp of Trondheim, Norway)
Eur J Vasc Endovasc Surg 44:267-272, 2012

Objectives.—To study incidence, handling and outcome of patients hospitalised with symptomatic and ruptured abdominal aortic aneurysm in Norway.

Design, Material and Methods.—Retrospective study of 1291 patients, between January 2008 and August 2010 using the National Patient Registry and a regional vascular surgery registry. We applied a stepwise logistic regression model to detect differences in regional in-hospital mortality.

Results.—385/711 (54%) patients hospitalised for aneurysm rupture, rAAA (ICD-10: I71.3), died. The odds of dying varied with a factor 2.3 between the extreme regions. 475/711 (67%) underwent repair, 323 survived, giving an in-hospital mortality rate of 32% after surgery. Older patients were significantly less likely to be transported for surgery. The overall incidence for patients aged >50 was 16.6 rAAA per 100 000 person-years. There was remarkable variation across counties with rates between 7.7 and 26.8. A total of 580 patients were hospitalised with suspected symptomatic aneurysms (ICD-10:I71.4, acute admission); 224 (39%) were treated with aneurysm repair, 356 (61%) were discharged without repair without a significant difference across health regions.

Conclusions.—For rAAA, we found substantial geographical variations in incidence, surgery and patient outcome. These results highlight the need for increased awareness about the condition and suggest ways to improve care trajectories to reduce delay to surgery, thereby minimising rupture mortality (Fig 2, Table 2).

▶ Have you ever had a feeling that certain geographies within your own region of practice have higher incidences of different types of vascular disease, whether it be infrainguinal disease in farming communities or diabetes in areas of depressed economic status?

These authors from Norway looked at the incidence, handling, and outcomes of patients presenting with symptomatic and ruptured abdominal aortic aneurysms from 1291 patients in a Norwegian National Patient Registry. Most of the patients with rupture were treated with open surgery, so the mortality rate was high.

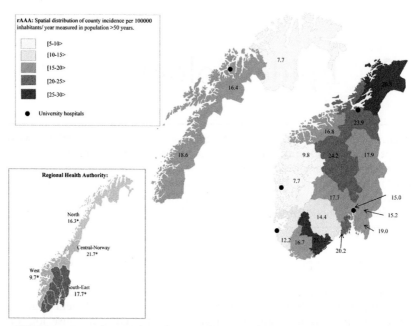

FIGURE 2.—Geographic variation in the reported incidence of ruptured AAA (rAAA) by county *Incidence rates by Regional Health Authority. All incidence rates calculated over population age ≥50 per 100 000 person-years, standardized to 2009 population (according to patient's county of residence). (Reprinted from European Journal of Vascular and Endovascular Surgery. Brattheim BJ, Eikemo TA, Altreuther M, et al. Regional disparities in incidence, handling and outcomes of patients with symptomatic and ruptured abdominal aortic aneurysms in Norway. *Eur J Vasc Endovasc Surg.* 2012;44:267-272, Copyright 2012, with permission from European Society for Vascular Surgery.)

TABLE 2.—Ruptured AAA (rAAA) In-Hospital Mortality Odds Ratios: Health Regional Disparities ($N = 711$)

Variables	Model 1 Odds Ratio	(95% CI)	Model 2 Odds Ratio	(95% CI)	Model 3 Odds Ratio	(95% CI)
Regional Health Authority						
North	1		1		1	
South-East	**2.11**	**(1.25–3.55)**	**2.13**	**(1.22–3.73)**	**2.28**	**(1.15–4.52)**
West	1.81	(0.95–3.45)	1.69	(0.85–3.37)	2.16	(0.96–4.86)
Central-Norway	**2.28**	**(1.27–4.10)**	**2.07**	**(1.09–3.90)**	1.37	(0.61–3.06)
Demographics						
Men			1.00	(0.69–1.46)	1.43	(0.90–2.27)
Age <70			1		1	
Age 70–79			**3.26**	**(2.03–5.22)**	**3.25**	**(1.86–5.66)**
Age >79			**9.70**	**(6.01–15.68)**	**6.11**	**(3.46–10.79)**
Surgery						
Surgical rate					1	
No surgery					**33.3**	**(16.7–50.0)**
−2LL[a](chi-square test)	973.8 (p < 0.000)		858.6 (p < 0.000)		647.3 (p < 0.000)	

Model 1: logistic regression on Regional Health Authority, Model 2: including demographic data, Model 3: including surgery.
Note: Significant estimates shown in bold.
[a]Log-Likelihood.

Interestingly, when regions of Norway were considered, the odds of dying after surgery were 2.28 times higher in central Norway compared with the odds for northern Norway (Table 2).

The incidence of ruptured abdominal aortic aneurysm also varied significantly (Fig 2) among regions, suggesting a potential favorable impact of screening programs in those areas most affected by higher prevalence of disease. I believe this article should serve as a model for targeted health care delivery and resource utilization.

B. W. Starnes, MD

No increased mortality with early aortic aneurysm disease
Mell M, on behalf of the Stanford Abdominal Aortic Aneurysm Specialized Center of Clinically Oriented Research (SCCOR) Investigators (Stanford Univ, CA)
J Vasc Surg 56:1246-1251, 2012

Objective.—In addition to increased risks for aneurysm-related death, previous studies have determined that all-cause mortality in abdominal aortic aneurysm (AAA) patients is excessive and equivalent to that associated with coronary heart disease. These studies largely preceded the current era of coronary heart disease risk factor management, however, and no recent study has examined contemporary mortality associated with early AAA disease (aneurysm diameter between 3 and 5 cm). As part of an ongoing natural history study of AAA, we report the mortality risk associated with presence of early disease.

Methods.—Participants were recruited from three distinct health care systems in Northern California between 2006 and 2011. Aneurysm diameter, demographic information, comorbidities, medication history, and plasma for biomarker analysis were collected at study entry. Survival status was determined at follow-up. Data were analyzed with t-tests or χ^2 tests where appropriate. Freedom from death was calculated via Cox proportional hazards modeling; the relevance of individual predictors on mortality was determined by log-rank test.

Results.—The study enrolled 634 AAA patients; age 76.4 ± 8.0 years, aortic diameter 3.86 ± 0.7 cm. Participants were mostly male (88.8%), not current smokers (81.6%), and taking statins (76.7%). Mean follow-up

---

TABLE 3.—Survival Comparison

Time period	Observed Cohort[a] (95% CI)	Estimate of Cohort[b] (95% CI)
1 year	98.2% (96.8%-99.0%)	93.8% (93.5%-94.1%)
2 years	95.8% (93.7%-97.2%)	87.6% (87.0%-88.2%)
3 years	90.9% (87.0%-93.7%)	81.5% (80.6%-82.4%)

CI, Confidence interval.
[a]Kaplan-Meier method.
[b]Estimate based on 2006 National Vital Statistics and adjusted for age, gender, and ethnicity.

was 2.1 ± 1.0 years. Estimated 1- and 3-year survival was 98.2% and 90.9%, respectively. Factors independently associated with mortality included larger aneurysm size (hazard ratio, 2.12; 95% confidence interval, 1.26-3.57 for diameter >4.0 cm) and diabetes (hazard ratio, 2.24; 95% confidence interval, 1.12-4.47). After adjusting for patient-level factors, health care system independently predicted mortality.

Conclusions.—Contemporary all-cause mortality for patients with early AAA disease is lower than that previously reported. Further research is warranted to determine important factors that contribute to improved survival in early AAA disease (Table 3).

▶ This is the first prospective US study of its kind in the era of cardiovascular risk management to report all-cause mortality for patients with small abdominal aortic aneurysms (AAAs). The authors have shown that patients with small AAAs can achieve comparable survival to that of the population at large (Table 3). This is a finding that certainly challenges some of the earlier studies that suggested that patients with small AAAs had a higher all-cause mortality compared with those without an AAA. In fact, prospective studies have shown that individuals with an AAA greater than 3.0 cm in diameter have a 2-fold increase in 5-year mortality compared with controls (65.1 vs 32.8 deaths per 1000 person-years).[1,2]

The authors attribute at least some of their results to a lower rate of smoking and higher rates of statin use in California. The authors also interestingly identified differing mortality rates between different health care systems within the same region, suggesting that institutional factors may also contribute to survival in early AAA disease.

B. W. Starnes, MD

References

1. Forsdahl SH, Solberg S, Singh K, Jacobsen BK. Abdominal aortic aneurysms, or a relatively large diameter of non-aneurysmal aortas, increase total and cardiovascular mortality: the Tromsø study. *Int J Epidemiol.* 2010;39:225-232.
2. Newman AB, Arnold AM, Burke GL, O'Leary DH, Manolio TA. Cardiovascular disease and mortality in older adults with small abdominal aortic aneurysms detected by ultrasonography: the cardiovascular health study. *Ann Intern Med.* 2001;134:182-190.

Racial Differences in Risks for First Cardiovascular Events and Noncardiovascular Death: The Atherosclerosis Risk in Communities Study, the Cardiovascular Health Study, and the Multi-Ethnic Study of Atherosclerosis

Feinstein M, Ning H, Kang J, et al (Northwestern Univ, Chicago, IL; et al)
Circulation 126:50-59, 2012

Background.—No studies have compared first cardiovascular disease (CVD) events and non-CVD death between races in a competing risks framework, which examines risks for numerous events simultaneously.

Methods and Results.—We used competing Cox models to estimate hazards for first CVD events and non-CVD death within and between races in 3 multicenter, National Heart, Lung, and Blood Institute—sponsored cohorts. Of 14 569 Atherosclerosis Risk in Communities (ARIC) study participants aged 45 to 64 years with mean follow-up of 10.5 years, 11.6% had CVD and 5.0% had non-CVD death as first events; among 4237 Cardiovascular Health Study (CHS) study participants aged 65 to 84 years and followed for 8.5 years, these figures were 43.2% and 15.7%, respectively. Middle-aged blacks were significantly more likely than whites to experience any CVD as a first event; this disparity disappeared by older adulthood and after adjustment for CVD risk factors. The pattern of results was similar for Multi-Ethnic Study of Atherosclerosis (MESA) participants. Traditional Cox and competing risks models yielded different results for coronary heart disease risk. Black men appeared somewhat more likely than white men to experience coronary heart disease with use of a standard Cox model (hazard ratio 1.06; 95% CI 0.90, 1.26), whereas they appeared less likely than white men to have a first coronary heart disease event with use of a competing risks model (hazard ratio, 0.77; 95% CI, 0.60, 1.00).

Conclusions.—CVD affects blacks at an earlier age than whites; this may be attributable in part to elevated CVD risk factor levels among blacks. Racial disparities in first CVD incidence disappear by older adulthood. Competing risks analyses may yield somewhat different results than traditional Cox models and provide a complementary approach to examining risks for first CVD events.

▶ Racial disparity research has rapidly proliferated in the clinical research realm. Indeed, a standard literature search on PubMed in 2012 demonstrated logarithmic growth in the subject since just 2000. Although in many medical circles, disparity research has become synonymous with access (like primary care and later oncologic diagnosis), the scope of disparity research for cardiovascular disease (CVD) is more complex and involves access, acuity, and diagnosis concurrently. This article demonstrates that health disparity research into CVD can be greatly altered by including the risks for non-CVD death that compete with CVD death simultaneously. Indeed, when such methodology is applied, the early onset disparate risk for CVD in blacks vs whites disappears, yet for both, CVD was a first event. Similarly, racial disparity, even in standard Cox model comparisons, disappears with aging when competing risks are coexamined. In effect, a competing risk model provides a more accurate real-time assessment of first CVD for patients and their doctors to consider.

J. Black, MD

Effect of a Single, Oral, High-dose Vitamin D Supplementation on Endothelial Function in Patients with Peripheral Arterial Disease: A Randomised Controlled Pilot Study

Stricker H, Tosi Bianda F, Guidicelli-Nicolosi S, et al (Ospedale La Carità, Locarno, Switzerland; et al)
Eur J Vasc Endovasc Surg 44:307-312, 2012

Objective.—Apart from its role in bone metabolism, vitamin D may also influence cardiovascular disease. The objective of this study was: (1) to determine the effect of a single, oral, high-dose vitamin D supplementation on endothelial function and arterial stiffness in patients with peripheral arterial disease (PAD) and (2) to investigate the impact of this supplementation on coagulation and inflammation parameters.

Methods.—In this double-blind, placebo-controlled, interventional pilot study, we screened 76 Caucasian patients with PAD for vitamin D deficiency. Sixty-two were randomised to receive a single, oral supplementation of 100 000 IU vitamin D3 or placebo. At baseline and after 1 month, we measured serum vitamin D and parathormone levels, and surrogate parameters for cardiovascular disease.

Results.—Sixty-five of 76 patients (86%) had low 25-hydroxyvitamin D levels (<30 ng ml^{-1}); of those, 62 agreed to participate in the study. At baseline, only parathormone was related to vitamin D. In supplemented patients, vitamin D levels increased from 16.3 ± 6.7 to 24.3 ± 6.2 ng ml^{-1} ($P < 0.001$), with wide variations between single patients; in the placebo group vitamin levels did not change. Seasonal factors accounted for a decrease of vitamin D levels by 8 ng ml^{-1} between summer and winter. After 1 month, none of the measured parameters was influenced by vitamin substitution.

Conclusion.—In this pilot study, most patients with PAD were vitamin D deficient. Vitamin D supplementation increased serum 25-hydroxyvitamin D without influencing endothelial function, arterial stiffness, coagulation and inflammation parameters, although the study was underpowered for definite conclusions.

▶ This study identified an 86% prevalence of vitamin D deficiency in a small group of patients with peripheral arterial disease (PAD). In this randomized, placebo-controlled pilot study, vitamin D supplementation was not associated with significant effects on arterial stiffness, endothelial function, microcirculation, inflammation, or coagulation parameters. Normal vitamin D levels were achieved in less than 20% of participants randomly assigned to supplementation with significant variation in individual responses, however, suggesting that an alternative dosing or administration protocol might be considered for future studies. When it comes to medical management and risk factor reduction for patients with PAD, vitamin D supplementation is not a part of the routine checklist for most practitioners. These results do not imply that vitamin D supplementation will reduce cardiovascular events or mortality, but the high prevalence of vitamin D deficiency in this study suggests that screening might be worthwhile in patients with PAD for overall health maintenance and prevention of associated skeletal complications.

M. A. Corriere, MD, MS

Prognostic Usefulness of Clinical and Subclinical Peripheral Arterial Disease in Men With Stable Coronary Heart Disease
Bouisset F, Bongard V, Ruidavets J-B, et al (Toulouse Rangueil Univ Hosp, France; Université de Toulouse III, France)
Am J Cardiol 110:197-202, 2012

The prognostic value of symptomatic peripheral arterial disease (PAD) in patients with coronary heart disease (CHD) is well documented, but few reports differentiating between symptomatic and asymptomatic forms of PAD are available. We investigated the respective prognostic effect of clinical and subclinical PAD on long-term all-cause mortality in patients with stable CHD. We analyzed 710 patients with stable CHD referred for hospitalization for CHD evaluation and management. As a part of the study, they completed questionnaires on medical history, underwent a standardized clinical examination, including ankle-brachial index (ABI) measurement, and provided a fasting blood sample. Three groups of patients were individualized: no PAD (no history of PAD and ABI > 0.9 but ≤1.4); subclinical PAD (no history of PAD but abnormal ABI [i.e., ≤0.9 or >1.4); and clinical PAD (history of claudication, peripheral arterial surgery, or amputation due to PAD). Clinical and subclinical PAD was present in 83 (11.7%) and 181 (25.5%) patients, respectively.

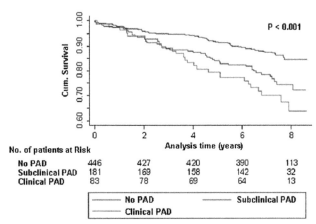

FIGURE.—Kaplan-Meier survival estimates according to absence (*blue line*) or presence of subclinical PAD (*red line*) or clinical PAD (*green line*). For Interpretation of the references to color in this figure legend, the reader is referred to web version of this article. (Reprinted from the American Journal of Cardiology. Bouisset F, Bongard V, Ruidavets J-B, et al. Prognostic usefulness of clinical and subclinical peripheral arterial disease in men with stable coronary heart disease. *Am J Cardiol.* 2012;110:197-202, Copyright 2012, with permission from Elsevier.)

After a median follow-up of 7.2 years, 130 patients died. On multivariate analysis adjusted for age, hypertension, diabetes, dyslipidemia, smoking, left ventricular ejection fraction, CHD duration, heart rate, history of stroke or transient ischemic attack, and coronary revascularization, previous clinical PAD (hazard ratio 2.11, 95% confidence interval 1.28 to 3.47) and subclinical PAD (hazard ratio 1.65, 95% confidence interval 1.11 to 2.44) were significantly associated with increased all-cause mortality. In conclusion, our study has demonstrated that the detection of subclinical PAD by ABI in patients with stable CHD provides additional information for long-term mortality risk evaluation (Fig).

▶ Peripheral arterial disease (PAD) is known to carry significant risk, and indeed its mere presence is considered a coronary equivalent to recommend the initiation of aggressive medical therapies for antiplatelet agents and low-density lipoprotein targeting. These authors open our eyes to the occurrence of asymptomatic PAD in the population of patients with overt coronary artery disease (CAD). Although close to 40% of CAD patients have PAD based on their ankle-brachial index criteria, nearly 70% are asymptomatic from their PAD. Their long-term survival is far worse than those without PAD and approximates those with symptomatic PAD (Fig). As vascular surgeons, we should look at those patients as residing in the sweet spot for strengthened vascular care. In such patients, ultrasound screening for abdominal aortic aneurysm and carotid disease may lend greatly toward improving their survival. Ignorance to PAD issues among cardiologists managing CAD will not be blissful, and educational outreach may shift the tide to demonstrate the benefit of multidisciplinary cooperative patient care teams for all facets of cardiovascular disease.

J. Black, MD

An integrated biochemical prediction model of all-cause mortality in patients undergoing lower extremity bypass surgery for advanced peripheral artery disease
Owens CD, Kim JM, Hevelone ND, et al (Univ of California, San Francisco; Brigham and Women's Hosp, Boston, MA)
J Vasc Surg 56:686-695, 2012

Background.—Patients with advanced peripheral artery disease (PAD) have a high prevalence of cardiovascular (CV) risk factors and shortened life expectancy. However, CV risk factors poorly predict midterm (<5 years) mortality in this population. This study tested the hypothesis that baseline biochemical parameters would add clinically meaningful predictive information in patients undergoing lower extremity bypass operations.

Methods.—This was a prospective cohort study of patients with clinically advanced PAD undergoing lower extremity bypass surgery. The Cox proportional hazard model was used to assess the main outcome of all-cause mortality. A clinical model was constructed with known CV risk factors, and the incremental value of the addition of clinical chemistry, lipid

Malnutrition (albumin < 3.5mg/dl)   Renal impairment (eGFR <60 ml/min)

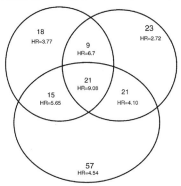

Inflammation (hsCRP> 5mg/L)

FIGURE 2.—A Venn diagram demonstrates the overlap among subsets of patients with malnutrition, renal impairment, and inflammation and shows the synergism of different mechanisms for the hazard ratio (*HR*) of death. Of 225 patients in this study, 74 (33%) had an estimated glomerular filtration rate (*eGFR*) <60 mL/min/1.73 m², 63 (28%) had an albumin concentration of <3.5 mg/dL, and 80 (36%) had high-sensitivity C-reactive protein (*hs*CRP) concentration of >5.0 mg/L. The 21 patients (9%) located within the intersection of all three circles have an HR for death of 9.08. (Reprinted from the Journal of Vascular Surgery. Owens CD, Kim JM, Hevelone ND, et al. An integrated biochemical prediction model of all-cause mortality in patients undergoing lower extremity bypass surgery for advanced peripheral artery disease. *J Vasc Surg*. 2012;56:686-695, Copyright 2012, with permission from The Society for Vascular Surgery.)

assessment, and a panel of 11 inflammatory parameters was investigated using the C statistic, the integrated discrimination improvement index, and Akaike information criterion.

Results.—The study monitored 225 patients for a median of 893 days (interquartile range, 539-1315 days). In this study, 50 patients (22.22%) died during the follow-up period. By life-table analysis (expressed as percent surviving ± standard error), survival at 1, 2, 3, 4, and 5 years, respectively, was 90.5% ± 1.9%, 83.4% ± 2.5%, 77.5% ± 3.1%, 71.0% ± 3.8%, and 65.3% ± 6.5%. Compared with survivors, decedents were older, diabetic, had extant coronary artery disease, and were more likely to present with critical limb ischemia as their indication for bypass surgery ($P < .05$). After adjustment for the above, clinical chemistry and inflammatory parameters significant (hazard ratio [95% confidence interval]) for all-cause mortality were albumin (0.43 [0.26-0.71]; $P = .001$), estimated glomerular filtration rate (0.98 [0.97-0.99]; $P = .023$), high-sensitivity C-reactive protein (hsCRP; 3.21 [1.21-8.55]; $P = .019$), and soluble vascular cell adhesion molecule (1.74 [1.04-2.91]; $P = .034$). Of the inflammatory molecules investigated, hsCRP proved most robust and representative of the integrated inflammatory response. Albumin, eGFR, and hsCRP improved the C statistic and integrated discrimination improvement index beyond that of the clinical model and produced a final C statistic of 0.82.

Conclusions.—A risk prediction model including traditional risk factors and parameters of inflammation, renal function, and nutrition had excellent discriminatory ability in predicting all-cause mortality in patients with clinically advanced PAD undergoing bypass surgery (Fig 2).

▶ Identification of widely available biomarkers that would predict mortality among patients with advanced peripheral arterial disease (PAD) is an attractive concept, particularly if an intervention to affect the pathophysiology identified by a laboratory test can potentially improve survival. The biochemical prediction modeling for this study combined clinical factors with standard chemistry and lipid biomarker data (widely obtainable for the average health care provider) as well as a panel of relatively exotic inflammatory biomarkers representing the coagulation and fibrinolytic system, soluble adhesion molecules and receptors, and inflammatory cytokines and pentaxins. The median follow-up of 893 days is reasonably long given the exceptionally high mortality rates associated with critical limb ischemia, which was the preoperative diagnosis for 59% of the study population. Interestingly, the only inflammatory biomarker included in the final Cox proportional hazard mortality model was high-sensitivity C-reactive protein, which contributed a smaller relative increase in discriminatory risk classification than the albumin or epidermal growth factor receptor. The results of this sophisticated and well-designed study, therefore, leave us with a predictive model that includes a number of commonly accepted clinical and laboratory risk factors plus a single inflammatory biomarker, none of which are readily modifiable. The study does, however, identify an alarming synergy between inflammation, renal failure, and malnutrition (Fig 2); patients with all 3 of these factors had a mortality hazard ratio of 9.08 (95% confidence interval, 4.85–17.01).

The authors suggest that identification of a high-risk patient may encourage the health care practitioner to choose an endovascular approach over bypass, but it is likely that many of the participants in this nonrandomized study were considered for endovascular management but underwent bypass in the absence of a durable or technically advisable endovascular alternative. Because bypass in the setting of advanced PAD is undertaken for symptomatic relief or limb salvage rather than midterm mortality reduction, many high-risk patients may receive significant benefit from revascularization despite significant midterm mortality. Although direct translation of these results into clinical practice modifications or changes in patient selection likely to impact mortality is, therefore, challenging, several interesting hypotheses are raised regarding potential benefits of anti-inflammatory, nutritional, and resistive training (none of which are currently considered routine components of cardiovascular risk reduction in PAD).

M. A. Corriere, MD, MS

3 Vascular Laboratory and Imaging

Isokinetic Strength and Endurance in Proximal and Distal Muscles in Patients With Peripheral Artery Disease
Câmara LC, Ritti-Dias RM, Menêses AL, et al (Univ of São Paulo, Brazil; Univ of Pernambuco, Brazil)
Ann Vasc Surg 26:1114-1119, 2012

Background.—The objective of this study was to analyze the muscle strength and endurance of the proximal and distal lower-extremity muscles in peripheral artery disease (PAD) patients.

Methods.—Twenty patients with bilateral PAD with symptoms of intermittent claudication and nine control subjects without PAD were included in the study, comprising 40 and 18 legs, respectively. All subjects performed an isokinetic muscle test to evaluate the muscle strength and endurance of the proximal (knee extension and knee flexion movements) and distal (plantar flexion and dorsiflexion movements) muscle groups in the lower extremity.

Results.—Compared with the control group, the PAD group presented lower muscle strength in knee flexion (-14.0%), dorsiflexion (-26.0%), and plantar flexion (-21.2%) movements $(P < 0.05)$ but similar strength in knee extension movements $(P > 0.05)$. The PAD patients presented a 13.5% lower knee flexion/extension strength ratio compared with the control subjects $(P < 0.05)$, as well as lower muscle endurance in dorsiflexion (-28.1%) and plantar flexion (-17.0%) movements $(P < 0.05)$. The muscle endurance in knee flexion and knee extension movements was similar between PAD patients and the control subjects $(P > 0.05)$.

Conclusion.—PAD patients present lower proximal and distal muscle strength and lower distal muscle endurance than control patients. Therefore, interventions to improve muscle strength and endurance should be prescribed for PAD patients.

▶ Historically, clinical research involving peripheral artery disease has centered on hemodynamic successes and direct imaging of the vascular territory. Indeed, rigorous reporting standards have emerged from the Society for Vascular Surgery that have solidified the primacy of data-driven examination. As we now enter the era of cost effectiveness, truly patient-centered outcomes will clearly assail the paradigm of ankle-brachial index, restenosis criteria, and other numerical estimates. In this context, this small study by Câmara et al enlightens a more functional, patient-centric assessment. The novelty of the study is reflected in the overall weakness of the claudicant vs control—reflecting deconditioning as a central event of our patients. Secondly, there exists an imbalance of anterior and posterior muscle groups, thus yielding a risk for falls. If we desire to improve our patients, Câmara et al suggest we consider the interface of muscle function as we do for vessel anatomy.

J. Black, MD

Maximal Venous Outflow Velocity: An Index for Iliac Vein Obstruction
Jones TM, Cassada DC, Heidel RE, et al (Univ of Tennessee Med Ctr, Knoxville)
Ann Vasc Surg 26:1106-1113, 2012

Leg swelling is a common cause for vascular surgical evaluation, and iliocaval obstruction due to May–Thurner syndrome (MTS) can be difficult to diagnose. Physical examination and planar radiographic imaging give anatomic information but may miss the fundamental pathophysiology of MTS. Similarly, duplex ultrasonographic examination of the legs gives little information about central impedance of venous return above the inguinal ligament. We have modified the technique of duplex ultrasonography to evaluate the flow characteristics of the leg after tourniquet-induced venous engorgement, with the objective of revealing iliocaval obstruction characteristic of MTS. Twelve patients with signs and symptoms of MTS were compared with healthy control subjects for duplex-derived maximal venous outflow velocity (MVOV) after tourniquet-induced venous engorgement of the leg. The data for healthy control subjects were obtained from a previous study of asymptomatic volunteers using the same MVOV maneuvers. The tourniquet-induced venous engorgement mimics that caused during vigorous exercise. A right-to-left ratio of MVOV was generated for patient comparisons. Patients with clinical evidence of MTS had a mean right-to-left MVOV ratio of 2.0, asymptomatic control subjects had a mean ratio of 1.3, and MTS patients who had undergone endovascular treatment had a poststent mean ratio of 1.2 ($P = 0.011$). Interestingly, computed tomography and magnetic resonance imaging results, when available, were interpreted as positive in only 53% of the patients with MTS according to both our MVOV criteria and confirmatory venography. After intervention, the right-to-left MVOV ratio in the MTS patients was found to be reduced similar to asymptomatic control subjects, indicating a relief of central venous obstruction by stenting the compressive MTS anatomy. Duplex-derived MVOV measurements are helpful for detection of iliocaval venous obstruction, such as MTS. Right-to-left MVOV ratios and postengorgement spectral analysis are helpful adjuncts to duplex imaging for leg swelling. The MVOV maneuvers are well tolerated by patients and yields physiological data regarding central venous obstruction that computed tomography and magnetic resonance imaging fail to detect.

▶ Iliofemoral venous obstruction can be difficult to diagnose with noninvasive testing. Although duplex ultrasound scan is readily available and effective in evaluating venous valve function in the legs, direct insonation of the iliocaval junction can be difficult related to body habitus and bowel gas pattern. Duplex-derived maximum venous outflow velocity (MVOV) is generated by inducing venous engorgement in the leg with a cuff inflated to 140 mm Hg for 2 minutes, having the patient take a deep breath and momentarily hold, followed by simultaneous rapid deflation and forced expiration during which velocity curve in the femoral vein is recorded. In this study, right-to-left MVOV ratios seem to be a reasonably reliable indirect marker for left iliac vein compression from May-Thurner syndrome. Adding this measurement to standard venous duplex examination should be considered, especially in those patients with a high index of suspicion, as well as for identifying patients who may have concomitant iliac vein compression and venous reflux.

M. A. Passman, MD

4 Perioperative Considerations

Greater saphenous vein evaluation from computed tomography angiography as a potential alternative to conventional ultrasonography

Johnston WF, West JK, Lapar DJ, et al (Univ of Virginia, Charlottesville)

J Vasc Surg 56:1331-1337.e1, 2012

Objective.—Autologous greater saphenous vein (GSV) graft is frequently used as a conduit during arterial bypass. Preoperative vein mapping has been traditionally used to assess conduit adequacy and define GSV anatomy, thereby decreasing operative time and reducing wound complications. The purpose of this study was to determine whether GSV mapping using computed tomography angiography (CTA) closely correlated with that of traditional duplex ultrasonography (US).

Methods.—From August 2009 through June 2011, 88 limbs from 51 patients underwent CTA of the lower extremities for the purpose of defining arterial anatomy with concurrent US for preoperative vein mapping. GSV diameters were measured by two blinded reviewers on CTA (both antero-posterior [AP] and lateral dimensions) and compared with US-based measurements at levels of the proximal thigh, mid-thigh, knee, mid-calf, and ankle. CTA and US measurements were compared at each anatomic level using linear regression. Statistical analysis was performed using SPSS software. Charge reduction was calculated based on technical and professional fees for each imaging study.

Results.—GSV diameter sequentially decreased from the proximal thigh to the mid-calf and then increased to the ankle as measured by CTA and US. CTA-based measurements of the GSV significantly correlated with US GSV diameters ($R = 0.927$ [lateral dimension], 0.922 [AP dimension]; $P < .005$). The strongest degree of correlation occurred in measurements at the proximal thigh, followed by the mid-thigh, mid-calf, knee, and ankle. GSV measurement by CTA was over 90% sensitive and accurate for detecting appropriate GSV diameter for bypass (diameter > 2.0 mm). Eliminating preoperative US vein mapping for the study patients at our institution would have resulted in charge reductions of $49,316 over the study period.

Conclusions.—Indirect venography by CTA correlates well with US for GSV mapping in the lower extremity and offers significant reduction in imaging-related preoperative charges. CTA is sensitive and accurate for detecting GSVs that are appropriate for bypass. Furthermore, CTA allows

AP and lateral evaluation of the GSV throughout its anatomic course. As CTA is often performed prior to arterial bypass, indirect evaluation of the GSV using preoperative CTA should be considered a promising alternative to the use of US.

▶ Successful lower extremity autogenous bypass grafting is dependent on adequate quality of the autogenous conduit. Duplex ultrasound scan is frequently used for vein mapping to assess greater saphenous vein quality. The expanded use of computed tomography (CT) angiography to evaluate lower extremity atherosclerotic occlusive disease and operative planning are opportunities for additional evaluation of greater saphenous vein adequacy. This study shows that indirect venography by CT angiography correlates well with ultrasound mapping. This free look at the greater saphenous vein should offer opportunity to limit duplex ultrasound scan to selective patients if there is unclear imaging based on poor venous phase timing of the CT angiogram and to patients who may need additional mapping for alternative autogenous conduit, thereby decreasing added cost of care.

M. A. Passman, MD

Common Carotid Intima-Media Thickness Measurements in Cardiovascular Risk Prediction: A Meta-analysis
Den Ruijter HM, Peters SAE, Anderson TJ, et al (Univ Med Ctr Utrecht, the Netherlands; Univ of Calgary, Alberta, Canada; et al)
JAMA 308:796-803, 2012

Context.—The evidence that measurement of the common carotid intima-media thickness (CIMT) improves the risk scores in prediction of the absolute risk of cardiovascular events is inconsistent.

Objective.—To determine whether common CIMT has added value in 10-year risk prediction of first-time myocardial infarctions or strokes, above that of the Framingham Risk Score.

Data Sources.—Relevant studies were identified through literature searches of databases (PubMed from 1950 to June 2012 and EMBASE from 1980 to June 2012) and expert opinion.

Study Selection.—Studies were included if participants were drawn from the general population, common CIMT was measured at baseline, and individuals were followed up for first-time myocardial infarction or stroke.

Data Extraction.—Individual data were combined into 1 data set and an individual participant data meta-analysis was performed on individuals without existing cardiovascular disease.

Results.—We included 14 population-based cohorts contributing data for 45 828 individuals. During a median follow-up of 11 years, 4007 first-time myocardial infarctions or strokes occurred. We first refitted the risk factors of the Framingham Risk Score and then extended the model with common CIMT measurements to estimate the absolute 10-year risks to develop a first-time myocardial infarction or stroke in both models. The C statistic of both models was similar (0.757; 95% CI, 0.749-0.764; and 0.759; 95% CI, 0.752-0.766). The net reclassification improvement with the addition of common CIMT was small (0.8%; 95% CI, 0.1%-1.6%). In those at intermediate risk, the net reclassification improvement was 3.6% in all individuals (95% CI, 2.7%-4.6%) and no differences between men and women.

Conclusion.—The addition of common CIMT measurements to the Framingham Risk Score was associated with small improvement in 10-year risk prediction of first-time myocardial infarction or stroke, but this improvement is unlikely to be of clinical importance.

▶ This is an interesting meta-analysis of high-quality studies performed to assess the value of the addition of routine common carotid intima-media thickness (CIMT) screening for cardiovascular (CV) risk prediction. Finding the ideal surrogate marker and risk prediction scoring system for the development of CV disease is crucial to prevent future adverse CV events. However, several elaborate scoring systems combined with ultrasound examination of CIMT or measurement of ankle-brachial indices to determine presence or absence of peripheral arterial disease have limitations. Furthermore, the addition of imaging adds expense. So the major question still exists: what is the best way to assess an individual's CV risk in order to maximize his or her health benefits and for vascular surgeons to prepare the patient for a major procedure without unanticipated outcomes?

This analysis specifically looked at studies adding common CIMT to Framingham risk scores and assessed the utility of doing so. The reclassification of a person's risk with the addition of common CIMT was not widespread among the more than 45 000 individuals studied. The conclusion is that this additional data point (common CIMT) should not be routinely gathered as it adds no clinical importance to risk prediction. Furthermore, as someone who has performed CIMT measurements, I find article is timely as the measurement takes a significant amount of time for a vascular technician to perform, but the question remains as to which area of the carotid artery should be used for risk prediction. Also, there is currently no third-party reimbursement for doing these studies. In these days of health care cost-consciousness, it is refreshing to have a study that informs practitioners that there is actually a test that is of limited utility that should not be routinely done.

R. L. Bush, MD, MPH

5 Grafts and Graft Complications

Systematic review and meta-analysis of vein cuffs for below-knee synthetic bypass
Twine CP, Williams IM, Fligelstone LJ (Morriston Hosp, Swansea, UK; Univ Hosp of Wales, Cardiff, UK)
Br J Surg 99:1195-1202, 2012

Background.—The aim was to investigate the possible benefit of vein cuffs for femoral to below-knee popliteal and femorodistal vessel synthetic bypass grafts.

Methods.—PubMed, the Cochrane library, Embase and ClinicalTrials.gov were searched for all studies on any clinical effect of vein cuffs on synthetic grafts. Outcomes were selected based on inclusion in two or more studies: primary patency and limb survival. The data were subjected to meta-analysis by outcome.

Results.—Three cohort and two randomized studies were selected for inclusion, involving 885 patients. Meta-analysis of five studies examining below-knee popliteal bypass showed a significant improvement for primary patency in cuffed grafts at 2 years, but not at 1 or 3 years (odds ratio at 2 years 0·46, 95 per cent confidence interval 0·22 to 0·97; $P = 0·04$). Limb salvage was significantly improved in cuffed grafts up to 2 years. Limb survival was also improved for cuffed distal grafts at 2 years (odds ratio 0·29, 0·11 to 0·75; $P = 0·01$) but showed no difference at any other time interval. Study quality was generally poor, with conflicting results.

Conclusion.—There was a small but significant benefit for vein cuffs on synthetic grafts used for femoral to below-knee popliteal anastomoses, but little benefit for femorodistal anastomoses (Fig 4).

▶ Meta-analyses critically depend on the quality of the available evidence to answer the study hypothesis. Unfortunately, meta-analyses are most commonly employed to comingle study populations from heterogeneous patient profiles, noncontemporary timeframes, and nonrandomized patient allocations. Simply put, they are "garbage in, garbage out" (or at least "clean garbage"). This study used the meta-analysis technique to determine the benefit of vein cuffs for below-knee revascularization. To the authors' credit, only randomized patient groups and cohort studies were used, yet when the SCIAMOS cohort trial (which refuted the utility of cuffs and also carried 41% of the weight of the

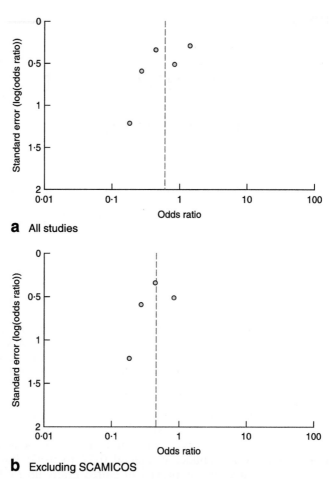

a All studies

b Excluding SCAMICOS

FIGURE 4.—Funnel plots for below-knee popliteal bypass primary patency at 1 year: **a** all studies ($I^2 = 66$ per cent, $P = 0.02$) and **b** excluding the Scandinavian Miller Collar Study (SCAMICOS) ($I^2 = 0$ per cent, $P = 0.43$). (Reprinted from Twine CP, Williams IM, Fligelstone LJ. Systematic review and meta-analysis of vein cuffs for below-knee synthetic bypass. *Br J Surg.* 2012;99:1195-1202, © 2012, British Journal of Surgery Society Ltd. Reproduced with permission. Permission is granted by John Wiley & Sons Ltd on behalf of the BJSS Ltd.)

population) was revealed to markedly increase the heterogeneity of conclusions favoring cuffs, it was excluded (Fig 4). The final conclusion seems delicate but sensible: vein cuffs can help with femoropopliteal anastomoses but remain unproven for femorodistal targets. As a surgeon, I admit to not changing my practice because of this study, knowing the answer will always be beyond us because a properly powered randomized controlled trial of vein cuffs on tibial targets is not in vogue during this endovascular era.

J. Black, MD

Vein graft neointimal hyperplasia is exacerbated by CXCR4 signaling in vein graft-extrinsic cells

Zhang L, Brian L, Freedman NJ (Duke Univ Med Ctr, Durham, NC)

J Vasc Surg 56:1390-1397, 2012

Objective.—Because vein graft neointimal hyperplasia engenders vein graft failure, and because most vein graft neointimal cells derive from outside the vein graft, we sought to determine whether vein graft neointimal hyperplasia is affected by activity of the CXC chemokine receptor-4 (CXCR4), which is important for bone marrow-derived cell migration.

Methods.—In congenic $Cxcr4^{-/+}$ and wild-type (WT) recipient mice, we performed interposition grafting of the common carotid artery with the inferior vena cava (IVC) of either $Cxcr4^{-/+}$ or WT mice to create four surgically chimeric groups of mice (n ≥ 5 each), characterized by vein graft donor/recipient: WT/WT; $Cxcr4^{-/+}$/WT; WT/$Cxcr4^{-/+}$; and $Cxcr4^{-/+}$/$Cxcr4^{-/+}$; vein grafts were harvested 6 weeks postoperatively.

Results.—The agonist for CXCR4 is expressed by cells in the arterializing vein graft. Vein graft neointimal hyperplasia was reduced by reducing CXCR4 activity in vein graft-extrinsic cells, but not in vein graft-intrinsic cells: the rank order of neointimal hyperplasia was WT/WT ≈ $Cxcr4^{-/+}$/WT > WT/$Cxcr4^{-/+}$ ≈ $Cxcr4^{-/+}$/$Cxcr4^{-/+}$; CXCR4 deficiency in graft-extrinsic cells reduced neointimal hyperplasia by 39% to 47% ($P < .05$). Vein graft medial area was equivalent in all grafts except $Cxcr4^{-/+}$/$Cxcr4^{-/+}$, in which the medial area was 60% ± 20% greater ($P < .05$). Vein graft re-endothelialization was indistinguishable among all three vein graft groups. However, the prevalence of medial leukocytes was 40% ± 10% lower in $Cxcr4^{-/+}$/$Cxcr4^{-/+}$ than in WT/WT vein grafts ($P < .05$), and the prevalence of smooth muscle actin-positive cells was 45% ± 20% higher ($P < .05$).

Conclusions.—We conclude that CXCR4 contributes to vein graft neointimal hyperplasia through mechanisms that alter homing to the vein graft of graft-extrinsic cells, particularly leukocytes.

Clinical Relevance.—The utility of autologous vein grafts is severely reduced by neointimal hyperplasia, which accelerates subsequent graft atherosclerosis. Our study demonstrates that vein graft neointimal hyperplasia is aggravated by activity of the cell-surface "CXC" chemokine receptor-4 (CXCR4), which is critical for recruitment of bone marrow-derived cells to sites of inflammation. Our model for CXCR4 deficiency used mice with heterozygous deficiency of $Cxcr4$. Consequently, our results suggest the possibility that a CXCR4 antagonist—like plerixafor, currently in clinical use—could be applied to vein grafts periadventitially, and perhaps achieve beneficial effects on vein graft neointimal hyperplasia.

▶ Saphenous vein grafts remain the most commonly used conduit for arterial bypass surgery but are associated with poor long-term patency rates: approximately 28% fail within 1 year of surgery and approximately 75% are either occluded or atherosclerotic within 10 years of surgery. The limited formation of intimal hyperplasia in the graft wall is considered an important component of successful adaptation; however, when this hyperplasia becomes excessive because of uncontrolled adaptation, it can lead to graft failure and clinical complications. Because there has been relatively no change in the 30% to 50% 5-year vein graft failure rates over the last several decades, it is essential that we gain a better understanding of the mechanisms leading to abnormal adaptation and graft failure. It is well documented that circulating progenitor cells, most of which originate from the bone marrow, play an important role in vascular remodeling, and CXC chemokine receptor-4 (CXCR4), the receptor for stromal cell–derived factor-1 (SDF-1), is a key modulator for the mobilization and recruitment of bone marrow–derived cells. This interesting article uses a genetic approach in mice to reduce CXCR4 activity in vein grafts to test the hypothesis that CXCR4 activity, particularly in vein graft-extrinsic cells, contributes to vein graft neointimal hyperplasia. Their results show that vein graft neointimal hyperplasia is exacerbated by CXCR4 activity in vein graft-extrinsic cells. Their work also suggests that an SDF-1/CXCR4 signaling system promotes inflammation associated with vein graft arterialization by showing that $Cxcr4^{-/+}$ vein graft recipients have fewer leukocytes in the vein graft media. Despite the fact that this study does not mimic all of the hemodynamic parameters that are obtained in vein grafts, it does highlight the therapeutic potential of CXCR4 antagonism to achieve clinically beneficial effects to reduce the vein graft failure rates. The CXCR4 antagonist plerixafor (AMD3100) is already safely used in humans, and, as the authors suggest, it could conceivably be used to treat vein grafts focally at the time of transplantation.

J. Cullen, PhD

Ezetimibe reduces intimal hyperplasia in rabbit jugular vein graft
Maekawa T, Komori K, Morisaki K, et al (Nagoya Univ Graduate School of Medicine, Japan; et al)
J Vasc Surg 56:1689-1697, 2012

Background.—The selective cholesterol transport inhibitor ezetimibe is widely used to prevent development of atherosclerosis in patients with hypercholesterolemia. However, whether this agent inhibits intimal hyperplasia in autologous vein grafts is unknown. The present study was undertaken to clarify if ezetimibe reduces cell proliferation and intimal hyperplasia in vein grafts.

Methods.—Forty-four rabbits were randomly divided into two groups: one group received ezetimibe (0.6 mg/kg/d), and the control group did not. Ezetimibe administration was started 1 week before rabbits underwent interposition reversed autologous jugular vein grafts. The proliferative cells and apoptotic cells were counted in the vein grafts 14 days after implantation, and changes in acetylcholine-induced relaxation and endothelial intracellular concentration of Ca^{2+} ($[Ca^{2+}]_i$) were examined at 28 days.

Results.—Ezetimibe reduced serum cholesterol and triglyceride. There were fewer proliferating cells in the ezetimibe group (5.7% ± 0.2%, n = 7) than in the control group (12.8% ± 0.5%, n = 7; $P < .0001$) and more apoptotic cells in the ezetimibe group (5.3% ± 0.2%, n = 7) than in the control group (2.3% ± 0.2%, n = 7; $P < .0001$). Intimal hyperplasia was less in the ezetimibe group (46.1 ± 6.0 μm, n = 7) than in the control group (76.0 ± 2.5 μm, n = 7; $P < .01$). Acetylcholine-produced endothelium-dependent relaxation was observed only in the ezetimibe group, which was blocked by the nitric oxide (NO) synthase inhibitor N^{ω}- nitro-L-arginine. Acetylcholine increased $[Ca^{2+}]_i$ only in the ezetimibe group.

Conclusions.—Ezetimibe reduced cell proliferation and enhanced cell apoptosis, thus inhibiting intimal hyperplasia in rabbit autologous vein grafts. Ezetimibe restored the acetylcholine-induced increase in $[Ca^{2+}]_i$ in endothelial cells and improved endothelium-dependent NO-mediated relaxation in the vein graft. Our results suggest that ezetimibe enhances the function of endothelial NO through an increase in endothelial $[Ca^{2+}]_i$, thus reducing vein graft intimal hyperplasia.

▶ Despite major advances in surgical techniques and postoperative care, vein graft failure rates remain high, with an observed incidence of vein graft occlusion at 30% to 50% after 5 years, and graft failure can lead to recurrent angina, myocardial infarction, additional revascularization procedures, and premature death. It is thought that these changes may be caused by the fact that the venous implants are subjected to increased shear stress, loss of endothelial cells, migration and invasion of inflammatory cells, and migration and proliferation of smooth muscle cells. The results of multiple clinical trials suggest that ezetimibe, a potent inhibitor of sterol absorption, may reduce the intimal hyperplasia seen in autologous vein grafts. This study was undertaken to determine whether long-term administration of ezetimibe was able to inhibit intimal hyperplasia in rabbit autologous vein grafts and to investigate the function of endothelial cells, which are suggested to play an essential role in regulation of intimal growth in vein grafts through the synthesis and release of nitric oxide (NO). Their results showed that ezetimibe treatment inhibited intimal hyperplasia because of reduction of cell proliferation and enhancement of cell apoptosis and by enhancing the function of endothelium-derived NO. Given that the 5-year vein graft failure rates have remained largely unchanged over the last several decades, it is important that the mechanisms involved and potential therapies are explored. These promising results suggest that ezetimibe has promising potential for reducing vein graft failure and warrants further investigation.

J. Cullen, PhD

Rosuvastatin improves vascular function of arteriovenous fistula in a diabetic rat model
Roan J-N, Fang S-Y, Chang S-W, et al (Natl Cheng Kung Univ, Tainan, Taiwan)
J Vasc Surg 56:1381-1389.e1, 2012

Objective.—This study investigates the pathogenesis of arteriovenous (AV) fistula failure in patients with diabetes mellitus (DM) and tests the vascular protective effect of rosuvastatin on the fistulous communication of diabetic rats.

Methods.—DM was induced in rats by a single injection of streptozotocin. One week later, a fistula was created in the descending aorta and the adjacent inferior vena cava (aortocaval [AC] fistula). Rats were then randomly assigned to receive placebo or rosuvastatin (15 mg/kg/d) in chow for 2 weeks. Blood flow in the aortic segments of the fistula was measured. Circulating CD34+/KDR+ endothelial progenitor cells (EPCs) were determined 2 weeks after creation of the AC fistulas using flow cytometry. Vascular function of the AC fistulas was assessed by isometric force testing. The expression of proinflammatory genes and generation of superoxide anions in the fistulas were examined.

Results.—The number of EPCs was reduced in diabetic rats, and rosuvastatin significantly increased the number of circulating EPCs. Reduced blood flow and impaired endothelium-dependent relaxation in the AC fistula of animals with diabetes was significantly potentiated after treatment with rosuvastatin. Rosuvastatin also attenuated the expression of inducible nitric oxide synthase and nicotinamide adenine dinucleotide phosphate oxidase and generation of superoxide anions in the fistula tissues isolated from diabetic rats.

Conclusions.—We provide the first evidence demonstrating that rosuvastatin improves blood flow and endothelial function of AC fistulas in rats with DM by attenuating the activity of proinflammatory genes and generation of superoxide anions in the remodeled vasculature.

Clinical Relevance.—Arteriovenous (AV) fistula is the most common vascular access for hemodialysis in patients with end-stage renal disease. Studies have shown that blood flow in the AV fistula is significantly reduced in patients with diabetes and the period for maturation of an AV fistula is longer in these patients. The underlying mechanisms of AV fistula failure in diabetes are still poorly understood and there are limited therapeutic approaches that can increase the lifespan of these fistulas. The present study demonstrates that oral administration rosuvastatin improves blood flow and endothelial function of AC fistulas in rats with diabetes, which results from attenuating the activity of proinflammatory genes in the remodeled vasculature, thereby reducing the generation of tissue superoxide anions. Our results may thus enhance our ability to prevent and manage vascular access failure in patients with diabetes with chronic renal disease.

▶ Hemodialysis vascular access failure is a significant challenge for health care professionals who care for patients in chronic renal failure. Although arteriovenous (AV) fistulas are the preferred method of vascular access with fewer complications, their failure remains a huge problem. The procedures for creating the AV fistula and treatment of the related complications account for more than 20% of hospitalizations of patients receiving dialysis and cost about 100 million US dollars annually. To date, limited studies have found an association between diabetes and AV fistula failure, and these authors utilize a rat model to investigate the potential therapeutic effects of rosuvastatin in maintaining a healthy, usable fistula. The results show that oral administration of rosuvastatin improves blood flow and endothelial function of aortocaval fistulas in rats with diabetes, which results from attenuating the activity of proinflammatory genes in the remodeled vasculature, thereby reducing the generation of tissue superoxide anions. The identification of the mechanisms involved in AV fistula failure is important in the management of vascular access, and although these results are from an animal model, they offer great insight because due to a lack of controlled, randomized prospective clinical trials, it remains clinically controversial whether statins could provide therapeutic benefits in the outcomes of AV access, particularly in patients with diabetes.

J. Cullen, PhD

A pilot study of a triple antimicrobial-bonded Dacron graft for the prevention of aortic graft infection
Aboshady I, Raad I, Shah AS, et al (Texas Heart Inst at St Luke's Episcopal Hosp, Houston; Univ of Texas Health Science Ctr, Houston; et al)
J Vasc Surg 56:794-801, 2012

Objective.—Perioperative infection of an aortic graft is one of the most devastating complications of vascular surgery, with a mortality rate of 10% to 30%. The rate of amputation of the lower limbs is generally > 25%, depending on the graft material, the location of the graft and infection, and the bacterial virulence. In vitro studies suggest that an antibiotic-impregnated graft may help prevent perioperative graft infection. In a pilot animal study, we tested a locally developed technique of bonding Dacron aortic grafts with three antimicrobial agents to evaluate the ensuing synergistic preventive effect on direct perioperative bacterial contamination.

Methods.—We surgically implanted a 6-mm vascular knitted Dacron graft in the infrarenal abdominal aorta of six Sinclair miniature pigs. Two pigs received unbonded, uninoculated grafts; two received unbonded, inoculated grafts; and two received inoculated grafts that were bonded with chlorhexidine, rifampin, and minocycline. Before implantation, the two bonded grafts and the two unbonded grafts were immersed for 15 minutes in a 2-mL bacterial solution containing 1 to 2×10^7 colony-forming units (CFU)/mL of *Staphylococcus aureus* (ATCC 29213). Two weeks after graft implantation, the pigs were euthanized, and the grafts were surgically excised for clinical, microbiologic, and histopathologic study.

Results.—The two bonded grafts treated with *S aureus* showed no bacterial growth upon explant, whereas the two unbonded grafts treated with *S aureus* had high bacterial counts (6.25×10^6 and 1.38×10^7 CFU/graft). The two control grafts (unbonded and untreated) showed bacterial growth (1.8×10^3 and 7.27×10^3 CFU/graft) that presumably reflected direct, accidental perioperative bacterial contamination; *S cohnii ssp urealyticus* and *S chromogenes*, but not *S aureus*, were isolated. The histopathologic and clinical data confirmed the microbiologic findings. Only pigs that received unbonded grafts showed histopathologic evidence of a perigraft abscess.

Conclusions.—Our results suggest that bonding aortic grafts with this triple antimicrobial combination is a promising method of reducing graft infection resulting from direct postoperative bacterial contamination for at least 2 weeks. Further studies are needed to explore the ability of this novel graft to combat one of the most feared complications in vascular surgery.

▶ One of the most challenging complications after any vascular procedure using a prosthetic implant is perioperative seeding infection of the graft. The mortality rate is high, as is the morbidity rate, which can include the need for many subsequent operative interventions, graft explantation, and, potentially, limb amputation. We as vascular surgeons take many prophylactic measures to prevent seeding of the implant during operation and afterward. One usually cannot identify any break in technique or postoperative instance in which seeding may have occurred unless the patient develops some other secondary infection such as pneumonia. Thus, this basic science study exploring the use of triple-antibiotic impregnated Dacron grafts is timely. Though using small animal cohorts (n = 2) to compare in this pilot study, it is clear that the treated grafts bonded with 3 antimicrobials acted in a synergistic manner to decrease bacterial counts. At 2 weeks after implantation and exposure to common staphylococcal bacterial strains, the treated grafts had no bacteria isolated, no evidence on gross or histologic analysis of abscess formation, and the animals did not exhibit signs of infection or sepsis before being euthanized.

I encourage the authors as well as other groups who study ways to combat perioperative vascular graft infections, to continue the work, to publish their results, to patent their techniques, and to partner with industry to provide improved techniques in the future that will decrease the horrible outcomes of graft infections by eliminating or decreasing the initial problem. It would be interesting to see these studies translate to clinical human studies, thus propagating the "bench to bedside research projects" that are designed to convert promising laboratory discoveries into new medical treatments. Improvement and new devices for combatting vascular graft infections may be one such medical treatment that would be ripe for external funding sources.

R. L. Bush, MD, MPH

6 Aortic Aneurysm

Effect of endovascular and open abdominal aortic aneurysm repair on thrombin generation and fibrinolysis

Abdelhamid MF, Davies RSM, Vohra RK, et al (Solihull Hosp, Birmingham, UK; Univ Hosp, Birmingham NHS Foundation Trust, UK)

J Vasc Surg 57:103-107, 2013

Background.—Abdominal aortic aneurysm (AAA) is associated with a prothrombotic diathesis that may increase the risk of cardiovascular events. This diathesis is exacerbated in the short term by open aneurysm repair (OAR) and endovascular aneurysm repair (EVAR). However, the effect of EVAR and OAR on coagulation and fibrinolysis in the medium and long term is poorly understood. The purpose of this study was to investigate the medium-term effects of EVAR and OAR on thrombin generation, neutralization, and fibrinolysis.

Methods.—Prothrombin fragment (PF)1 + 2, thrombin antithrombin (TAT) complex, plasminogen activator inhibitor (PAI) activity, and tissue-plasminogen activator (t-PA) antigen were measured in eight age-matched controls (AMCs), 29 patients with AAA immediately before (preoperatively) and 12 months after EVAR (post-EVAR), and in 11 patients at a mean of 16 months after OAR (post-OAR).

Results.—Preoperatively, PF1 + 2 levels were significantly higher in patients with AAAs than in AMC. PF1 + 2 levels post-EVAR and post-OAR were significantly lower than preoperative values and similar to AMC. There was no significant difference in TAT, PAI, or t-PA between AMC, AAA preoperatively, and post-EVAR. Post-OAR, PAI activity was significantly higher than in preoperative patients.

Conclusions.—AAA is associated with increased thrombin generation without upregulation of fibrinolysis. The prothrombotic, hypofibrinolytic diathesis observed in patients with AAA returns toward normal in the medium term after EVAR and OAR, although there is a trend toward decreased fibrinolysis post-OAR.

▶ The purpose of this study was to investigate, for the first time, the medium-term effects of endovascular aneurysm repair (EVAR) and open surgical repair (OSR) of abdominal aortic aneurysms on thrombin generation, neutralization, and fibrinolysis. The article is fairly self-explanatory with regard to grouping of patients and results. The major findings of this study were that the mere presence of an aortic aneurysm causes increased thrombin generation without upregulation of fibrinolysis. This prothrombotic state actually returns to normal after EVAR or

OSR (when compared with results for age-matched controls). The reasons for this prothrombotic condition are poorly understood but could be related to cigarette smoking, the presence of peripheral vascular disease, or the biologic activity of the aortic wall or intramural thrombus.

This is of particular interest to me because I treat a large number of patients who have ruptured aortic aneurysms and I have independently observed that the rate of endoleak in patients presenting with rupture is lower than in our elective population of EVARs. Could this be a result of an even more pronounced prothrombotic state in the population of ruptures? This is probably worth exploring further in a similar fashion as these authors have.

B. W. Starnes, MD

Remodelling of Vascular (Surgical) Services in the UK

Earnshaw JJ, Mitchell DC, Wyatt MG, et al (Gloucestershire Royal Hosp, UK; North Bristol Hosp, UK; Freeman Hosp, Newcastle upon Tyne, UK; et al)

Eur J Vasc Endovasc Surg 44:465-467, 2012

The last few years have seen major changes in the delivery of vascular services in the UK. An increasingly elderly population with greater expectations from their medical services has challenged established methods. It also became apparent that outcomes for low volume, high risk index vascular interventions such as abdominal aortic aneurysm repair were poor in the UK compared to the rest of Europe. Other ongoing challenges were the introduction of a national aortic aneurysm screening programme and the development of vascular surgery as a separate speciality. This article details the approach taken to modernise vascular services in the UK, using a quality framework agreed by vascular specialists, which drove the structural change to move vascular interventions into fewer, higher volume centres. The introduction of modern networks is designed to maintain services in surrounding hospitals without on site vascular inpatient services. The initial effects of this service remodelling are positive, with elective aortic aneurysm mortality rates falling nationally from 7.5 to 2.4 per cent.

▶ This article is an interesting historic review of the recent changes in vascular care across the United Kingdom.

In 2008, a European report suggested that the United Kingdom had the worst mortality rate in Europe for elective abdominal aortic aneurysm (AAA) repair (7.5% vs 3.5% European average). This event served as a call to action to completely overhaul and reorganize vascular service lines in the United Kingdom.

Restructuring included the shift and consolidation of complicated procedures from low-volume to high-volume centers, implementation of a national screening program for AAA, and a change in the training paradigm for vascular specialists. The results were dramatic. Mortality rates for elective AAA repair fell dramatically from 7.5% to 2.4%!

The past few years have seen great changes in vascular services in the United Kingdom, partly because of challenges such as poor surgical outcomes and the introduction of mass screening. These are endorsed by a group of vascular specialists who are attempting to improve quality and performance.

B. W. Starnes, MD

Low Density Lipoprotein Receptor Related Protein 1 and Abdominal Aortic Aneurysms
Wild JB, Stather PW, Sylvius N, et al (Univ of Leicester, UK)
Eur J Vasc Endovasc Surg 44:127-132, 2012

Objectives.—A recent GWAS demonstrated an association between low density lipoprotein receptor related protein 1 (LRP1) and Abdominal Aortic Aneurysm (AAA). This review aims to identify how LRP1 may be involved in the pathogenesis of abdominal aortic aneurysm.

Design and Materials.—A systematic review of the English language literature was undertaken in order to determine whether LRP1 and associated pathways were plausible candidates for contributing to the development and/or progression of AAA.

Methods and Results.—A comprehensive literature search of MEDLINE (since 1948), Embase (since 1980) and Health and Psychological Instruments (since 1985) was conducted in January 2012 identified 50 relevant articles. These studies demonstrate that LRP1 has a diverse range of biological functions and is a plausible candidate for playing a central role in aneurysmogenesis. Importantly, LRP1 downregulates MMP (matrix metalloproteinase) activity in vascular smooth muscle cells and regulates other key pathways involved in extracellular matrix remodelling and vascular smooth muscle migration and proliferation. Crucially animal studies have shown that LRP1 depletion leads to progressive destruction of the vascular architecture and aneurysm formation.

Conclusions.—Published evidence suggests that LRP1 may play a key role in the development of AAA.

▶ A recent genome-wide association study found a genetic association between LRP1 (Low density lipoprotein receptor related protein 1) and abdominal aortic aneurysms (AAA). These authors aimed to conduct a systematic review of the current literature regarding this association and to explain how LRP1 may be involved in the pathogenesis of AAA.

LRP1 is implicated in vascular smooth muscle cell migration and proliferation via the binding of specific growth factors, and LRP1 also binds matrix metalloproteinase 9 (MMP9), a protease capable of degrading collagen. Interestingly, there is compelling evidence from animal knockout studies in which mice with vascular smooth muscle cell–specific LRP1 knockout had diversely altered vascular histology and ultimately developed AAA.

This review highlights the current knowledge of LRP1 and its potential role in AAA development. LRP1 mutation is likely to be caused by a combination of genetic and environmental factors. The most significant environmental factor seems to be smoking, and it is likely that the damage to the cellular structure from cigarette smoking will interact with several underlying genetic aberrations, such as LRP1 mutation, thus allowing an aneurysm to form. LRP1 and its associated pathways appear to be a potential candidate target for the treatment of AAA.

B. W. Starnes, MD

Total Endovascular Debranching of the Aortic Arch
Yoshida RA, Kolvenbach R, Yoshida WB, et al (São Paulo State Univ UNESP, Botucatu, Brazil; Augusta Hosp and Catholic Clinics Dusseldorf, Germany)
Eur J Vasc Endovasc Surg 42:627-630, 2011

Background.—Significant morbidity and mortality are related to conventional aortic replacement surgery. Endovascular debranching techniques, fenestrated or branched endografts are time consuming and costly.

Objective.—We alternatively propose to use endovascular approach with parallel grafts for debranching of aortic arch.

Methods.—Under general anesthesia, 12 F sheaths were inserted in the femoral, axillary and common carotid arteries for vascular accesses. Via-Bahn grafts 10 − 15 cm in length were placed into the aortic arch from right common carotid, left common carotid and left axillary arteries, until the tip of each graft reached into the ascending aorta. Through one femoral artery, the aortic stent −graft was positioned and delivered. Soon after, the parallel grafts were sequentially delivered. Self-spanding Wallstents[R] were used for parallel grafts reinforcement. Ballooning was routinely used for parallel grafts and rarely for aortic graft.

Results.—This technique was used in 2 cases. The first one was a lady with 72 years old, with an aortic retrograde dissection from left subclavian artery and involving remaining arch branches. Through right common carotid artery a stent-graft was placed in the ascending aorta and through the left common carotid artery a ViaBahn was inserted parallel to the former. A thoracic endograft then covered all the aortic arch dissection extending into the ascending aorta close to the sinu −tubular junction. The second case was a 82 year old male patient with a 7 cm aortic arch aneurysm. Through both common carotid arteries ViaBahn grafts were introduced and positioned into the ascending aorta. Soon after, the deployment of the thoracic stent graft covered all parallel grafts of the aortic arch, excluding the aneurysm. Both cases did not have neurologic or cardiac complications and were discharged 10 days after the procedure.

Conclusions.—This technique may be a good minimal invasive off-the-shelf technical option for aortic arch "debranching". More data and further improvements are required before this promising technique can be widely advocated.

▶ The authors present 2 successful cases of complete aortic arch debranching utilizing chimney grafts. The easy response is that more research is needed in this area. The reality is that surgeons are increasingly choosing a compromised endovascular repair or an off-the-shelf repair over the surgical mortality associated with major aortic procedures. It is my belief that endovascular technology is capable of treating the entire spectrum of aortic aneurysmal disease; however, I do not believe that chimney grafts are the final solution.

The aortic arch lends itself to endovascular procedures because the branch vessels are surgically accessible prior to the end organ; this makes fenestrations, internal branches, and preloaded branches a simple reality. The aortic root, our proposed seal zone, is the most dynamic portion of the aorta; with each heart-beat, it distends 15% to 20% in diameter, elongates, and shifts axially toward the right chest. For these reasons, the endograft interface must be able to balance these forces. Too little interface results in an endoleak, and a rigid interface risks a retrograde dissection. Three Viabahn stent grafts and a thoracic stent graft in the aortic root increase the number of interfaces with the root that may result in intimal injury. In addition, the forces between the thoracic stent graft and the Viabahn stents are competing, which constantly places the branch vessels at risk for occlusion. The authors placed wall stents inside the Viabahn stents for this reason, but will it be enough?

Z. M. Arthurs, MD

A Multicentre Observational Study of the Outcomes of Screening Detected Sub-aneurysmal Aortic Dilatation

Wild JB, Stather PW, Biancari F, et al (Univ of Leicester, UK; Oulu Univ Hosp, Finland; et al)
Eur J Vasc Endovasc Surg 45:128-134, 2013

Objectives.—Currently most abdominal aortic aneurysm screening programmes discharge patients with aortic diameter of less than 30 mm. However, sub-aneurysmal aortic dilatation (25 mm—29 mm) does not represent a normal aortic diameter. This observational study aimed to determine the outcomes of patients with screening detected sub aneurysmal aortic dilatation.

Design and Methods.—Individual patient data was obtained from 8 screening programmes that had performed long term follow up of patients with sub aneurysmal aortic dilatation. Outcome measures recorded were the progression to true aneurysmal dilatation (aortic diameter 30 mm or greater), progression to size threshold for surgical intervention (55 mm) and aneurysm rupture.

Results.—Aortic measurements for 1696 men and women (median age 66 years at initial scan) with sub-aneurysmal aortae were obtained, median period of follow up was 4.0 years (range 0.1—19.0 years). Following Kaplan Meier and life table analysis 67.7% of patients with 5 complete years of surveillance reached an aortic diameter of 30 mm or greater however 0.9% had an aortic diameter of 54 mm. A total of 26.2% of patients with 10 complete years of follow up had an AAA of greater that 54 mm.

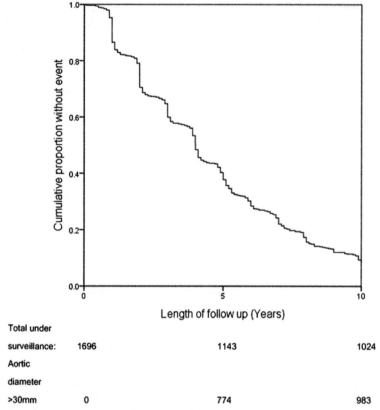

FIGURE 1.—Proportion of patients progressing from sub-aneurysmal aortic dilatation to an aortic diameter of >30 mm. Mean time to event 4.75 years (95% Confidence Interval 4.54–4.96) SE 0.11, median time to event 4.00 years (95% Confidence Interval 3.90–4.10) SE 0.49. (Reprinted from European Journal of Vascular and Endovascular Surgery. Wild JB, Stather PW, Biancari F, et al. A multicentre observational study of the outcomes of screening detected sub-aneurysmal aortic dilatation. *Eur J Vasc Endovasc Surg.* 2013;45:128-134, Copyright 2013, with permission from European Society for Vascular Surgery.)

Conclusion.—Patients with sub-aneurysmal aortic dilatation are likely to progress and develop an AAA, although few will rupture or require surgical intervention (Fig 1).

▶ We used to believe (and some still do) that an aortic diameter of 30 mm or less on screening ultrasound scan meant that no aneurysm was present, and patients were thus discharged from the screening event only to be lost to follow-up. But what about aortas that are clearly large on screening (25–29 mm) but NOT aneurysmal? That was the purpose of this well-conducted study from the United Kingdom.

Of 1696 patients with subaneurysmal aortas, 67.7% of patients reached a definition of aneurysm greater than 3 cm with 5 years of follow-up. A total of 26.2% of patients with 10 complete years of follow-up had a large abdominal aortic aneurysm of greater than 54 mm (Fig 1)!

Mean time from subaneurysmal aorta to development of a true aneurysm was 4.7 years with 96% developing an aneurysm by 10 years; 8.3% developed large aneurysms (> 54 mm) by a mean of 13.2 years.

Interestingly, of the 14 ruptures known to have occurred, the mean time from diagnosis of subaneurysmal aorta to rupture was 18.7 years.

These data would suggest that, for patients found to have subaneurysmal aortic diameters on screening that are clearly abnormal, screening should be repeated at least every 5 years.

B. W. Starnes, MD

Endovascular repair of ruptured infrarenal abdominal aortic aneurysm is associated with lower 30-day mortality and better 5-year survival rates than open surgical repair
Mehta M, Byrne J, Darling RC III, et al (Albany Med College, NY)
J Vasc Surg 57:368-375, 2013

Objective.—Endovascular aneurysm repair (EVAR) decreases 30-day mortality for patients with ruptured abdominal aortic aneurysms (r-AAAs) compared with open surgical repair (OSR). However, which patients benefit or whether there is any long-term survival advantage is uncertain.

Methods.—From 2002 to 2011, 283 patients with r-AAA underwent EVAR (n = 120 [42.4%]) or OSR (n = 163 [57.6%]) at Albany Medical Center. All data were collected prospectively. Patients were analyzed on an intention-to-treat basis, and outcomes were evaluated by a logistic regression multivariable model. Kaplan-Meier analysis was used to compare long-term survival.

Results.—The EVAR patients had a significantly lower 30-day mortality than did the OSR patients (29/120 [24.2%] vs 72/163 [44.2%]; $P < .005$) and better cumulative 5-year survival (37% vs 26%; $P < .005$). Men benefited more from EVAR (mortality: 20.9% for EVAR vs 44.3% for OSR; $P < .001$) than did women (mortality: 32.4% vs 43.9%; $P = .39$). Age ≥80 years was a significant predictor of death for EVAR (odds ratio [OR], 1.07; $P = .003$) but not for OSR (OR, 1.04; $P = .056$). Preexisting hypertension was a significant predictor of survival for both EVAR (OR, 0.17; $P < .001$) and OSR (OR, 0.48; $P = .021$). Almost one fourth of EVAR patients (21/91 [23.1%]) required secondary interventions. Survival advantage was maintained for EVAR patients to 5 years.

Conclusions.—For r-AAA, EVAR reduces the 30-day mortality and improves long-term survival up to 5 years. However, whereas open survivors require few graft-related interventions, up to 23% of EVAR patients will require reintervention for endoleaks or graft migration. Close follow-up of all EVAR survivors is mandatory (Figs 1 and 3).

▶ I chose this report for this year's VASCULAR YEAR BOOK because it represents the single largest institutional experience to date with endovascular repair of ruptured abdominal aortic aneurysms (REVAR). The Albany group championed

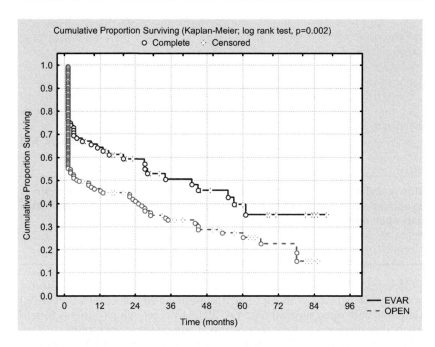

Interval Start	0	12	24	36	48	60	72	84
EVAR								
Number Entering	120	44	28	21	16	11	5	3
Cum. Prop. Surviving	1.00	0.62	0.57	0.48	0.43	0.37	0.33	0.29
Std. Err. Cum. Surv.		0.05	0.05	0.06	0.06	0.07	0.07	0.08
OPEN								
Number Entering	163	56	43	30	21	14	6	1
Cum. Prop. Surviving	1.00	0.44	0.40	0.31	0.28	0.26	0.21	0.12
Std. Err. Cum. Surv.		0.04	0.04	0.04	0.04	0.04	0.05	0.06

FIGURE 1.—Cumulative survivals for patients undergoing open surgical repair (*OPEN*) and endovascular aneurysm repair (*EVAR*) for ruptured abdominal aortic aneurysm (r-AAA). (Reprinted from the Journal of Vascular Surgery. Mehta M, Byrne J, Darling RC III, et al. Endovascular repair of ruptured infrarenal abdominal aortic aneurysm is associated with lower 30-day mortality and better 5-year survival rates than open surgical repair. *J Vasc Surg*. 2013;57:368-375, Copyright 2013, with permission from the Society for Vascular Surgery.)

an aggressive endovascular first strategy for treating patients with a model of pure catastrophic intra-abdominal hemorrhage. This is a 9.5-year experience with 283 patients or roughly 29 patients per year. The use of REVAR increased dramatically over time (Fig 3).

The important findings in this study were that (1) REVAR patients have a significantly lower 30-day and in-hospital mortality when compared with patients receiving open surgical repair, (2) REVAR patients have better long-term survival, and (3) in women, REVAR brought no statistically significant benefit.

Importantly, these authors showed for the first time that the initial mortality benefit is not short lived and extends beyond the midterm (Fig 1). This was

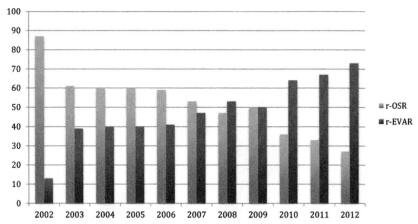

FIGURE 3.—Trends in management of ruptured abdominal aortic aneurysm (r-AAA) at Albany Medical Center from 2002 to 2012. Expressed as percentage of cases per year. *EVAR*, Endovascular aneurysmrepair; *OSR*, open surgical repair; *r*, ruptured. (Reprinted from the Journal of Vascular Surgery. Mehta M, Byrne J, Darling RC III, et al. Endovascular repair of ruptured infrarenal abdominal aortic aneurysm is associated with lower 30-day mortality and better 5-year survival rates than open surgical repair. *J Vasc Surg.* 2013;57:368-375, Copyright 2013, with permission from the Society for Vascular Surgery.)

not, however, without consequences. The REVAR patients required diligent follow-up, and a full 23% required some form of reintervention. The authors are to be congratulated on this series.

B. W. Starnes, MD

A modern experience with saccular aortic aneurysms
Shang EK, Nathan DP, Boonn WW, et al (Univ of Pennsylvania, Philadelphia)
J Vasc Surg 57:84-88, 2013

Objective.—Repair of saccular aortic aneurysms (SAAs) is frequently recommended based on a perceived predisposition to rupture, despite little evidence that these aneurysms have a more malignant natural history than fusiform aortic aneurysms.

Methods.—The radiology database at a single university hospital was searched for the computed tomographic (CT) diagnosis of SAA between 2003 and 2011. Patient characteristics and clinical course, including the need for surgical intervention, were recorded. SAA evolution was assessed by follow-up CT, where available. Multivariate analysis was used to examine potential predictors of aneurysm growth rate.

Results.—Three hundred twenty-two saccular aortic aneurysms were identified in 284 patients. There were 153 (53.7%) men and 131 women with a mean age of 73.5 ± 10.0 years. SAAs were located in the ascending aorta in two (0.6%) cases, the aortic arch in 23 (7.1%), the descending thoracic aorta in 219 (68.1%), and the abdominal aorta in 78 (24.2%).

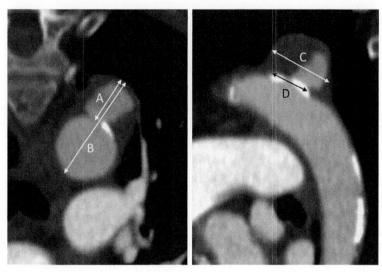

FIGURE 1.—Depiction of measurements obtained on individual saccular aneurysms. **A**, saccular aneurysm depth; **B**, maximum transaortic diameter; **C**, maximum saccular aneurysm size; **D**, aneurysm neck length. (Reprinted from the Journal of Vascular Surgery. Shang EK, Nathan DP, Boonn WW, et al. A modern experience with saccular aortic aneurysms. *J Vasc Surg.* 2013;57:84-88, Copyright 2013, with permission from the Society for Vascular Surgery.)

One hundred thirteen (39.8%) patients underwent surgical repair of SAA. Sixty-two patients (54.9%) underwent thoracic endovascular aortic repair, 22 underwent endovascular aneurysm repair (19.5%), and 29 (25.6%) required open surgery. The average maximum diameter of SAA was 5.0 ± 1.6 cm. In repaired aneurysms, the mean diameter was 5.4 ± 1.4 cm; in unrepaired aneurysms, it was 4.4 ± 1.1 cm ($P < .001$). Eleven patients (3.9%) had ruptured SAAs on initial scan. Of the initial 284 patients, 50 patients (with 54 SAA) had CT follow-up after at least 3 months (23.2 ± 19.0 months). Fifteen patients (30.0%) ultimately underwent surgical intervention. Aneurysm growth rate was 2.8 ± 2.9 mm/yr, and was only weakly related to initial aortic diameter ($R^2 = .19$ by linear regression, $P = .09$ by multivariate regression). Decreased calcium burden ($P = .03$) and increased patient age ($P = .05$) predicted increased aneurysm growth by multivariate analysis.

Conclusions.—While SAA were not found to have a higher growth rate than their fusiform counterparts, both clinical and radiologic follow-up is necessary, as a significant number ultimately require surgical intervention. Further clinical research is necessary to determine the optimal management of SAA (Fig 1).

▶ Saccular aneurysms have historically been perceived by vascular surgeons as possessing a greater rupture risk than their fusiform counterparts and, as a consequence, are often repaired at smaller diameters (Fig 1). Historically, the mere presence of a saccular aneurysm was considered an indication for repair.

Despite the common perception of a more malignant natural history of saccular aortic aneurysms, the true rupture risk of saccular aneurysms is not known. These authors attempted to characterize the growth rate and rupture risk in a large single-institution series.

The growth rate of saccular aneurysms in this study was roughly 2 to 3 mm/y, and when compared with other reports on growth rates of fusiform aneurysms, was not different.

The similarity with respect to growth rates and diameters between saccular and fusiform aneurysms suggests that saccular aneurysms are not necessarily more prone to rupture than fusiform aneurysms of the aorta.

B. W. Starnes, MD

Differences in readmissions after open repair versus endovascular aneurysm repair
Casey K, Hernandez-Boussard T, Mell MW, et al (Naval Med Ctr San Diego, CA; Stanford Univ Med Ctr, CA)
J Vasc Surg 57:89-95, 2013

Objective.—Reintervention rates after repair of abdominal aortic aneurysm (AAA) are higher for endovascular repair (EVAR) than for open repair, mostly due to treatment for endoleaks, whereas open surgical operations for bowel obstruction and abdominal hernias are higher after open repair. However, readmission rates after EVAR or open repair for nonoperative conditions and complications that do not require an intervention are not well documented. We sought to determine reasons for all-cause readmissions within the first year after open repair and EVAR.

Methods.—Patients who underwent elective AAA repair in California during a 6-year period were identified from the Health Care and Utilization Project State Inpatient Database. All patients who had a readmission in California ≤1 year of their index procedure were included for evaluation. Readmission rates and primary and secondary diagnoses associated with each readmission were analyzed and recorded.

Results.—From 2003 to 2008, there were 15,736 operations for elective AAA repair, comprising 9356 EVARs (60%) and 6380 open repairs (40%). At 1 year postoperatively, the readmission rate was 52.1% after open repair and 55.4% after EVAR ($P = .0003$). The three most common principal diagnoses associated with readmission after any type of AAA repair were failure to thrive, cardiac issues, and infection. When stratified by repair type, patients who underwent open repair were more likely to be readmitted with primary diagnoses associated with failure to thrive, cardiac complications, and infection compared with EVAR (all $P < .001$). Those who underwent EVAR were more likely, however, to be readmitted with primary diagnoses of device-related complications ($P = .05$), cardiac complications, and infection.

Conclusions.—Total readmission rates within 1 year after elective AAA repair are greater after EVAR than after open repair. Reasons for

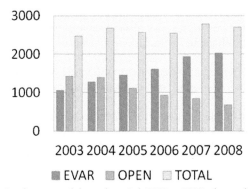

FIGURE 1.—During the course of the study period (2003 to 2008), the number of total aneurysms repaired in California remained relatively constant. Endovascular aneurysm repair (*EVAR*), however, replaced open repair (*OPEN*) as the treatment method of choice. (Reprinted from the Journal of Vascular Surgery. Casey K, Hernandez-Boussard T, Mell MW, et al. Differences in readmissions after open repair versus endovascular aneurysm repair. *J Vasc Surg*. 2013;57:89-95, Copyright 2013, with permission from the Society for Vascular Surgery.)

readmission vary between the two cohorts but are related to the magnitude of open surgery after open repair, device issues after EVAR, and the usual cardiac and infectious complications after either intervention. Systems-based analysis of these causes of readmission can potentially improve patient expectations and care after elective aneurysm repair (Fig 1).

▶ These authors examined readmission rates after either open aneurysm repair or endovascular repair (EVAR) in a statewide database in the state of California. A total of 15 736 operations were performed over a 6-year period. Of those, 9356 were EVAR (60%), and 6380 were open repairs (40%). The trends for aneurysm repair are shown in Fig 1. The results showed a small but highly significant difference in the rates of readmission between operative strategies (open = 52.1% and EVAR = 55.4%, P = .0003). The three primary reasons for readmission were (1) failure to thrive, (2) cardiac issues, and (3) infection.

Patients undergoing open repair of their aneurysm had a 6.7% operative mortality rate and were more likely to be readmitted within 30 and 90 days and, when readmitted, had much longer lengths of stay.

Not every readmission can be related to the method of repair. This underscores the fact that patients with aneurysmal disease have significant comorbidities and are of the age that they return to the hospital at high rates within the first year after surgery.

An interesting and surprising finding was that wound complications were high in the EVAR group, suggesting that lower readmission rates may be possible by focusing on purely percutaneous strategies along with endovascular repair.

B. W. Starnes, MD

Palliation of Abdominal Aortic Aneurysms in the Endovascular Era
Western CE, Carlisle J, McCarthy RJ, et al (Torbay Hosp, Torquay, UK)
Eur J Vasc Endovasc Surg 45:37-43, 2013

Objectives.—To establish outcome of patients with abdominal aortic aneurysm (AAA) deemed unfit for repair.
Design.—Retrospective non-randomised study.
Materials and Methods.—Identification of males with >5.5 cm or females with >5.0 cm AAA turned down for elective repair between 01/01/2006—24/07/2009 from a prospective database. Comorbidities, reasons for non-intervention, aneurysm size, survival, use of CPEX (cardio-pulmonary exercise) testing and cause of death were analysed. Although well-established at the time, patients unfit for open operation were not considered for endovascular repair.

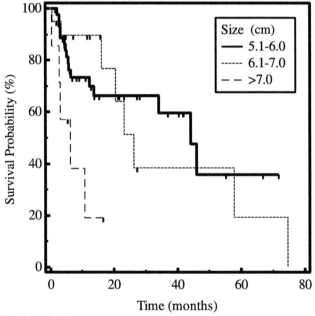

Number at risk:

5.1 - 6.0cm	45	15	8	2	0
6.1 - 7.0cm	20	6	2	1	0
> 7.0cm	7	0	0	0	0

FIGURE 4.—Survival when stratified according to aneurysm size. (Reprinted from European Journal of Vascular and Endovascular Surgery. Western CE, Carlisle J, McCarthy RJ, et al. Palliation of abdominal aortic aneurysms in the endovascular era. *Eur J Vasc Endovasc Surg.* 2013;45:37-43, Copyright 2013, with permission from European Society for Vascular Surgery.)

TABLE 2.—. Features of Non-Operated AAA When Stratified According to Size

Aneurysm Size	5.1–6.0 cm	6.1–7.0 cm	>7.0 cm
Number of patients	45	20	7
Median age (range, standard deviation)	79(58–93, SD 7.9)	83(67–91, SD 5.9)	84(75–94, SD 6.7)
Alive	29	12	2
Dead — rupture (%)	5 (11%)	4 (20%)	3 (43%)
Dead — non-rupture	11	4	2
Median survival: months (range)	44 (1.5–72)	26 (0.5–75)	6 (0.4–17)

Results.—Seventy two patients were unsuitable for AAA repair. Aneurysm size ranged from 5.3 cm to 12 cm. Functional status, comorbidity and patient preference determined decision to palliate. Sixty percent of patients were alive at study close. Aneurysm rupture was cause of death in 46%. CPEX testing was performed in 54%, whose mortality was 28%, vs. 54% in the non-CPEX group ($P < 0.05$). Median survival of patients with 5.1–6.0 cm AAA was 44 months and 11% died of rupture. Between 6.1 and 7.0 cm median survival was 26 months and 20% died of rupture. However, with >7 cm aneurysms, survival was 6 months and 43% ruptured.

Conclusion.—Under half the deaths in our comorbid cohort were due to rupture. However, decision to palliate may be revisited as risk-benefit ratio changes with aneurysm expansion (Fig 4, Table 2).

▶ It is extremely hard to come by a somewhat pure natural history study regarding aortic aneurysms. These authors in the United Kingdom were highly selective of their patients to undergo elective abdominal aortic aneurysm (AAA) repair. Despite the widespread availability of minimally invasive endovascular techniques for repair, if a patient was not a candidate for open repair, they were not offered endovascular repair! Of 194 patients presenting over a 3.5-year period, 72 (37%) were turned down for repair. These patients were then followed up until death. Aneurysm rupture was the cause of death in 46%.

These patients should not die in vain, and we can learn something from these natural history data (Table 2, Fig 4).

Median survival of patients with 5.1- to 6.0-cm AAA was 44 months, and 11% died of rupture. Between 6.1 and 7.0cm, median survival was 26 months, and 20% died of rupture. However, with aneurysms greater than 7 cm, survival was 6 months, and 43% ruptured.

Discussions to palliate are surgeon specific. These data are helpful to present to patients harboring AAAs so that they may participate as informed individuals in these decisions regarding treatment.

B. W. Starnes, MD

Technique of supraceliac balloon control of the aorta during endovascular repair of ruptured abdominal aortic aneurysms

Berland TL, Veith FJ, Cayne NS, et al (New York Univ Langone Med Ctr; et al)
J Vasc Surg 57:272-275, 2013

Endovascular aneurysm repair is being used increasingly to treat ruptured abdominal aortic aneurysms (RAAAs). Approximately 25% of RAAAs undergo complete circulatory collapse before or during the procedure. Patient survival depends on obtaining and maintaining supraceliac balloon control until the endograft is fully deployed. This is accomplished with a sheath-supported compliant balloon inserted via the groin contralateral to the side to be used for insertion of the endograft main body. After the main body is fully deployed, a second balloon is placed within the endograft, and the first balloon is removed so that extension limbs can be placed in the contralateral side. A third balloon can be placed via the contralateral side and ipsilateral extensions deployed as necessary. This technique of supraceliac balloon control is important to achieving good outcomes with RAAAs. In addition to minimizing blood loss, this technique minimizes visceral ischemia and maintains aortic control until the aneurysm rupture site is fully excluded (Fig).

▶ Ruptured abdominal aortic aneurysms (AAAs) represent a model of pure catastrophic intraabdominal hemorrhage. Rapid aortic control is essential for anyone who tries to treat a patient presenting with a ruptured aortic aneurysm. The mortality rate for patients presenting with ruptured AAA has plummeted with the use of endovascular techniques.[1] This is partly because of the implementation of structured protocols for treating these patients but, for the sickest patients, could be based on the rapid insertion of an aortic occlusion balloon (Fig).

The authors describe their technique in detail. I am absolutely convinced that this technique will be used increasingly by noninterventionalists to manage noncompressible torso hemorrhage in urban trauma centers and on the modern battlefield. If this is to happen, we need new devices to aid in the blind placement of these devices and a method of gaining rapid, accurate, and safe access to the femoral arteries. There are many exciting new developments in this area.

B. W. Starnes, MD

Reference

1. Starnes BW, Quiroga E, Hutter C, et al. Management of ruptured abdominal aortic aneurysm in the endovascular era. *J Vasc Surg*. 2010;51:9-18.

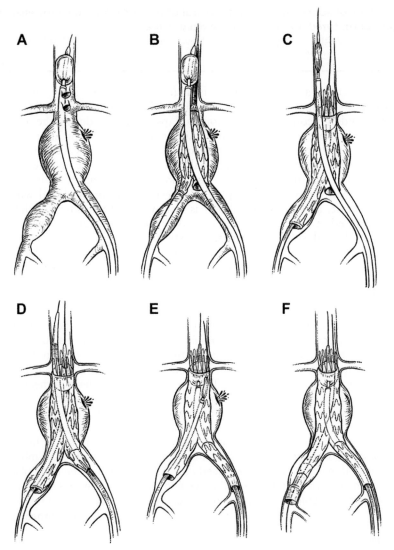

FIGURE.—A, Supraceliac balloon control via a large contralateral sheath. B, Main body of endograft is deployed via ipsilateral access. Slight temporary deflation of the balloon may be required to allow for passage of the tip of the device. C, After the endograft body and ipsilateral limb are deployed, a second balloon is placed via the ipsilateral groin and inflated within the main body of the graft, maintaining continuous aortic control. D, The contralateral gate is cannulated and the contralateral limb is deployed while maintaining balloon control from the ipsilateral side. E, To allow for extension of the ipsilateral limb without losing aortic control, a third balloon is placed through the contralateral groin, maintaining wire access on the ipsilateral side. F, With the third balloon still inflated via the contralateral groin, the ipsilateral limb is extended to allow for a distal seal. The balloon is then deflated and angiography is performed (see text for details). (Reprinted from the Journal of Vascular Surgery. Berland TL, Veith FJ, Cayne NS, et al. Technique of supraceliac balloon control of the aorta during endovascular repair of ruptured abdominal aortic aneurysms. *J Vasc Surg.* 2013;57:272-275, Copyright 2013, with permission from the Society for Vascular Surgery.)

Intraluminal abdominal aortic aneurysm thrombus is associated with disruption of wall integrity

Koole D, Zandvoort HJA, Schoneveld A, et al (Univ Med Ctr Utrecht, The Netherlands; et al)

J Vasc Surg 57:77-83, 2013

Objective.—An association of intraluminal thrombus (ILT) with abdominal aortic aneurysm (AAA) growth has been suggested. Previous in vitro experiments have demonstrated that aneurysm-associated thrombus may secrete proteolytic enzymes and may develop local hypoxia that might lead to the formation of tissue-damaging reactive oxygen species. In this study, we assessed the hypothesis that ventral ILT thickness is associated with markers of proteolysis and with lipid oxidation in the underlying AAA vessel wall.

Methods.—Ventral AAA tissue was collected from asymptomatic patients at the site of maximal diameter during open aneurysm repair. Segments were divided, one part for biochemical measurements and one for histologic analyses. We measured total cathepsin B, cathepsin S levels, and matrix metalloproteinase (MMP)-2 and MMP-9 activity. Myeloperoxidase and thiobarbituric acid reactive substances were determined as measures of lipid oxidation. Histologic segments were analyzed semiquantitatively for the presence of collagen, elastin, vascular smooth muscle cells (VSMCs), and inflammatory cells. Preoperative computed tomography angiography scans of 83 consecutive patients were analyzed. A three-dimensional reconstruction was obtained, and a center lumen line of the aorta was constructed. Ventral ILT thickness was measured in the anteroposterior direction at the level of maximal aneurysm diameter on the orthogonal slices.

Results.—Ventral ILT thickness was positively correlated with aortic diameter ($r = 0.25$; $P = .02$) and with MMP-2 levels ($r = 0.27$; $P = .02$).

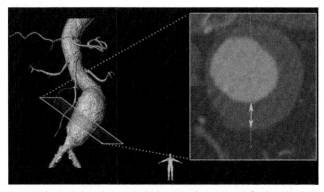

FIGURE 1.—Intraluminal thrombus (ILT) thickness (*red arrow*) is defined as the distance from the ventral aneurysm wall to the aortic lumen in the anteroposterior direction on the orthogonal slices. For Interpretation of the references to color in this figure legend, the reader is referred to web version of this article. (Reprinted from the Journal of Vascular Surgery. Koole D, Zandvoort HJA, Schoneveld A, et al. Intraluminal abdominal aortic aneurysm thrombus is associated with disruption of wall integrity. *J Vasc Surg.* 2013;57:77-83, Copyright 2013, with permission from the Society for Vascular Surgery.)

No biochemical correlations were observed with MMP-9 activity or cathepsin B and S expression. No correlation between ventral ILT thickness and myeloperoxidase or thiobarbituric acid reactive substances was observed. Ventral ILT thickness was negatively correlated with VSMCs (no staining, 18.5 [interquartile range, 12.0-25.5] mm; minor, 17.6 [10.7-22.1] mm; moderate, 14.5 [4.6-21.7] mm; and heavy, 8.0 [0.0-12.3] mm, respectively; $P = .01$) and the amount of elastin (no staining, 18.6 [12.2-30.0] mm; minor, 16.5 [9.0-22.1] mm; moderate, 11.7 [2.5-15.3] mm; and heavy 7.7 [0.0-7.7] mm, respectively; $P = .01$) in the medial aortic layer.

Conclusions.—ILT thickness appeared to be associated with VSMCs apoptosis and elastin degradation and was positively associated with MMP-2 concentrations in the underlying wall. This suggests that ILT thickness affects AAA wall stability and might contribute to AAA growth and rupture. ILT thickness was not correlated with markers of lipid oxidation (Fig 1).

▶ This study is quite interesting. These authors took 83 consecutive patients undergoing open repair for abdominal aortic aneurysm (AAA) and, at the time of operation, sampled the anterior aneurysm wall at the site of maximum diameter (presumably the weakest segment). They sent this tissue for both biologic and histologic analysis. They then evaluated the computed tomography scans of each patient and measured the intraluminal thrombus (ILT) at the site of biopsy (Fig 1).

ILT thickness appeared to be associated with vascular smooth muscle cell apoptosis and elastin degradation and was positively associated with matrix metalloproteinase—2 concentrations in the underlying wall. This suggests that ILT thickness affects AAA wall stability and might contribute to AAA growth and rupture. ILT thickness had no correlation with markers of lipid oxidation.

This study would be very interesting to repeat in a cohort of patients undergoing open repair of ruptured AAA.

B. W. Starnes, MD

Asymmetric expansion of aortic aneurysms on computed tomography imaging
Cronin P, Upchurch GR Jr, Patel HJ, et al (Univ of Michigan Med Ctr, Ann Arbor; Univ of Virginia Health System, Charlottesville)
J Vasc Surg 57:390-398.e3, 2013

Objective.—To investigate whether wall growth during aneurysm development spares the aortic wall between the intercostal or lumbar arteries or, alternatively, is uniform around the circumference.

Methods.—Computed tomography scans of 155 patients with aortic aneurysms (40 thoracic, 50 thoracoabdominal, and 65 abdominal) in a single hospital of a large academic institution were retrospectively inspected. Computed tomography studies of 100 control subjects (40 thoracic and 60

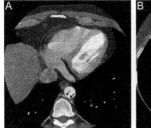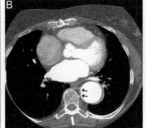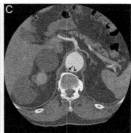

FIGURE 1.—Intravenous contrast material-enhanced computed tomographic scans. **A,** Lower thoracic aorta in a control subject. Note the normal-caliber aorta and the short interbranch arc length (ie, the arc length between the arterial origins of each paired intercostal artery; *black arrow*). **B,** Thoracic aorta in a patient with an aortic aneurysm. Note the increased diameter of the thoracic aorta but the relatively preserved short interbranch arc length (ie, the arc length between the arterial origins of each paired intercostal artery; *black arrow*). **C,** Abdominal aorta in a patient with an aortic aneurysm at the level of the celiac axis. Again, note the increased diameter of the abdominal aorta but the relatively preserved short interbranch arc length (ie, the arc length between the arterial origins of each paired lumbar artery; *black arrow*). (Reprinted from the Journal of Vascular Surgery. Cronin P, Upchurch Jr GR, Patel HJ, et al. Asymmetric expansion of aortic aneurysms on computed tomography imaging. *J Vasc Surg.* 2013;57:390-398.e3, Copyright 2013, with permission from the Society for Vascular Surgery.)

abdominal) were also reviewed. In all 255 patients, the ratio of the arc length between the origins of the intercostal or lumbar arteries (interbranch arc length) to the remainder of the aortic residual circumference was calculated. These ratios were compared between all subjects with aneurysms and the controls at each vertebral body level and between those with thoracic or thoracoabdominal or abdominal aneurysms and controls at each vertebral body level.

Results.—Interbranch arc lengths and residual aortic circumferences were larger in aneurysm patients than in control subjects, but the differences were statistically significant only at T4 and from T8 to L4 ($P = .009$ to $P < .001$) and from T4 to L4 ($P < .001$), respectively. The ratio of interbranch arc length to residual circumference in aneurysmal aortas was significantly smaller than that in controls at 12 out of 13 levels from T4 to L4 ($P = .004$ to $P < .001$). There was a statistically significant smaller ratio at 8 out of 9 levels for thoracic aneurysms ($P = .006$ to $P < .001$), 12 out of 13 levels for thoracoabdominal aneurysms ($P = .008$ to $P < .001$), and 3 out of 4 levels for abdominal aneurysms compared with controls ($P = .006$ to $P < .001$).

Conclusions.—Wall growth in aortic aneurysms is asymmetric, with greater aneurysmal growth in the anterior aorta wall and relative sparing of the portion of aortic wall between the intercostal or lumbar arteries. The mechanisms effecting this asymmetric growth have not been fully characterized (Fig 1).

▶ These authors' preliminary observations in 16 patients with descending thoracic aortic aneurysms supported a hypothesis that different regions of the aortic wall had differential expression of matrix metalloproteinases.[1] One hundred fifty computed tomography scans of patients with various aortic aneurysmal pathologies were analyzed and compared with those of 100 control subjects. Arc length measurements were determined between paired intercostal and lumbar arteries and compared with residual aortic wall circumference at each level between T4 and L4 (Fig 1).

Not surprisingly, the authors found a differential increased enlargement of the aortic wall anterior to the paired branch vessels compared with the aortic wall between the intercostal and lumbar artery origins. Because the intercostal arteries are a principal supply to the vasa vasorum, the aortic wall closest to the vessel origins may be better oxygenated and better nourished than the wall remote from them, that is, on the opposing aneurysm wall. These findings raise the question of whether other portions of the aortic wall, such as that bearing the left subclavian origin, might be similarly protected.

B. W. Starnes, MD

Reference

1. Sinha I, Bethi S, Cronin P, et al. A biologic basis for asymmetric growth in descending thoracic aortic aneurysms: a role for matrix metalloproteinase 9 and 2. *J Vasc Surg.* 2006;43:342-348.

Impact of chronic kidney disease on outcomes after abdominal aortic aneurysm repair
Patel VI, Lancaster RT, Mukhopadhyay S, et al (Massachusetts General Hosp, Boston)
J Vasc Surg 56:1206-1213, 2012

Objective.—Chronic kidney disease (CKD) is associated with increased morbidity and death after open abdominal aortic aneurysm (AAA) repair (OAR). This study highlights the effect of CKD on outcomes after endovascular AAA (EVAR) and OAR in contemporary practice.

Methods.—The National Surgical Quality Improvement Program (NSQIP) Participant Use File (2005-2008) was queried by Current Procedural Terminology (American Medical Association, Chicago, Ill) code to identify EVAR or OAR patients, who were grouped by CKD class as having mild (CKD class 1 or 2), moderate (CKD class 3), or severe (CKD class 4 or 5) renal disease. Propensity score analysis was performed to match OAR and EVAR patients with mild CKD with those with moderate or severe CKD. Comparative analysis of mortality and clinical outcomes was performed based on CKD strata.

Results.—We identified 8701 patients who were treated with EVAR (n = 5811) or OAR (n = 2890) of intact AAAs. Mild, moderate, and severe CKD was present in 63%, 30%, and 7%, respectively. CKD increased ($P < .01$) overall mortality, with rates of 1.7% (mild), 5.3% (moderate), and 7.7% (severe) in unmatched patients undergoing EVAR or OAR. Operative mortality rates in patients with severe CKD were as high as 6.2% for EVAR and 10.3% for OAR. Severity of CKD was associated with increasing

TABLE 4.—Postoperative Outcomes of Propensity-Matched Patients with Mild vs Moderate Chronic Kidney Disease (CKD) Undergoing Endovascular (*EVAR*) or Open (*OAR*) Abdominal Aortic Aneurysm (AAA) Repair

	EVAR (1:1 match n = 3460)			OAR (1:1 match n = 1740)		
Variable[a]	Mild (n = 1733)	Moderate (n = 1727)	P[b]	Mild (n = 867)	Moderate (n = 873)	P[b]
30-day mortality	1.9	3.2	.013	3.1	8.4	<.0001
Any complication	8.3	12.8	<.0001	25.2	32.4	.001
Wound complications	2.3	2.7	.5	5.0	4.9	.97
Pneumonia	1.9	2.4	.29	9.7	11.2	.29
Ventilation >48 hours	0.5	0.1	.018	10.6	14.3	.019
Acute renal failure	0.7	1.7	.005	2.5	6.0	.0004
Stroke	0.5	0.8	.2	1.0	1.4	.52
Myocardial infarction	0.4	0.5	.79	0.6	1.4	.091
Cardiac arrest	0.5	0.6	.65	1.9	2.1	.74
Bleeding (>4 units transfused)	0.6	1.0	.19	2.3	4.5	.013
Sepsis	1.1	1.5	.36	5.9	4.9	.38
Shock	0.9	1.9	.014	5.2	10.1	.0001

[a]Data are presented as percentage of the patients.
[b]Values of P < .05 are statistically significant.

frequency of risk factors; therefore, propensity matching to control for comorbidities was performed, resulting in similar baseline clinical and demographic features of patients with mild compared with those with moderate or severe disease. In propensity-matched cohorts, moderate CKD increased the risk of 30-day mortality for EVAR (1.9% mild vs 3.2% moderate; $P = .013$) and OAR (3.1% mild vs 8.4% moderate; $P < .0001$). Moderate CKD was also associated with increased morbidity in patients treated with EVAR (8.3% mild vs 12.8% moderate; $P < .0001$) or OAR (25.2% mild vs 32.4% moderate; $P = .001$). Similarly, severe CKD increased the risk of 30-day mortality for EVAR (2.6% mild vs 5.7% severe; $P = .0081$) and OAR (4.1% mild vs 9.9% severe; $P = .0057$). Severe CKD was also associated with increased morbidity in patients treated with EVAR (10.6% mild vs 19.2% severe; $P < .0001$) or OAR (31.1% mild vs 39.6% severe; $P = .04$).

Conclusions.—The presence of moderate or severe CKD in patients considered for AAA repair is associated with significantly increased mortality and therefore should figure prominently in clinical decision making. The high mortality of AAA repair in patients with severe CKD is such that elective repair in such patients is not advised, except in extenuating clinical circumstances (Table 4).

▶ Utilizing the National Surgical Quality Improvement Program (NSQIP), these authors examined 8701 patients undergoing either open surgical repair (n = 2890) or endovascular aortic repair (EVAR; n = 5811) and stratified the patients according to level of underlying chronic kidney disease (CKD; mild, stages 1 and 2, moderate, stage 3, and severe, stages 4 and 5). Mortality rates were significantly different between stratified groups (Table 4).

The robust clinical data available in the NSQIP data set allowed the authors to accurately determine estimated glomerular filtration rate and CKD severity using validated clinical data for all patients included in the study.

Bottom line and not surprisingly—there is increased morbidity and mortality associated with worsening renal function for both EVAR and open surgical repair. The authors boldly state that elective repair in patients with severe CKD has prohibitive operative risk and is not advised except in extenuating clinical circumstances.

B. W. Starnes, MD

An Association between Chronic Obstructive Pulmonary Disease and Abdominal Aortic Aneurysm beyond Smoking: Results from a Case—control Study

Meijer CA, Kokje VBC, van Tongeren RBM, et al (Leiden Univ Med Ctr, The Netherlands; Deventer Hosp, The Netherlands; et al)
Eur J Vasc Endovasc Surg 44:153-157, 2012

Objectives.—It is currently unclear whether the parallels between abdominal aortic aneurysms (AAAs) and chronic obstructive pulmonary disease (COPD) are explained by common risk factors alone, such as cigarette smoking, or by a predetermined cause. Given the persistent controversy with regard to the association between AAA and COPD, we studied this association in depth.

Methods.—We conducted a case—control study comparing patients with a small AAA (maximum infrarenal diameter $35-50$ mm, $n = 221$) with controls diagnosed with peripheral artery disease (PAD, $n = 87$). The controls were matched to the cases for lifetime cigarette smoking. Pulmonary function was measured by spirometry, and all subjects completed a questionnaire on medical history and smoking habits (current, former and never smokers).

Results.—Aneurysm patients were similar to controls with respect to gender ($p = 0.71$), lifetime cigarette smoking (39 vs. 34 pack years, $p = 0.23$) and history of cardiovascular disease (45% vs. 55%, $p = 0.12$). Aneurysm patients had more airway obstruction (forced expiratory volume in 1 s/forced vital capacity (FEV1/FVC) (0.69 ± 0.12 vs. 0.78 ± 0.11, $p < 0.001$)), which was most pronounced in never smokers (0.73 ± 0.07 vs. 0.86 ± 0.07, $p < 0.001$). COPD was more prevalent in aneurysm patients (44%; 98/221) than in controls (20%; 17/87) (adjusted odds ratio (OR) 3.0; 95% confidence interval (95% CI) 1.6-5.5, $p < 0.001$). In particular, a major proportion of AAA patients was newly diagnosed with COPD; only 40 of 98 patients (41%) with COPD (mild, moderate or severe/very severe) were known before with obstructive pulmonary defects and received treatment.

Conclusions.—This study confirms an association between AAA and COPD and shows that this association is independent from smoking.

TABLE 3.—Spirometry Outcome Measures in Cases with Abdominal Aortic Aneurysm and Controls[a]

	PAD $n = 87$	AAA $n = 221$	p
FVC (L)	3.23 ± 0.78	3.46 ± 0.83	0.024
FEV1 (L)	2.50 ± 0.69	2.39 ± 0.71	0.21
FEV1 % predicted	84.0 ± 17.8	80.4 ± 19.0	0.13
FEV1/FVC ratio	0.78 ± 0.11	0.69 ± 0.12	<0.001
Current smokers	0.75 ± 0.11	0.69 ± 0.14	0.013
Former smokers	0.79 ± 0.10	0.68 ± 0.12	<0.001
Never smokers	0.86 ± 0.07	0.73 ± 0.07	<0.001

FVC; forced vital capacity, FEV1; forced expiratory volume in 1 s, L; litre. FVC is slightly increased in aneurysm patients. Mean FEV1/FVC ratio is significantly reduced in aneurysm patients compared with controls, most pronounced in never smokers.

[a]Data are presented as mean ± SD.

Findings also demonstrate that COPD is under-diagnosed in AAA patients (Table 3).

▶ I chose this study for the VASCULAR YEAR BOOK for 2 specific reasons. (1) It supports my own internal bias that chronic obstructive pulmonary disease (COPD) is underdiagnosed in abdominal aortic aneurysms (AAA) patients. In fact, 59% of COPD cases were previously undetected in the AAA group. (2) There is relationship between AAA and COPD that is unexplained by smoking alone.

These authors took 221 patients with known small AAAs with complete spirometry data and compared them head to head with a control group of 87 patients with peripheral arterial disease (PAD) and no evidence of AAA (and complete spirometry data).

Most interestingly, aneurysm patients had more airway obstruction that was most pronounced in neversmokers (0.73 ± 0.007 vs 0.86 ± 0.07; $P < .001$; Table 3).

Several parallels exist between AAA and COPD with regard to risk factors and the underlying pathophysiology. The observations by these authors suggest that the relationship between AAA and COPD reflects a common susceptibility, a notion that is fully supported by converging pathophysiologic pathways to include neutrophil elastase and MMPs.[1,2]

B. W. Starnes, MD

References

1. Brusselle GG, Joos GF, Bracke KR. New insights into the immunology of chronic obstructive pulmonary disease. *Lancet*. 2011;378:1015-1026.
2. Lindeman JH, Abdul-Hussien H, Schaapherder AF, et al. Enhanced expression and activation of pro-inflammatory transcription factors distinguish aneurysmal from atherosclerotic aorta: IL-6- and IL-8-dominated inflammatory responses prevail in the human aneurysm. *Clin Sci (Lond)*. 2008;114:687-697.

Endovascular Treatment of Infected Aortic Aneurysms

Sedivy P, Spacek M, El Samman K, et al (Na Homolce Hosp, Prague, Czech Republic; General Univ Hosp, Prague, Czech Republic)
Eur J Vasc Endovasc Surg 44:385-394, 2012

Objective.—To report on the short- and long-term outcomes of patients with primary infected aortic aneurysm (IAA) treated by stent graft (SG) in two centers.

Material and Method.—Over a period of 15 years, 32 patients with IAA underwent endovascular treatment. None had undergone previous aortic surgery. The causal relationship was gastrointestinal infection in 9 patients (28%), endovascular diagnostic/therapeutic procedures/resuscitation in 6 (19%), wound infection after previous surgeries in 5 (16%), urinary infection in 4 (13%), urology or gastroenterology procedures in 3 (9%), pancreatitis in 2 (6%), endocarditis in 1 (3%) and phlebitis in 1 (3%) patient. We implanted 11 bifurcated, 10 tubular thoracic, 4 aorto-uni-iliac, 4 tubular abdominal and 1 iliac SG. Two other surgeries were hybrid procedures.

Results.—The etiological agent was identified in 28 (88%) patients. Twenty-six (81%) patients survived the 30-day postoperative period. Sixteen (50%) survived to 1-year follow-up and 13 (40.6%) survived to 3-year follow-up. Three patients have survived for less than 1 year and a further 3 for less than 3 years, so far. Among patients with aneurysms situated in central parts of the thoracic and infrarenal aorta there was a better death/survival ratio than among patients with a proximal or distal aneurysm location.

Conclusion.—The implantation of a SG may be an alternative to open surgery in selected groups of patients with primary IAA. Aneurysms of the central part of the thoracic or abdominal aorta have a more favorable prognosis with endovascular treatment (Fig 5).

▶ The endovascular management of patients presenting with mycotic aortic aneurysms has been increasingly popular with little or no good evidence of safety and effectiveness and certainly no clinical randomized trials. Primarily infected aortic aneurysms are rare, but when they do present, clinicians are often left with a challenging situation in a patient unsuitable for a very complex open surgical procedure. Naturally, an easier way to manage these patients would be attractive to most surgeons and interventionalists when the outcome for these patients has been so dismal.

We can learn some important lessons from this relatively large experience with mycotic aneurysms: (1) Patients who are actively septic should probably *never* be treated, because in this series the mortality rate was 100%. (2) An aggressive attempt must be made, prior to initiation of antimicrobial therapy, to identify the infectious agent and guide the choice of antibiotics. (3) Patients should be treated a minimum of 3 to 7 days with appropriate antibiotics before endovascular repair.

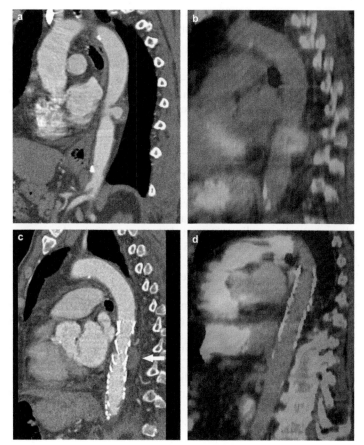

FIGURE 5.—a. Saccular aneurysm of descending aorta with inflammatory infiltration lining on CT. Salmonella was captured in hemocultures, infection originated from urinary tract, anamnesis duration 56 days. CT scan. b. Significant metabolic activity typical of infected aneurysm on FDG/PET CT. c. CT scan, the same view 1 week after tubular SG implantation. Arrow points at the thrombosed aneurysms. d. FDG/PET CT after 1 year: metabolic activity disappeared, no signs of aneurysm or residual inflammation. (Reprinted from European Journal of Vascular and Endovascular Surgery. Sedivy P, Spacek M, El Samman K, et al. Endovascular treatment of infected aortic aneurysms. *Eur J Vasc Endovasc Surg.* 2012;44:385-394, Copyright 2012, with permission from the European Society for Vascular Surgery.)

Forty-one percent of these patients survived more than 3 years without any additional therapy. This is an impressive statistic, and the role of this therapy serving as a bridge is called into question.

Another interesting aspect to this series involves the use of 18-fluorodeoxy-glucose—positron emission tomography scanning for the diagnosis and surveillance of these patients (Fig 5). There is an evolving body of literature suggesting that this method of diagnosis has utility.

The major drawback of this study is that the authors present a separate cohort of patients managed with open surgery during the same time interval, but unfortunately they do not offer the same mortality statistics at 30 days, 1 year, and 3 years. This information would obviously be useful.

B. W. Starnes, MD

Effects of Statin Therapy on Abdominal Aortic Aneurysm Growth: A Meta-analysis and Meta-regression of Observational Comparative Studies
Takagi H, Yamamoto H, Iwata K, et al (Shizuoka Med Ctr, Japan)
Eur J Vasc Endovasc Surg 44:287-292, 2012

Objective.—To determine whether statin therapy reduces the growth rate of small abdominal aortic aneurysms (AAAs).

Design.—A meta-analysis and a meta-regression of comparative studies.

Materials.—Eligible studies were randomized controlled trials or observational comparative studies of statin therapy versus placebo or no statin, enrolling individuals with small (<55 mm in diameter) AAAs and reporting AAA growth rate as an outcome.

Methods.—Study-specific estimates (standardized mean differences [SMDs]) were combined in the fixed- and random-effects model.

Results.—Seven adjusted and 4 unadjusted observational comparative studies enrolling 4647 patients with a small AAA were identified. Pooled analysis of all 11 studies suggested a significant reduction in AAA growth rate among patients assigned to statin therapy versus no statin (SMD, −0.420; 95% confidence interval [CI], −0.651 to −0.189). Combining the 7 high-quality studies providing adjusted data for growth rates generated an attenuated but still statistically significant result favoring statin therapy (SMD, −0.367; 95% CI, −0.566 to −0.168). The meta-regression coefficient for the baseline diameter was statistically significant (−0.096; 95% CI, −0.132 to −0.061).

Conclusion.—Statin therapy is likely effective in prevention of the growth of small AAAs, and may be more beneficial as the baseline diameter increases (Fig 3).

▶ It is highly unlikely that a prospective, randomized, controlled trial will ever again be conducted comparing statin therapy with placebo or no statin therapy. This is because statins have already been shown in multiple studies to be beneficial for just about everything related to cardiovascular health.

These authors conducted a meta-analysis of 4 unadjusted low-quality and 7 adjusted high-quality studies comparing patients receiving statin with patients receiving no statin therapy and the effects on growth rates of small aortic aneurysms.[1-11] There were no randomized, controlled trials found in the literature.

A total of 4647 patients formed the group of interest with 1347 patients receiving statins and 3300 not. Primary meta-analysis, sensitivity analysis, and meta-regression analysis all showed significant reductions in the growth rate of aortic aneurysms greater than 36 mm with a more significant reduction in larger aneurysms (Fig 3).

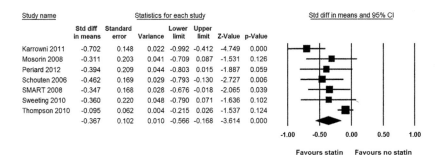

FIGURE 3.—Forest plot of growth rates of abdominal aortic aneurysm among patients assigned to statin therapy versus no statins from the 7 high-quality studies providing adjusted data. (Reprinted from European Journal of Vascular and Endovascular Surgery. Takagi H, Yamamoto H, Iwata K, et al. Effects of statin therapy on abdominal aortic aneurysm growth: a meta-analysis and meta-regression of observational comparative studies. *Eur J Vasc Endovasc Surg.* 2012;44:287-292, Copyright 2012, with permission from European Society for Vascular Surgery.)

Statin therapy is expected to prevent abdominal aortic aneurysm (AAA) development because the pleiotropic effect of statins includes an anti-inflammatory effect, an anti-oxidative effect, and reduction of matrix metalloproteinase secretion. The major message from this review: If possible, all AAA patients benefit from statin therapy!

B. W. Starnes, MD

References

1. Badger SA, Jones C, McClements J, Lau LL, Young IS, Patterson CC. Surveillance strategies according to the rate of growth of small abdominal aortic aneurysms. *Vasc Med.* 2011;16:415-421.
2. Ferguson CD, Clancy P, Bourke B, et al. Association of statin prescription with small abdominal aortic aneurysm progression. *Am Heart J.* 2010;159:307-313.
3. Karlsson L, Bergqvist D, Lindbäck J, Pärsson H. Expansion of small-diameter abdominal aortic aneurysms is not reflected by the release of inflammatory mediators IL-6, MMP-9 and CRP in plasma. *Eur J Vasc Endovasc Surg.* 2009;37:420-424.
4. Karrowni W, Dughman S, Hajj GP, Miller FJ Jr. Statin therapy reduces growth of abdominal aortic aneurysms. *J Investig Med.* 2011;59:1239-1243.
5. Mosorin M, Niemelä E, Heikkinen J, et al. The use of statins and fate of small abdominal aortic aneurysms. *Interact Cardiovasc Thorac Surg.* 2008;7:578-581.
6. Periard D, Guessous I, Mazzolai L, Haesler E, Monney P, Hayoz D. Reduction of small infrarenal abdominal aortic aneurysm expansion rate by statins. *Vasa.* 2012;41:35-42.
7. Schouten O, van Laanen JH, Boersma E, et al. Statins are associated with a reduced infrarenal abdominal aortic aneurysm growth. *Eur J Vasc Endovasc Surg.* 2006;32:21-26.
8. Schlösser FJ, Tangelder MJ, Verhagen HJ, et al. Growth predictors and prognosis of small abdominal aortic aneurysms. *J Vasc Surg.* 2008;47:1127-1133.
9. Sukhija R, Aronow WS, Sandhu R, Kakar P, Babu S. Mortality and size of abdominal aortic aneurysm at long-term follow-up of patients not treated surgically and treated with and without statins. *Am J Cardiol.* 2006;97:279-280.
10. Sweeting MJ, Thompson SG, Brown LC, Greenhalgh RM, Powell JT. Use of angiotensin converting enzyme inhibitors is associated with increased growth rate of abdominal aortic aneurysms. *J Vasc Surg.* 2010;52:1-4.
11. Thompson AR, Cooper JA, Ashton HA, Hafez H. Growth rates of small abdominal aortic aneurysms correlate with clinical events. *Br J Surg.* 2010;97:37-44.

Derivation and validation of a practical risk score for prediction of mortality after open repair of ruptured abdominal aortic aneurysms in a U.S. regional cohort and comparison to existing scoring systems

Robinson WP, Schanzer A, Li Y, et al (Univ of Massachusetts Med School and UMass Memorial Med Ctr, Worcester; et al)
J Vasc Surg 57:354-361, 2013

Objective.—Scoring systems for predicting mortality after repair of ruptured abdominal aortic aneurysms (RAAAs) have not been developed or tested in a United States population and may not be accurate in the endovascular era. Using prospectively collected data from the Vascular Study Group of New England (VSGNE), we developed a practical risk score for in-hospital mortality after open repair of RAAAs and compared its performance to that of the Glasgow aneurysm score, Hardman index, Vancouver score, and Edinburg ruptured aneurysm score.

Methods.—Univariate analysis followed by multivariable analysis of patient, prehospital, anatomic, and procedural characteristics identified significant predictors of in-hospital mortality. Integer points were derived from the odds ratio (OR) for mortality based on each independent predictor in order to generate a VSGNE RAAA risk score, which was internally validated using bootstrapping methodology. Discrimination and calibration of all models were assessed by calculating the area under the receiver-operating characteristic curve (C-statistic) and applying the Hosmer-Lemeshow test.

Results.—From 2003 to 2009, 242 patients underwent open repair of RAAAs at 10 centers. In-hospital mortality was 38% (n = 91). Independent

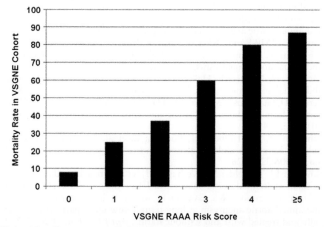

FIGURE 1.—Mortality rate according to the Vascular Study Group of New England (*VSGNE*) ruptured abdominal aortic aneurysm (*RAAA*) risk score. (Reprinted from the Journal of Vascular Surgery. Robinson WP, Schanzer A, Li Y, et al. Derivation and validation of a practical risk score for prediction of mortality after open repair of ruptured abdominal aortic aneurysms in a U.S. regional cohort and comparison to existing scoring systems. *J Vasc Surg.* 2013;57:354-361, Copyright 2013, with permission from the Society for Vascular Surgery.)

TABLE 5.—Multivariable Predictors of in-Hospital Mortality

Variable	OR	95% CI	P Value
Age >76	5.3	2.8-10.1	<.0001
Cardiac arrest	4.3	1.6-12.0	.0048
Loss of consciousness	2.7	1.2-6.0	.018
Suprarenal aortic clamp	2.4	1.3-4.6	.0057

CI, Confidence interval; OR, odds ratio.

TABLE 6.—Calculation of VSGNE RAAA Risk Score

Variable	OR	Integer Points
Age >76	5.3	2
Cardiac arrest	4.3	2
Loss of consciousness	2.7	1
Suprarenal clamp	2.4	1
VSGNE RAAA risk score[a] 0-6		

OR, Odds ratio; RAAA, ruptured abdominal aortic aneurysm; VSGNE, Vascular Study Group of New England.

[a]Sample case demonstrating calculation of the VSGNE RAAA risk score in an 80-year-old man who had loss of consciousness but no cardiac arrest and was repaired with suprarenal clamping of the aorta:

Age >76: 2 points
Cardiac arrest: 0 points.
Loss of consciousness: 1 point.
Suprarenal clamp: 1 point.
VSGNE RAAA risk score = 2 + 0 + 1 + 1 = 4.

predictors of mortality included age > 76 years (OR, 5.3; 95% confidence interval [CI], 2.8-10.1), preoperative cardiac arrest (OR, 4.3; 95% CI, 1.6-12), loss of consciousness (OR, 2.6; 95% CI, 1.2-6), and suprarenal aortic clamp (OR, 2.4; 95% CI, 1.3-4.6). Patient stratification according to the VSGNE RAAA risk score (range, 0-6) accurately predicted mortality and identified those at low and high risk for death (8%, 25%, 37%, 60%, 80%, and 87% for scores of 0, 1, 2, 3, 4, and ≥5, respectively). Discrimination (C = .79) and calibration ($\chi^2 = 1.96$; $P = .85$) were excellent in the derivation and bootstrap samples and superior to that of existing scoring systems. The Glasgow aneurysm score, Hardman index, Vancouver score, and Edinburg ruptured aneurysm score correlated with mortality in the VSGNE cohort but failed to identify accurately patients with a risk of mortality > 65%.

Conclusions.—Existing scoring systems predict mortality after RAAA repair in this cohort but do not identify patients at highest risk. This parsimonious VSGNE RAAA risk score based on four variables readily assessed at the time of presentation allows accurate prediction of in-hospital mortality after open repair of RAAAs, including identification of those patients at highest risk for postoperative mortality (Fig 1, Tables 5 and 6).

▶ This is another useful study from the Vascular Study Group of New England (VSGNE) evaluating a practical new risk score to predict mortality after open repair of ruptured abdominal aortic aneurysm (AAA). Independent predictors of mortality were age greater than 76 years, preoperative cardiac arrest, loss of consciousness, and need for a suprarenal cross-clamp (Table 5).

Based on these 4 variables, a score was created with 2 integer points each for age greater than 76 years and cardiac arrest and one each for loss of consciousness and suprarenal clamp (Table 6). Mortality rates correlated well with this scoring system and were validated using bootstrapping methodology (Fig 1).

It would be interesting to apply this scoring system to a similar cohort of patients undergoing endovascular repair and to substitute need for an aortic occlusion balloon with the need for suprarenal cross-clamp!

B. W. Starnes, MD

Cost—Effectiveness at Two Years in the VA Open versus Endovascular Repair Trial

Lederle FA, for the Open Versus Endovascular Repair (OVER) Veterans Affairs Cooperative Study Group (Veterans Affairs Med Ctr, Minneapolis, MN; et al)
Eur J Vasc Endovasc Surg 44:543-548, 2012

Background.—Long-term clinical outcomes have been similar for endo-vascular and open repair of abdominal aortic aneurysm (AAA), increasing the importance of comparing cost—effectiveness.

Methods.—We compared data to two years from a multicenter random-ized trial of 881 patients. Quality-adjusted life years (QALYs) were calculated from EQ-5D questionnaires. Healthcare utilization data were obtained from patients and from national VA and Medicare sources. VA costs were obtained using methods previously developed by the VA Health Economics Resource Center. Costs for non-VA care were determined from Medicare or billing data.

Results.—Mean life-years were 1.78 in the endovascular and 1.74 in the open repair group ($P = 0.29$), and mean QALYs were 1.462 in the endovas-cular and 1.461 in the open group ($P = 0.78$). Although graft costs were higher in the endovascular group (\$14,052 vs. \$1363; $P < 0.001$), length of stay was shorter (5.0 vs. 10.5 days; $P < 0.001$), resulting in lower cost of AAA repair hospitalization in the endovascular group (\$37,068 vs. \$42,970; $P = 0.04$). Costs remained lower after 2 years in the endovascular group but the difference was no longer significant (−\$5019; 95% CI: −\$16,720 to \$4928; $P = 0.35$). The probability that endovascular repair was both more effective and less costly was 70.9% for life-years and 51.4% for QALYs.

Interpretation.—Endovascular repair is a cost-effective alternative to open repair in the US VA healthcare system for at least the first two years.

► This analysis by the OVER Veterans Affairs cooperative study group provides an updated perspective on cost effectiveness of open vs endovascular abdominal aortic aneurysm repair with findings that are distinct from previous analyses based on similar randomized trials from outside the United States. The analysis takes advantage of the VA Decision Support System National Data Extracts and Medical SAS® datasets in combination with Medicare data, thereby providing a unique and relatively comprehensive perspective of total health care costs. In contrast to the results of the United Kingdom Endovascular Aneurysm Repair (EVAR) and Dutch Randomized Endovascular Management (DREAM) trials, which found endovascular repair to be more costly,[1,2] this study identified endovascular repair as a cost-effective alternative to open repair with a nonsignificant difference in cost at 2 years. The authors suggest differences in inpatient hospitalization costs between the US and Europe as a possible (and quite plausible) explanation for these findings as well as a number of other factors related to differences in health care delivery systems and screening. Because the cost estimates from this study are based on a postoperative interval of 2 years, it will be interesting to see if the cost neutrality is maintained as costs associated with surveillance imaging and reintervention continue to unfold over time. It is also important to note that within this randomized trial, all endovascular repairs were performed within strict anatomic criteria and compliance with device instructions for use. These results, therefore, cannot be generalized to off-label endovascular repairs performed with less strict anatomic inclusion criteria, where differences in procedure-associated costs as well as survival and repeat intervention would potentially have a significant negative impact on cost effectiveness.

M. A. Corriere, MD, MS

References

1. Prinssen M, Buskens E, de Jong SE, et al. Cost-effectiveness of conventional and endovascular repair of abdominal aortic aneurysms: results of a randomized trial. *J Vasc Surg.* 2007;46:883-890.
2. Greenhalgh RM, Brown LC, Powell JT, et al. Endovascular versus open repair of abdominal aortic aneurysm. *N Engl J Med.* 2010;362:1863-1871.

Expression of cytoskeleton and energetic metabolism-related proteins at human abdominal aortic aneurysm sites

Modrego J, López-Farré AJ, Martínez-López I, et al (Hosp Clníco San Carlos, Madrid, Spain)
J Vasc Surg 55:1124-1133, 2012

Objective.—The purpose of this study was to evaluate the expression of proteins related to cytoskeleton and energetic metabolism at abdominal aortic aneurysm (AAA) sites using proteomics. Several remodeling-related mechanisms have been associated with AAA formation but less is known about the expression of proteins associated with cytoskeleton and energetic metabolism in AAAs.

Methods.—AAA samples (6.73 ± 0.40 cm size) were obtained from 13 patients during elective aneurysm repair. Control abdominal aortic samples were obtained from 12 organ donors. Proteins were analyzed using two-dimensional electrophoresis and mass spectrometry.

Results.—The expression of filamin was increased in the AAA site compared to control abdominal aortic samples while microfibril-associated glycoprotein-4 isotype 1, annexin A5 isotype 1, and annexin A2 were reduced compared with control abdominal aortic samples. The reduction in expression level of energetic metabolism-associated proteins such as triosephosphate isomerase, glyceraldehyde 3-phosphate dehydrogenase, and cytosolic aldehyde dehydrogenase was also observed in AAAs compared to controls. Reduction of triosephosphate isomerase expression was also observed by Western blot, which was accompanied by diminished triosephosphate isomerase activity. At the AAA site, pyruvate dehydrogenase expression was reduced and the content of both lactate and pyruvate was increased with respect to controls without changes in lactate dehydrogenase activity.

Conclusions.—The present results suggest that an anaerobic metabolic state may be favored further to reduce the expression of cytoskeleton-related proteins. The better knowledge of molecular mechanism involved in AAAs may favor development of new clinical strategies.

▶ Abdominal aortic aneurysms (AAAs) are histopathologically characterized by the extensive degeneration of the aortic extracellular matrix, but besides the well-characterized elastolysis and collagenolysis, little is known about the changes in other proteins. With recent advances in vascular biology, the cellular and molecular pathways involved in AAA formation are being evaluated with the hope of the development of a noninvasive therapeutic approach for AAA treatment. The field of proteomics has grown exponentially over the past 10 years, and various methods have been developed that allow us to identify proteins in biologic samples. Proteomics gives a much better understanding of an organism than genomics, as the level of transcription of a gene gives only a rough estimate of its level of expression in a protein. The task of studying the proteome is quite daunting, because approximately 20 000 genes in the human genome can code for at least 10 times as many proteins.

This study evaluated the expression of proteins related to cytoskeleton and energetic metabolism at AAA sites using proteomics. The results show that at the AAA site there is a different level of expression of proteins associated with the cytoskeleton and with the glycolytic pathway than those observed in control abdominal aortic samples. These proteins include annexin A2 and A5, both of which have been associated with antithrombotic properties. Therefore, a reduction in their levels in AAAs may promote the presence of intraluminal mural thrombus in AAAs, which has been associated with AAA ruptures.

Evidence has suggested that maintenance of vascular function is particularly dependent on vascular energetic metabolism, and the current results demonstrate that an anaerobic metabolic state may be favored at the AAA site. Although the study design did not allow for an assessment of the clinical relevance of the findings, the results are interesting and could help uncover the molecular mechanisms associated with AAAs and may favor the development of new clinical strategies.

J. Cullen, PhD

Free-radical scavenger edaravone inhibits both formation and development of abdominal aortic aneurysm in rats
Morimoto K, Hasegawa T, Tanaka A, et al (Kobe Univ Graduate School of Medicine, Japan)
J Vasc Surg 55:1749-1758, 2012

Objective.—An ideal pharmaceutical treatment for abdominal aortic aneurysm (AAA) is to prevent aneurysm formation and development (further dilatation of pre-existing aneurysm). Recent studies have reported that oxidative stress with reactive oxygen species (ROS) is crucial in aneurysm formation. We hypothesized that edaravone, a free-radical scavenger, would attenuate vascular oxidative stress and inhibit AAA formation and development.

Methods.—An AAA model induced with intraluminal elastase and extraluminal calcium chloride was created in 42 rats. Thirty-six rats were divided three groups: a low-dose (group LD; 1 mg/kg/d), high-dose (group HD; 5 mg/kg/d), and control (group C, saline). Edaravone or saline was intraperitoneally injected twice daily, starting 30 minutes before aneurysm preparation. The remaining six rats (group DA) received a delayed edaravone injection (5 mg/kg/d) intraperitoneally, starting 7 days after aneurysm preparation to 28 days. AAA dilatation ratio was calculated. Pathologic examination was performed. ROS expression was semi-quantified by dihydroethidium staining and the oxidative product of DNA induced by ROS, 8-hydroxydeoxyguanosine (8-OHdG), by immunohistochemical staining.

Results.—At day 7, ROS expression and 8-OHdG-positive cells in aneurysm walls were decreased by edaravone treatment (ROS expression: 3.0 ± 0.5 in group LD, 1.7 ± 0.3 in group HD, and 4.8 ± 0.7 in group C; 8-OHdG-positive cells: 106.2 ± 7.8 cells in group LD, 64.5 ± 7.7 cells in group HD, and 136.6 ± 7.4 cells in group C; $P < .0001$), compared with group C. Edaravone treatment significantly reduced messenger RNA expressions of cytokines and matrix metalloproteinases (MMPs) in aneurysm walls (MMP-2: 1.1 ± 0.5 in group LD, 0.6 ± 0.1 in group HD, and 2.3 ± 0.4 in group C; $P < .001$; MMP-9: 1.2 ± 0.1 in group LD, 0.2 ± 0.6 in group HD, and 2.4 ± 0.2 in group C; $P < .001$). At day 28, aortic walls in groups LD and HD were less dilated, with increased wall thickness and elastin content than those in group C (dilatation ratio: $204.7\% \pm 16.0\%$ in group C, $156.5\% \pm 6.6\%$ in group LD, $136.7\% \pm 2.0\%$ in group HD; $P < .0001$). Delayed edaravone administration significantly prevented further aneurysm dilatation, with increased elastin content ($155.2\% \pm 2.9\%$ at day 7, $153.1\% \pm 11.6\%$ at day 28; not significant).

Conclusions.—Edaravone inhibition of ROS can prevent aneurysm formation and expansion in the rat AAA model. Free-radical scavenger edaravone might be an effective pharmaceutical agent for AAA in clinical practice.

▶ Abdominal aortic aneurysms (AAA) are characterized by localized remodeling and vessel dilation attributable to the degeneration of elastin and collagen in the aortic wall. Oxidative stress has been implicated in multiple disease pathologies ranging from atherosclerosis to Parkinson disease. Reactive oxygen species (ROS) are abundantly produced during inflammatory processes, and their production in vessel walls has been linked to degradation of the extracellular matrix. Indeed, emerging evidence suggests that ROS are associated with AAA formation in both animal models and in humans. There are currently no effective approaches to prevent AAA, except invasive surgical or endovascular therapies, and because it remains a complex multifactorial disease with still unknown etiology, effective pharmaceutical treatment has not yet been established clinically. However, experimental studies have found that genetic and pharmacologic inhibition of ROS production can inhibit aneurysm formation. In this study, the authors investigate the effect of edaravone, a free-radical scavenger, on both AAA formation and development using a rat AAA model induced with intraluminal elastase and extraluminal calcium chloride. The results show that the free-radical scavenger edaravone decreases the influx of inflammatory cells that could account for decreased oxygen radical damage and cytokine and matrix metalloproteinase expression, leading to prevention of AAA formation. In addition, another interesting finding was that delayed edaravone treatment also prevents further dilatation of pre-existing AAAs. This may be of great importance, as effective AAA pharmacotherapy might be of significant benefit to many patients with small AAAs or who are refused surgical procedures because of poor general condition. A limitation of the study is the animal model that is used; however, it must be pointed out that there is no ideal animal model for AAA that mirrors the pathology of the human disease, and there are advantages and disadvantages associated with each of the wide variety of models used for AAA research. These promising results suggest that edaravone has promising potential for AAA pharmacotherapy and warrants further investigation in other animal models of AAA.

J. Cullen, PhD

Comparison of 18F-fluoro-deoxy-glucose, 18F-fluoro-methyl-choline, and 18F-DPA714 for positron-emission tomography imaging of leukocyte accumulation in the aortic wall of experimental abdominal aneurysms
Sarda-Mantel L, Alsac J-M, Boisgard R, et al (Institut National de la Santé et de la Recherche Médicale, Paris, France; Service Hospitalier Frédéric Joliot, Paris, France; et al)
J Vasc Surg 56:765-773, 2012

Objective.—Abdominal aortic aneurysm (AAA) is a frequent form of atherothrombotic disease, whose natural history is to enlarge and rupture. Indicators other than AAA diameter would be useful for preventive surgery decision-making, including positron-emission tomography (PET) methods permitting visualization of aortic wall leukocyte activation relevant to prognostic AAA evaluation. In this study, we compare three PET tracers of activated leukocytes, 18F-fluoro-deoxy-glucose (FDG), 18F-fluoro-methyl-choline (FCH), and 18F-DPA714 (a peripheral benzodiazepine receptor antagonist) for in vivo PET quantification of aortic wall inflammation in rat experimental AAAs, in correlation with histopathological studies of lesions.

Methods.—AAAs were induced by orthotopic implantation of decellularized guinea pig abdominal aorta in 46 Lewis rats. FDG-PET (n = 20), FCH-PET (n = 8), or both (n = 12) were performed 2 weeks to 4 months after the graft, 1 hour after tracer injection (30 MBq). Six rats (one of which had FDG-PET) underwent 18F-DPA714-PET. Rats were sacrificed after imaging; AAAs and normal thoracic aortas were cut into axial sections for quantitative autoradiography and histologic studies, including ED1 (macrophages) and CD8 T lymphocyte immunostaining. Ex vivo staining of AAAs and thoracic aortas with 18F-DPA714 and unlabeled competitors was performed.

Results.—AAAs developed in 35 out of 46 cases. FCH uptake in AAAs was lower than that of FDG in all cases on imaging, with lower AAA-to-background maximal standardized uptake value (SUV_{max}) ratios (1.78 ± 0.40 vs 2.71 ± 0.54; $P < .01$ for SUV_{max} ratios), and lower AAA-to-normal aorta activity ratios on autoradiography (3.52 ± 1.26 vs 8.55 ± 4.23; $P < .005$). FDG AAA-to-background SUV_{max} ratios correlated with the intensity of CD8 + ED1 staining ($r = .76$; $P < .03$). FCH AAA-to-background SUV_{max} ratios correlated with the intensity of ED1 staining ($r = .80$; $P < .03$). 18F-DPA714 uptake was similar in AAAs and in normal aortas, both in vivo and ex vivo.

Conclusions.—In rat experimental AAA, characterized by an important aortic wall leukocytes activity, FDG-PET showed higher sensitivity than FCH-PET and 18F-DPA714-PET to detect activated leukocytes. This enhances potential interest of this tracer for prognostic evaluation of AAA in patients.

▶ Aneurysm rupture represents a catastrophic event with a mortality rate of 90%. Currently the decision for preventative surgery is based on clinical signs and anatomic criteria. Because abdominal aortic aneurysm (AAA) progression is not linear and growth acceleration usually precedes rupture, indicators of lesion development, other than AAA diameter, would be useful for surgical decision making.

The authors investigated if indicators other than AAA diameter would be useful for preventive surgery decision making, including positron emission tomography (PET) methods permitting visualization of aortic wall leukocyte activation relevant to prognostic AAA evaluation. In this study, they compared three PET tracers of activated leukocytes, 18F-fluoro-deoxy-glucose (FDG), 18F-fluoro-methyl-choline (FCH), and 18F-DPA714 (a peripheral benzodiazepine receptor antagonist) using an experimental rat model of AAA. Imaging was performed 2 weeks to 4 months after graft and histologic studies were conducted to stain for macrophages and CD8$^+$ lymphocytes. Their results demonstrate that in their model, characterized by an important aortic wall leukocytes activity, FDG-PET showed higher sensitivity than FCH-PET and 18F-DPA714-PET to detect activated leukocytes. These data suggest that because of its higher sensitivity of detection, FDG is a good candidate for activated leukocyte imaging in AAA. It is well documented that human AAA lesions are richer in inflammatory cells, including lymphocytes, which can produce elastases that aid the progression and rupture of AAA. Therefore, it is possible that early detection of these inflammatory cells in the aortic wall may indicate the need for preventative surgery. Although this animal study has yielded exciting results, investigation into the pathobiology of human AAA lesions and a better understanding of pathophysiologic mechanisms underlying initiation and progression of aneurysmal degeneration, especially the involvement of leukocytes, is required before this tracer could be used for the prognostic evaluation of AAA in patients.

J. Cullen, PhD

Changes in thrombin generation, fibrinolysis, platelet and endothelial cell activity, and inflammation following endovascular abdominal aortic aneurysm repair

Abdelhamid MF, Davies RSM, Adam DJ, et al (Univ Dept of Vascular Surgery, Birmingham, UK; et al)
J Vasc Surg 55:41-46, 2012

Background.—Abdominal aortic aneurysm (AAA) is a chronic inflammatory condition associated with a prothrombotic, hypofibrinolytic diathesis that may increase the risk of cardiovascular events. The effect of endovascular aneurysm repair (EVAR) on this prothrombotic diathesis is not fully understood, especially over the medium and long term. A better understanding of these postintervention changes may improve the risk of cardiovascular complications in the long term. The purpose of this study was to examine thrombin generation, fibrinolysis, platelet and endothelial activation, and the inflammatory response during the 12 months following EVAR.

Methods.—Twenty-nine patients (mean age, 76.9 years) undergoing EVAR for AAA (mean diameter 6.9 cm) had prothrombin fragment (PF) 1 + 2, thrombin-antithrombin complex (TAT), plasminogen activator inhibitor (PAI) activity, tissue plasminogen activator (t-PA) activity and antigen, soluble P- and E-selectin, and highly sensitive C-reactive protein (hsCRP) measured before and at 24 hours, and 1, 6, and 12 months after surgery.

Results.—PF1 + 2 were markedly elevated prior to EVAR and remained so at 24 hours and 1 month, but had decreased significantly at 6 and 12 months. TAT was also elevated prior to EVAR and increased still further by 24 hours, but fell to below baseline levels thereafter. PAI activity and t-PA antigen were normal prior to EVAR, increased significantly at 24 hours, and then fell to baseline levels. t-PA activity was only detectable at 1 and 6 months; there was a significant rise in soluble P- and E-selectin after EVAR, which was sustained for 12 months. hsCRP increased transiently in response to EVAR but returned to preoperative levels by 1 month.

Conclusions.—The prothrombotic, hypofibrinolytic diathesis associated with AAA is normalized 12 months after EVAR. This beneficial systemic

TABLE 2.—Changes in Different Markers Over Time (Median and IQR)

	Preoperative Median (IQR)	24 Hours Median (IQR)	1 Month Median (IQR)	6 Months Median (IQR)	12 Months Median (IQR)
Prothrombin fragment 1 + 2 (0.4-1.1 nmol/L)	2.1 (1.5-3.7)	2 (1.4-2.9)	2.1 (1.6-3.4)	1.9 (1.2-2.5)[a]	1 (0.7-2)[a]
Thrombin-antithrombin complex (1-4.1 µg/L)	6.2 (4.4-15.6)	14 (11-24.6)[a]	8.1 (5.4-14.3)	8.9 (5.1-11.6)	7 (5.1-11)
Plasminogen activator inhibitor activity (1-7 U/mL)	4.9 (0.3-6.8)	8.5 (0.3-10.6)[a]	0.3 (0.3-3)[a]	0.3 (0.3-4)[a]	5.7 (3.8-7.7)
Tissue plasminogen activator antigen (2-8 ng/mL)	3.4 (2.6-4.4)	5.1 (3.1-6.4)[a]	3.5 (2.4-5.4)	1.2 (1-2.2)[a]	3.4 (2.4-4.5)
Tissue plasminogen activator activity (0 U/mL) mean (±SD)	0 (0)	0 (0)	0.046 (0.09)[a]	0.023 (0.06)[a]	0 (0)
sP-selectin (92-212 ng/mL)	71 (61-86)	80 (61-93)	113 (80-141.5)[a]	110 (73.5-139.5)[a]	87 (61-116)[a]
E-selectin (17.5-88.1 ng/mL)	14 (9-18)	24.5 (12.5-42.5)[a]	15 (9-22)	52 (23.5-59.5)[a]	38 (24-42)[a]
Highly sensitive C-reactive protein (mg/L)	4.3 (1.5-12.75)	82.2 (53-105.5)[a]	7 (3.3-19)	4.3 (2.1-16.3)	2.7 (1.2-11.6)

IQR, Interquartile range; *SD*, standard deviation.
[a]$P < .05$ against preoperative values.

effect of EVAR for AAA disease may help protect patients against future thromboembolic cardiovascular events (Table 2).

▶ Endovascular repair of abdominal aortic aneurysms (AAA) is considered the standard of care in properly selected patients. A number of studies have found that arterial diseases, including AAA, have pathophysiologically an inflammatory set of events leading to a diseased state of the artery. In addition, endothelial dysfunction and prothrombotic states are a result of a complex process in arterial disease. Prothrombotic assays evaluating prothrombin fragment (PF) 1 + 2 and thrombin-antithrombin complex (TAT) and fibrinolytic assays assessing plasminogen activator inhibitor-1 (PAI-1) and tissue plasminogen activator (tPA) can be measured when determining a patient's prothrombotic and fibrinolytic states, respectively. In addition, platelet and endothelial activation can be assessed by measuring soluble P- and E-selectins, respectively, and generalized inflammation by highly sensitive C-reactive protein (hs-CRP). Both open and endovascular (EVAR) repair of AAA are associated with increased thrombin generation and relative hypofibrinolysis in the immediate perioperative period, and these conditions have been postulated to potentially be responsible for the increased perioperative thrombotic complications. In this study of 29 patients undergoing EVAR, the authors measured thrombotic and fibrinolytic markers before implantation of EVAR and after and at 1 year follow-up. Before EVAR, patients with AAA had significantly elevated PF 1 + 2 and TAT, indicating a prothrombotic state, which reduced significantly to normal levels at 12 months after EVAR. In addition, PAI-1 and tPA were normal before EVAR, rapidly increased, and then decreased to baseline levels at 12 months, whereas the tPA activity increased at 1 and 6 months (Table 2). Inflammation as measured by hs-CRP, increased immediately after surgery and then normalized, indicative of acute trauma. In addition, there was sustained activation of platelets and the endothelium after EVAR. Interestingly, aneurysm size did not correlate with coagulation, fibrinolytic, or inflammatory markers pre- or postoperatively. The combination of no increase in thrombin generation (measured by PF 1 + 2) and increased thrombin neutralization (measured by TAT) after EVAR may be protective against cardiovascular complications and thromboembolic disorders in this group of patients. The significant increase in platelet activity, as represented by elevated soluble P-selectin during the first postoperative year, may justify giving dual antiplatelet therapy to patients after EVAR, especially during the first year after the operation; however, this recommendation would have to be tested prospectively and be weighed against the risk of bleeding and costs. Taken together, this small study would indicate that there is a prothrombotic and hypofibrinolytic diathesis associated with AAA that normalizes 12 months after EVAR. This beneficial systemic effect of EVAR for AAA disease may help protect patients against future thromboembolic cardiovascular events. Future studies with larger sample size, with adjustment for age and comorbidities and outcome measures of thromboembolic cardiovascular events, will be necessary to confirm these very interesting data.

J. D. Raffetto, MD

7 Abdominal Aortic Endografting

Fractured superior mesenteric artery stents after fenestrated endovascular aneurysm repair
Canavati R, How TV, Brennan JA, et al (Royal Liverpool Univ Hosp, UK; Univ of Liverpool, UK)
J Vasc Surg 57:511-514, 2013

Stent fracture after fenestrated endovascular aneurysm repair is a recognized complication. In this report, we record the occurrence of superior mesenteric artery stent fractures in our series and describe the management of embolized stent fragments during secondary intervention (Figs 1 and 2).

▶ Now that fenestrated endovascular aneurysm repair (FEVAR) is becoming a mainstream option, reported complications are emerging from individual case series. In this report, an experienced group evaluated their experience with FEVAR. Eighty-one patients underwent stenting of 165 visceral arteries in conjunction with FEVAR. The authors noted 4 superior mesenteric artery stent fractures, 2 of which serve as the basis for this report. In each of the 2 re-interventions, the aortic portion of the fractured stent embolized into the iliac limbs of the aortic stent graft, requiring additional stenting to remedy (Figs 1 and 2).

In each of the cases of stent fracture, a Palmaz Genesis (Cordis, Roden, The Netherlands) stent was used. The Palmaz Genesis stent is a closed-cell, balloon-expandable stent. Its high rigidity may make the stent more prone to fatigue fracture when it is exposed to repetitive stresses. Currently, there are no reporting standards for FEVAR from the Society for Vascular Surgery, and there is a forming committee to address these standards from a panel of experts. It is important to address the reporting of the different types of stents used in visceral vessels, as some may not be compatible with FEVAR. It is clear that the Palmaz Genesis stent is one such example.

B. W. Starnes, MD

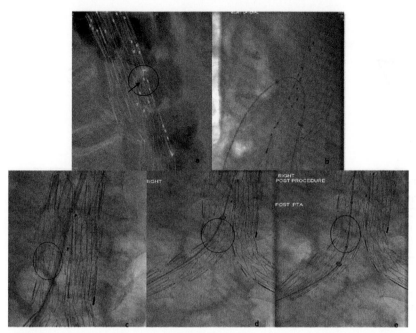

FIGURE 1.—a, Lateral abdominal radiograph showing fractured superior mesenteric artery (SMA) stent with the aortic portion at the level of the fenestration (*arrow*). b, Fluoroscopic image showing a guidewire and balloon catheter in the SMA. The aortic fragment of the SMA stent is no longer visible and has embolized. c, Aortic portion of the Palmaz Genesis stent shown in the right limb of the bifurcated graft (*circle*). d, Aortic portion well aligned with the stent graft. e, Aortic portion of the Palmaz Genesis stent apposing the iliac segment securely after ballooning. SMA, Superior mesenteric artery. (Reprinted from the Journal of Vascular Surgery. Canavati R, How TV, Brennan JA, et al. Fractured superior mesenteric artery stents after fenestrated endovascular aneurysm repair. *J Vasc Surg*. 2013;57:511-514, Copyright 2013, with permission from The Society for Vascular Surgery.)

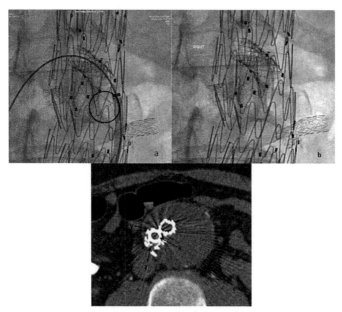

FIGURE 2.—a, Fractured superior mesenteric artery (SMA) stent with the aortic portion lying at the level of the right renal stent (*circle*). b, The aortic portion of the stent has embolized. c, Axial computed tomography (CT) image showing the crushed stent fragment (z) between the graft limb (y) and the Wall-stent (x). (Reprinted from the Journal of Vascular Surgery. Canavati R, How TV, Brennan JA, et al. Fractured superior mesenteric artery stents after fenestrated endovascular aneurysm repair. *J Vasc Surg.* 2013;57:511-514, Copyright 2013, with permission from The Society for Vascular Surgery.)

A meta-analysis of outcomes of endovascular abdominal aortic aneurysm repair in patients with hostile and friendly neck anatomy

Antoniou GA, Georgiadis GS, Antoniou SA, et al (Central Manchester Univ Hosps, UK; Democritus Univ of Thrace, Alexandroupolis, Greece; Philipps Univ Marburg, Germany)
J Vasc Surg 57:527-538, 2013

Background.—An increasing number of abdominal aortic aneurysms with unfavorable proximal neck anatomy are treated with standard endograft devices. Skepticism exists with regard to the safety and efficacy of this practice.

Methods.—A systematic review of the literature was undertaken to identify all studies comparing the outcomes of endovascular aneurysm repair (EVAR) in patients with hostile and friendly infrarenal neck anatomy. Hostile neck conditions were defined as conditions that were not consistent with the instructions for use of the endograft devices employed in the selected studies. Outcome data were pooled, and combined overall effect sizes were calculated using fixed or random effects models.

Results.—Seven observational studies reporting on 1559 patients (hostile anatomy group, 714 patients; friendly anatomy group, 845 patients) were

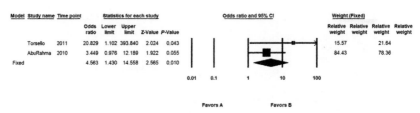

FIGURE 8.—Differences in the incidence of type I endoleak at 1 year between the hostile and friendly anatomy groups (A = hostile anatomy group; B = friendly anatomy group). *CI*, Confidence interval. (Reprinted from the Journal of Vascular Surgery. Antoniou GA, Georgiadis GS, Antoniou SA, et al. A meta-analysis of outcomes of endovascular abdominal aortic aneurysm repair in patients with hostile and friendly neck anatomy. *J Vasc Surg*. 2013;57:527-538, Copyright 2013, with permission from the Society for Vascular Surgery.)

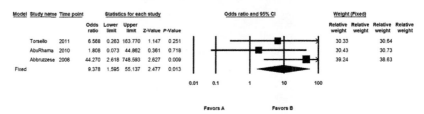

FIGURE 10.—Differences in aneurysm-related mortality rates at 1 year between the hostile and friendly anatomy groups (A = hostile anatomy group; B = friendly anatomy group). *CI*, Confidence interval. (Reprinted from the Journal of Vascular Surgery. Antoniou GA, Georgiadis GS, Antoniou SA, et al. A meta-analysis of outcomes of endovascular abdominal aortic aneurysm repair in patients with hostile and friendly neck anatomy. *J Vasc Surg*. 2013;57:527-538, Copyright 2013, with permission from the Society for Vascular Surgery.)

included. Patients with hostile anatomy required an increased number of adjunctive procedures to achieve proximal seal compared with patients with friendly anatomy (odds ratio [OR], 3.050; 95% confidence interval [CI], 1.884-4.938). Although patients with unfavorable neck anatomy had an increased risk of developing 30-day morbidity (OR, 2.278; 95% CI, 1.025-5.063), no significant differences in the incidence of type I endoleak and reintervention rates within 30 days of treatment between the two groups were identified (OR, 2.467 and 1.082; 95% CI, 0.562-10.823 and 0.096-12.186). Patients with hostile anatomy had a fourfold increased risk of developing type I endoleak (OR, 4.563; 95% CI, 1.430-14.558) and a ninefold increased risk of aneurysm-related mortality within 1 year of treatment (OR, 9.378; 95% CI, 1.595-55.137).

Conclusions.—Insufficient high-level evidence for or against performing standard EVAR in patients with hostile neck anatomy exists. Our analysis suggests EVAR should be cautiously used in patients with anatomic neck constraints (Figs 8 and 10).

▶ This meta-analysis evaluated 7 low-quality observational studies reporting on 1559 patients treated with endovascular aneurysm repair (EVAR) with either friendly aortic neck anatomy (n = 845) or hostile aortic neck anatomy (n = 714). Insufficient clinical information currently exists to provide strong evidence for or against the safety of EVAR in patients presenting with hostile aortic neck anatomy.

Most of the studies reviewed in this analysis had low methodologic quality mostly because of patient or control selection biases and inadequate reporting of nonresponders. Nonetheless, it should come as no surprise what the outcome of this analysis was. There was no significant difference in the incidence of type 1 endoleak and reintervention rates within 30 days between the 2 groups. Patients with hostile neck anatomy had a 4-fold increased risk of type 1 endoleak development and a 9-fold increased risk of aneurysm-related mortality within 1 year of treatment (Figs 8 and 10).

The authors concluded that there is insufficient high-level evidence for or against performing standard EVAR in patients with hostile neck anatomy. Message—follow the instructions for use!

B. W. Starnes, MD

Transcatheter Embolisation of Type 1 Endoleaks after Endovascular Aortic Aneurysm Repair with Onyx: When No Other Treatment Option is Feasible
Chun J-Y, Morgan R (St George's Hosp, London, UK)
Eur J Vasc Endovasc Surg 45:141-144, 2013

Type 1 endoleaks following endovascular aortic aneurysm repair are associated with poor outcomes and re-intervention is recommended as soon as possible after diagnosis. When standard endovascular or surgical treatment options are unsuitable due to severe co-morbidity or adverse anatomic factors, patients can be treated by transcatheter embolisation of the endoleak itself. We describe six such patients with proximal and distal type 1 endoleaks, who have been successfully treated by transcatheter embolisation with Onyx. The embolisation technique, advantages of using this relatively novel liquid embolic agent and potential pitfalls are discussed (Fig 1).

▶ I chose this article for review in the VASCULAR YEAR BOOK as an introduction to a technique for the management of endoleaks after endovascular aortic repair.

The authors describe 6 cases of successful management of type 1 endoleaks using Onyx, a novel nonadhesive liquid embolic agent that is most commonly used to treat intracranial arteriovenous malformations. It is comprised of ethylene vinyl alcohol dissolved in dimethyl sulfoxide and suspended in micronized tantalum powder to provide contrast (Fig 1).

What is most interesting to me about this is that 4 of the 6 patients described were originally treated outside the Instructions for Use (IFU) for the original device! The more innovative procedures we see to treat aortic pathology with purely endovascular techniques, the more complications we see that lead to more innovative solutions for treating the complications. This seems backward to me. How about we select our patients appropriately for the intended procedure and not push the boundaries far beyond that which the literature supports?

One prediction is clear: the more off-label use we see of these devices, the more agents and devices we will see to attempt to solve the problems associated with

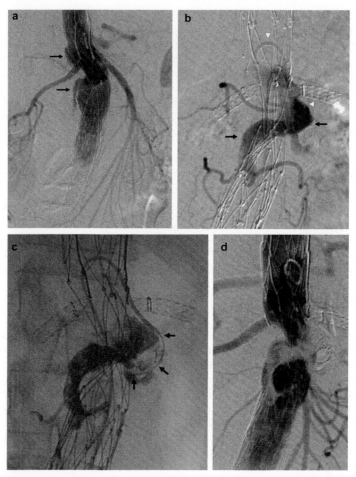

FIGURE 1.—(a) Completion angiogram following placement of Ventana fenestrated aortic endograft shows a proximal type 1 endoleak (arrows) and occluded left renal fenestration. (b) Entry into the proximal type 1 endoleak was achieved with a sidewinder catheter (white arrowheads). Selective angiography demonstrated the extent of the endoleak cavity (black arrows). (c) A more stable position was obtained within the endoleak cavity with a microcatheter (black arrows). Onyx was injected slowly into the deepest component of the endoleak initially and the microcatheter tip was subsequently withdrawn gradually during further slow injection. (d) Completion angiogram shows no residual endoleak after embolisation with 7 ml of Onyx. (Reprinted from European Journal of Vascular and Endovascular Surgery. Chun J-Y, Morgan R. Transcatheter embolisation of type 1 endoleaks after endovascular aortic aneurysm repair with onyx: when no other treatment option is feasible. *Eur J Vasc Endovasc Surg.* 2013;45:141-144, Copyright 2013, with permission from European Society for Vascular Surgery.)

these practice patterns. Onyx is nifty—and it works in some cases—but if we had better, more capable devices, we shouldn't need it!

B. W. Starnes, MD

Outcomes after endovascular abdominal aortic aneurysm repair are equivalent between genders despite anatomic differences in women
Dubois L, Novick TV, Harris JR, et al (London Health Sciences Centre and Western Univ, Ontario, Canada)
J Vasc Surg 57:382-389.e1, 2013

Objective.—Prior work confirms gender-specific anatomic differences in patients undergoing endovascular aneurysm repair, but the clinical implications remain ill defined. The purpose of this study was to compare gender-specific early outcomes after endovascular aneurysm repair using a large international registry.

Methods.—Over the 2-year period ending in 2011, 1,262 patients (131 women, 10.4%; 1,131 men, 89.6%) with infrarenal aneurysms treated with the Endurant stent graft were prospectively enrolled in the ENGAGE registry and followed clinically and radiographically.

Results.—Women were older (75.5 ± 7.0 vs 72.8 ± 8.1; $P=.0003$) and had smaller aneurysms (57.8 ± 9.5 vs 60.6 ± 11.9 mm; $P=.01$). Women's infrarenal aortic necks were of narrower diameter (21.8 ± 3.4 vs 24.0 ± 3.5 mm; $P<.0001$), shorter length (24.3 ± 11.8 vs 27.3 ± 12.4 mm; $P=.009$), and greater angulation (37.7 ± 26.2° vs 29.4 ± 23.3°; $P=.0002$). More women had an infrarenal neck angle > 60° (19.2% vs 9.1%; $P=.001$). Technical success was achieved in equal numbers of women and men (97.7% vs 99.2%; $P=.10$). On completion angiography, the incidence of any endoleak (21.5% vs 15.4%; $P=.08$) and type I endoleak (1.5% vs 1.1%; $P=.60$) did not differ between genders. At the 1-month follow-up, there were no differences between women and men with respect to endograft occlusion (2.5% vs 1.9%; $P=.70$), and differences observed in any endoleak (17.2% vs 11.4%; $P=.08$) and type I endoleaks (3.3% vs 1.2%; $P=.08$) did not reach statistical significance. Freedom from major adverse events was similar for women and men at 30 days (98.5% vs 95.8%; $P=.23$) and 1 year (85% vs 89.8%; $P=.40$). Survival at 30 days (100% vs 98.6%) and 1 year (92.5% vs 91.6%; $P=.99$) was similar for women and men.

Conclusions.—This large multinational registry confirms the previously observed prevalence of suboptimal neck anatomy in women. Even though

TABLE 2.—Anatomic Characteristics

Characteristic	Men ($n=1131$)	Women ($n=131$)	P Value
Size of aneurysm (mm)	60.6 ± 11.9[a]	57.8 ± 9.5	.01
Infrarenal proximal aortic neck diameter (mm)	24.0 ± 3.5	21.8 ± 3.4	<.001
Length of aortic neck (mm)	27.3 ± 12.4	24.3 ± 11.8	<.001
Diameter of right common iliac artery (mm)	14.3 ± 3.5	12.9 ± 3.5	<.001
Diameter of left common iliac artery (mm)	13.9 ± 3.6	12.5 ± 2.9	<.001
Infrarenal aortic neck angle (°)	29.4 ± 23.3	37.7 ± 26.2	<.001
Infrarenal neck angle greater than 60° (%, m/n)	9.1% (100/1095)[b]	19.2% (25/130)	.001

[a]Mean ± standard deviation.
[b]% (m/n).

women have shorter and more angulated infrarenal necks, their technical outcomes at 30 days and clinical outcomes at 1 year were similar to those of men. Much longer follow-up is necessary to determine whether these outcomes proved durable (Table 2).

▶ This is a large real-world experience showing yet again that women present unique challenges to aortic stent grafting, yet their attendant outcomes are exactly the same as those of men. The ENGAGE registry followed up 1262 patients (1131 men and 131 women) with detailed anatomic measurements (Table 2).

Women had smaller diameter, shorter length, and more angulated aortic necks than men, yet their outcomes with the Endurant stent graft were exactly the same. I'm not sure what this study adds to what we already know other than in the current era, aortic stent grafting is finally just as safe in women as it is in men.

B. W. Starnes, MD

Early Results from the ENGAGE Registry: Real-world Performance of the Endurant Stent Graft for Endovascular AAA Repair in 1262 Patients

Stokmans RA, Teijink JAW, Forbes TL, et al (Catharina Hosp, Eindhoven, The Netherlands; Univ of Western Ontario, London, Canada; et al)
Eur J Vasc Endovasc Surg 44:369-375, 2012

Objective.—The ENGAGE registry was undertaken to examine the real-world outcome after endovascular abdominal aortic aneurysm (AAA) repair (EVAR) with the Endurant Stent Graft in a large, contemporary, global series of patients.

Methods.—From March 2009 to April 2011, 1262 AAA patients (89.6% men; mean age 73.1 years, range 43—93 years) were enrolled from 79 sites in 30 countries and treated with Endurant. Results are described following the reporting standards for EVAR. Follow-up data were tabulated for all 1262 patients at a 30-day follow-up and for the first 500 patients at a 1-year follow-up.

Results.—Intra-operative technical success was achieved in 99.0% of cases. Within 30 days, adverse events were reported in 3.9% of patients, including a 1.3% mortality rate. Type-I or —III endoleaks were identified in 1.5% of cases. Estimated overall survival, aneurysm-related survival and freedom from secondary interventions at 1 year were 91.6%, 98.6% and 95.1%, respectively. At 1 year, aneurysm size increased ≥5 mm in 2.8% and decreased ≥5 mm in 41.3% of cases.

Conclusion.—Early results from this real world, global experience are promising and indicate that endovascular AAA repair with the Endurant Stent Graft is safe and effective across different geographies and standards of practice. Longer-term follow-up is necessary to assess durability of these results (Fig 1).

▶ This is an interesting report of a 2-year experience with the Medtronic Endurant stent graft under "real-world" conditions. As reported in the article, 1262

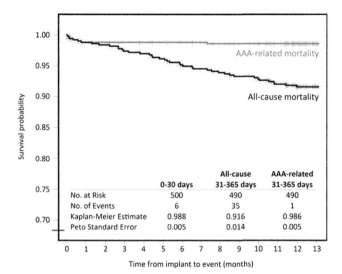

FIGURE 1.—Kaplan—Meier estimates for all-cause mortality & AAA-related mortality. (Reprinted from European Journal of Vascular and Endovascular Surgery. Stokmans RA, Teijink JAW, Forbes TL, et al. Early results from the ENGAGE registry: real-world performance of the Endurant Stent Graft for endovascular AAA repair in 1262 patients. *Eur J Vasc Endovasc Surg.* 2012;44:369-375, Copyright 2012, with permission from European Society for Vascular Surgery.)

abdominal aortic aneurysm (AAA) patients were enrolled from 79 sites in 30 countries. Interestingly, 17.9% of the patients (n = 226) were treated outside the instructions for use (IFU) for various reasons, hence the "real-world" mantra.

What this article shows, more than anything, is the power of international registries. Now, like no other time in history, we are able to obtain useful data on a large number of patients in a very short period of time (Fig 1).

The Endurant stent graft IFU allow for treatment of short necks (< 10 mm), yet the average neck length in this large series was 27 ± 12.4 mm. I remain disappointed that outcomes were not further stratified for those patients undergoing treatment with neck lengths between 10 and 15 mm or for those 17.9% of patients treated outside the IFU.

B. W. Starnes, MD

Comparison of fenestrated endovascular and open repair of abdominal aortic aneurysms not suitable for standard endovascular repair

Canavati R, Millen A, Brennan J, et al (Royal Liverpool Univ Hosp, UK)
J Vasc Surg 57:362-367, 2013

Background.—Abdominal aortic aneurysms that are unsuitable for a standard endovascular repair (EVAR) could be considered for fenestrated endovascular repair (f-EVAR). The aim of this study was to conduct a risk-adjusted retrospective concurrent cohort comparison of f-EVAR and open repair for such aneurysms.

Methods.—All patients who underwent repair of an abdominal aortic aneurysm that was unsuitable for a standard EVAR due to inadequate neck within one institution between January 2006 and December 2010 were identified. Case notes were retrieved for clinical data, Vascular Physiological and Operative Severity Score for enUmeration of Mortality and Morbidity (V-POSSUM) score, and aneurysm morphology. Computed tomography scans were reviewed to establish aneurysm morphology.

Results.—A total of 107 patients were identified. The open surgery cohort included 54 patients (35 men) who were a median age of 72 years (interquartile range [IQR], 9.5; range, 60-86 years). The aortic cross-clamp was infrarenal in 20 patients, suprarenal or above in 21, and inter-renal in eight. Postoperatively, 63 major complications were noted in 30 patients, nine of whom required 16 reinterventions. Cumulative hospital stay of the cohort was 1170 days (median, 12; IQR, 13; range, 1-205 days) of which 234 days (median, 28; IQR, 36; range, 1-77 days) were in the intensive therapy unit (ITU). Perioperative mortality was 9.2% (n = 5), exactly as estimated by V-POSSUM. The f-EVAR cohort included 53 patients (47 men) who were a median age of 76 years (IQR, 11.50; range, 55-87 years). Two

TABLE 3.—Postoperative Complications

Complication	Open Repair		f-EVAR	
	Events, No.	Pts, No. (%)	Events, No.	Pts, No. (%)
Cardiovascular	17	13 (24)	10	7 (13)
Myocardial infarction	6		3	
Dysrhythmia	7		4	
Cardiac failure	4		3	
Respiratory	17	15 (27)	8	7 (13.2)
Pleural effusion	2		0	
Chest infection	9		8	
Respiratory failure	2		0	
ARDS	1		0	
Tracheostomy	3		0	
Gastrointestinal	10	9 (17)	3	3 (5.6)
Mesenteric ischemia/bleeding	4		1	
Pancreatitis	1		0	
Diarrhea	1		1	
Upper gastrointestinal bleeding	1		0	
Bowel fistula	2		0	
Compartment syndrome	1		0	
Peritonitis	0		1	
Renal	9	9 (17)	8	8 (15)
AKI (>50% basal creatinine)	9		8	
Temporary dialysis		3 (5.5)		1 (1.8)
Neurologic				
Transient ischemic attack	0		1	
Other				
Acute limb ischemia	1		1	
Wound problems	4		2	
Retroperitoneal bleed	1		0	
Graft infection	1		1	
Heparin-induced thrombocytopenia	0		2	

AKI, Acute kidney injury; *ARDS*, acute respiratory distress syndrome; *f-EVAR*, fenestrated endovascular aneurysm repair; *Pts*, patients.

fenestrations and one scallop was the most frequent configuration (n = 31). Postoperatively, 37 major complications were noted in 18 patients, six requiring reintervention. Hospital stay was 559 days (median, 7; IQR, 4.5; range, 4-64 days), of which 31 days (median, 4; IQR, 10.5; range, 1-15 days) were in the ITU. Two patients died perioperatively (3.7%), resulting in an observed crude absolute risk reduction of 5.5% compared with open repair. The V-POSSUM estimated perioperative death in five patients (9.4%) in the f-EVAR cohort. In a hypothetic scenario of the f-EVAR cohort undergoing open repair, V-POSSUM estimated seven deaths (13.2%), resulting in an estimated risk-adjusted absolute risk reduction due to f-EVAR of 9.5%.

Conclusions.—In this group of patients, f-EVAR reduced mortality and morbidity substantially compared with open repair and also reduced total hospital stay and ITU utilization (Table 3).

▶ This is the first study to date to compare a single-institution experience of open surgery with a fenestrated endovascular aneurysm repair (FEVAR) in patients with aneurysm neck anatomy that is unsuitable for standard endovascular repair. The results are not surprising. FEVAR trumped open repair with regard to 30-day and in-hospital mortality and reintervention rates. The 30-day mortality rate was 9.2% in the open group vs 3.7% in the FEVAR group. Postoperative complications were twice as high in the open group (Table 3).

What may be even more relevant here are cost considerations. Cost is not reported. However, the open group was in the hospital a total of 1170 days with 234 in the intensive care unit (ICU) compared with a total of 559 days in the hospital for FEVAR patients with 31 days in the ICU. This is a marked and not unexpected difference.

This is a retrospective study, and the profound results call into question whether a prospective, randomized trial should even be done. Long-term reporting of target vessel loss will be important in the next several years. Fortunately, no patient in the FEVAR group ruptured while waiting for the customized graft to be shipped from Australia.

B. W. Starnes, MD

Temporary axillobifemoral bypass during fenestrated aortic aneurysm repair
Constantinou J, Giannopoulos A, Cross J, et al (Univ College, London, UK)
J Vasc Surg 56:1544-1548, 2012

Objective.—Fenestrated endovascular aortic aneurysm repair (f-EVAR) of juxtarenal aneurysms requiring cannulation of the superior mesenteric artery and renal arteries is technically challenging, has a long operating time, and requires bilateral large-caliber sheath insertion into the femoral arteries. Consequently, the risk of lower limb ischemia and subsequent reperfusion injury is increased. We describe the use of an adjunct temporary axillobifemoral bypass graft (TABFBG) for f-EVAR and propose that it be used as a strategy to avoid ischemia—reperfusion injury in patients anticipated as being at increased risk.

Methods.—Consecutive patients from a tertiary referral center undergoing f-EVAR, between October 2008 and August 2011, were retrospectively analyzed. Patients with lower limb arterial occlusive disease and those with difficult anatomy had an adjunct TABFBG.

Results.—All patients presenting with a juxtarenal aortic aneurysm were treated endovascularly, regardless of aneurysm anatomy and technical difficulties. There were 37 patients without TABFBG (group 1) and 27 with TABFBG (group 2). No patients required open conversion. Sex and age were not significantly different between the groups. The median ankle-brachial pressure index was significantly higher in group 1 ($P = .0001$). The groups had similar median blood loss, percentage of target vessel cannulation, and median stay in the intensive therapy unit. Morbidities were similar in both groups. There were no significant differences in cardiac, renal, or respiratory complications between the groups. The 30-day mortality was 10.8% ($n = 4$) in group 1 and 0% in group 2 ($P = .046$).

Conclusions.—Our series has demonstrated a significant reduction in mortality (10.8% absolute risk reduction) and no increase in morbidity with the use of a TABFBG for fenestrated grafts. This is likely a result of the reduction in ischemia and ischemia—reperfusion injury in these patients. We therefore recommend the use of TABFBG in patients with proximal severe stenotic or occlusive disease and those in whom an operative time of >4 hours is predicted (typically those for whom three or more target fenestrations is planned) (Table 2).

► In my opinion, this is one of the most important contributions to the VASCULAR YEAR BOOK this year. Fenestrated endovascular repair (FEVAR) is becoming mainstream, especially with the introduction of new devices on the market. There are inexperienced operators who will need to traverse the learning curve for these procedures and will clearly run into cases with long procedure times. These patients simply do not tolerate long periods of ischemia to the lower extremities. Furthermore, when large-bore femoral sheaths are removed at the end of the procedure and those ischemic limbs are reperfused, the result is hypotension,

TABLE 2.—Procedural Data

Variable[a]	Group 1 (n = 37)	Group 2 (n = 27)	P
Procedural time, min	294 (210-660)	319 (240-660)	.12
Blood loss, mL	1205 (200-5000)	1919 (240-4000)	.53
Target vessels			
Total number	86	75	.16
Cannulation	100	97.3	.42
Length of stay, days			
Intensive therapy unit	5 (1-35)	6 (1-38)	.47
Hospital	11 (2-54)	11.5 (4-100)	.52
30-day mortality	10.8	0	.046

[a]Continuous data are presented as median (range) and categoric data as percentage or as indicated.

which may cause a vicious spiral toward more and more complications to include the most feared: paraplegia.

These authors had a mortality rate of 10.8% with their first 37 FEVARs and then implemented a standard of performing extracorporeal temporary axillobifemoral bypass during the conduct of the fenestrated procedure. The subsequent 27 patients were managed with this technique (adding only 25 minutes to the average operative time) and had a 0% mortality (Table 2).

This is an important article and for those surgeons dipping their toes into the waters of FEVAR—best take heed of this sage advice!

B. W. Starnes, MD

Cost–Effectiveness at Two Years in the VA Open versus Endovascular Repair Trial

Lederle FA, for the Open Versus Endovascular Repair (OVER) Veterans Affairs Cooperative Study Group (Veterans Affairs Med Ctr, Minneapolis, MN; et al)

Eur J Vasc Endovasc Surg 44:543-548, 2012

Background.—Long-term clinical outcomes have been similar for endovascular and open repair of abdominal aortic aneurysm (AAA), increasing the importance of comparing cost–effectiveness.

Methods.—We compared data to two years from a multicenter randomized trial of 881 patients. Quality-adjusted life years (QALYs) were calculated from EQ-5D questionnaires. Healthcare utilization data were obtained from patients and from national VA and Medicare sources. VA costs were obtained using methods previously developed by the VA Health Economics Resource Center. Costs for non-VA care were determined from Medicare or billing data.

Results.—Mean life-years were 1.78 in the endovascular and 1.74 in the open repair group ($P = 0.29$), and mean QALYs were 1.462 in the endovascular and 1.461 in the open group ($P = 0.78$). Although graft costs were higher in the endovascular group ($14,052 vs. $1363; $P < 0.001$), length of stay was shorter (5.0 vs. 10.5 days; $P < 0.001$), resulting in lower cost of AAA repair hospitalization in the endovascular group ($37,068 vs. $42,970; $P = 0.04$). Costs remained lower after 2 years in the endovascular group but the difference was no longer significant (−$5019; 95% CI: −$16,720 to $4928; $P = 0.35$). The probability that endovascular repair was both more effective and less costly was 70.9% for life-years and 51.4% for QALYs.

Interpretation.—Endovascular repair is a cost-effective alternative to open repair in the US VA healthcare system for at least the first two years (Fig 1).

▶ The OVER (Open vs Endovascular Repair) trial is, to date, the most comprehensive randomized, controlled clinical trial comparing open repair with endovascular aneurysm repair (EVAR) for those abdominal aortic aneurysm (AAA) patients deemed suitable for both modes of therapy.

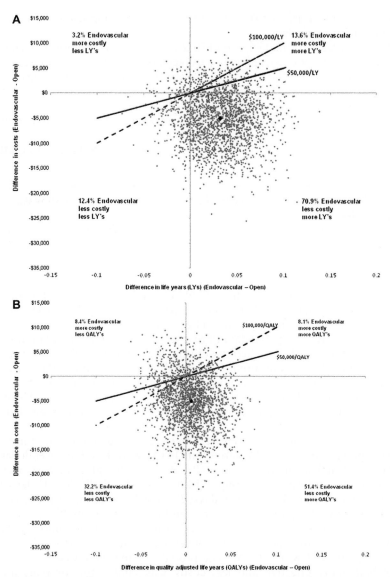

FIGURE 1.—Cost—effectiveness planes. Bootstrap replications showing the differences in costs and/or life-years (LYs) (A) or quality-adjusted life year (QALYs) (B) on the cost—effectiveness plane between patients randomized to endovascular or open repair at 2 years of follow-up. The large dot indicates the point estimate from the study. (Reprinted from the European Journal of Vascular and Endovascular Surgery. Lederle FA, for the Open Versus Endovascular Repair (OVER) Veterans Affairs Cooperative Study Group. Cost—effectiveness at two years in the VA open versus endovascular repair trial. *Eur J Vasc Endovasc Surg.* 2012;44:543-548, Copyright 2012, with permission from the European Society for Vascular Surgery.)

It continues to perplex me that educated individuals continue to use trials such as these to say that both modes of therapy have equivalent outcomes. This is nonsense. In fact, the OVER trial proves that EVAR is better than open surgical repair for AAA! With a perioperative mortality rate that is 6 times higher with open repair (3.0% vs 0.5% with EVAR), who in their right mind would want an open repair?

Population-based studies now show that patients undergoing open aneurysm repair are 12 times as likely to undergo laparotomy and lysis of adhesions for small bowel obstruction. In the OVER trial, patients undergoing open repair were just as likely to require secondary intervention for laparotomy-related complications, such as ventral hernia repair, and hospitalization for bowel obstruction. It is inaccurate to state that EVAR is costlier than open repair. In this study, the initial cost of EVAR was significantly less compared with that of open repair. However, at 2 years, the cost was still lower but not significantly so. Furthermore, quality of life was not significantly different between the 2 treatments.

These cost-effectiveness data are extremely helpful in shining new light on the superiority of EVAR over open surgical repair (Fig 1).

B. W. Starnes, MD

Duplex ultrasound factors predicting persistent type II endoleak and increasing AAA sac diameter after EVAR

Beeman BR, Murtha K, Doerr K, et al (Pennsylvania Hosp, Philadelphia)
J Vasc Surg 52:1147-1152, 2010

Objective.—While the significance of type II endoleaks (T2ELs) on the long-term outcome of endovascular abdominal aneurysm repair (EVAR) to repair abdominal aortic aneurysms (AAAs) is debatable, duplex ultrasonography (DU) parameters have been suggested to be predictive of their closure or persistence. The purpose of this study was to determine which, if any, of these variables was associated with persistent T2EL or increased AAA sac diameter.

Methods.—Between 1998 and 2009, 278 patients underwent EVAR and post-operative DU surveillance during long-term follow-up (1-11 years) in our accredited non-invasive vascular laboratory by one of three experienced technologists. DU measured intra-sac flow velocity (IFV), spectral doppler waveform (SDW) patterns, post-EVAR sac diameter, and number of T2ELs.

Results.—T2ELs developed in 14% (38/278) of patients post-EVAR. Fourteen patients had T2ELs that resolved, and sac diameter decreased or remained the same: the average IFV was 42 cm/second; SDW patterns were monophasic in five, biphasic in seven and bidirectional in two; and multiple T2ELs were not present (0%) in any patient. Twelve patients had T2ELs that persisted, but sac diameter decreased or remained the same: the average IFV was 47 cm/second; SDW patterns were monophasic in one, biphasic in five, bidirectional in five, and undetermined in one; and multiple T2ELs were found in 17% (2) of patients. Twelve patients had T2ELs that persisted and were associated with increased sac diameter: the

TABLE 1.—Doppler Ultrasonography Results of Post-endovascular Abdominal Aneurysm Repair

	Group 1	Group 2	Group 3
Number of patients	14	12	12
Intrasac flow velocity (cm/sec) (mean)	42	47	43
Spectral Doppler waveform			
Monophasic	5	1	1
Biphasic	7	5	2
Bidirectional	2	5	9
Unknown	0	1	0
Type 2 endoleak			
Number with 1 type 2 endoleak	14	10	3
Number with multiple type 2 endoleaks	0	2	9
Follow-up, months (mean)	38	31	65
Abdominal aortic aneurysm sac diameter			
Decreased	10	3	0
No change	4	9	0
Increased	0	0	12

Group 1, resolution of type 2 endoleak, no sac enlargement; Group 2, persistent type 2 endoleak, no sac enlargement; Group 3, persistent type 2 endoleak, sac enlargement.

average IFV was 43 cm/second, SDW patterns were monophasic in one, biphasic in two, and bidirectional in nine; and multiple T2ELs were identified in 75% (9) of patients. None of the 38 patients with T2ELs treated with selective surgical or endovascular intervention for enlarging sac diameters (11/12) experienced a ruptured aneurysm.

Conclusion.—Contrary to previous smaller reports of T2ELs and DU surveillance, parameters such as IFV did not correlate with increased post-EVAR sac diameter. The presence of multiple T2ELs and bidirectional SDW may be the strongest factors predictive of increased sac diameter (Table 1).

▶ Type 2 endoleaks are the most common endoleaks occurring after endovascular abdominal aneurysm repair (EVAR). The utility of which duplex ultrasound parameters predict endoleak closure is of great interest in an era of cost containment and increasing focus on patient safety. These authors sought to characterize which factors easily obtained on any duplex examination after EVAR would be most predictive of increasing sac diameter.

Of 278 EVAR patients followed up with duplex surveillance over 10 years, the authors found 38 patients with type 2 endoleaks (14%). They evaluated the following parameters:

1. Intrasac flow velocity (IFV)
2. Spectral doppler waveform patterns (SDW)
3. Post-EVAR sac diameter
4. Number of type 2 endoleaks

Of the 38 type 2 endoleak patients, the observations are listed in Table 1. Although the literature has suggested that IFV greater than 80 cm/s correlates with increased type 2 endoleak persistence, the authors did not observe this. Instead, they found that the presence of multiple type 2 endoleaks and bidirectional SDW were the strongest predictors for sac diameter increase.

B. W. Starnes, MD

Endovascular aneurysm repair in nonagenarians is safe and effective
Goldstein LJ, Halpern JA, Rezayat C, et al (Univ of Miami Jackson Memorial Med Ctr, FL; Weill Med College of Cornell Univ, NY)
J Vasc Surg 52:1140-1146, 2010

Objectives.—Advanced age is a significant risk factor that has traditionally steered patients away from open aneurysm repair and toward expectant management. Today, however, the reduced morbidity and mortality of aortic stent grafting has created a new opportunity for aneurysm repair in patients previously considered too high a risk for open surgery. Here we report our experience with endovascular aneurysm repair (EVAR) in nonagenarians.

Methods.—Retrospective chart review identified all patients >90-years-old undergoing EVAR over a 9-year period at our institution. Collected data included preoperative comorbidities, perioperative complications, endoleaks, reinterventions, and long-term survival.

Results.—24 patients underwent EVAR. The mean age was 91.5 years (range 90-94) among 15 (63%) males and 9 (37%) females. Mean abdominal aortic aneurysm diameter was 6.3 ± 1.1 cm. Eight patients (33%) were symptomatic (pain or tenderness). There were no ruptures. Fourteen patients (58%) had general anesthesia while 10 (42%) had local or regional anesthesia. Mean postoperative length of stay was 3.2 ± 2.4 days (2.8 ± 1.9 days for asymptomatic vs 4.1 ± 3.2 days for symptomatic, $P = .29$). There was one perioperative mortality (4.2%). There were two local groin seromas (8.3%) and six systemic complications (25%). One patient required reintervention for endoleak (4.2%). There were no aneurysm related deaths beyond the 30-day postoperative period. Mean survival beyond 30 days was 29.7 ± 18.0 months for patients expiring during follow-up. Cumulative estimated 12, 24, and 36-month survival rates were 83%, 64%, and 50%, respectively. Linear regression analysis demonstrated an inverse relationship between the number of preoperative comorbidities and postoperative survival in our cohort ($R^2 = 0.701$), with significantly decreased survival noted for patients presenting with >5 comorbidities. Those still alive in follow-up have a mean survival of 36.1 ± 16.0 months.

Conclusion.—This is the largest reported EVAR series in nonagenarians. Despite their advanced age, these patients benefit from EVAR with low morbidity, low mortality, and mean survival exceeding 2.4 years. Survival appears best in those patients with ≤5 comorbidities. With or without

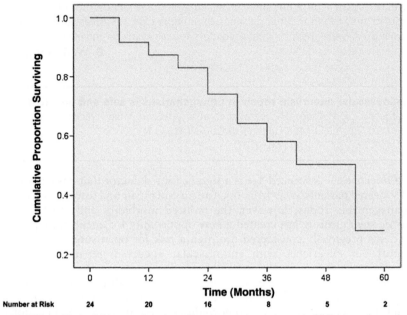

FIGURE 1.—Kaplan-Meier curve for estimated long-term postoperative survival following endovascular aneurysm repair (EVAR) in nonagenarians. (Reprinted from the Journal of Vascular Surgery. Goldstein LJ, Halpern JA, Rezayat C, et al. Endovascular aneurysm repair in nonagenarians is safe and effective. *J Vasc Surg.* 2010;52:1140-1146, Copyright 2010, with permission from the Society for Vascular Surgery.)

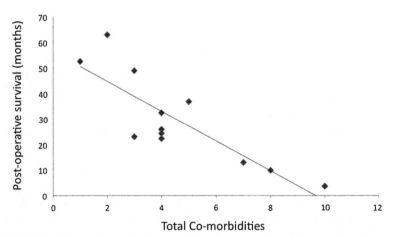

FIGURE 2.—Postoperative survival vs comorbidities in nonagenarians following endovascular aneurysm repair (EVAR). Linear regression of preoperative comorbidities vs postoperative survival (*months*) in patients reaching endpoint of death, $R^2 = 0.701$. (Reprinted from the Journal of Vascular Surgery. Goldstein LJ, Halpern JA, Rezayat C, et al. Endovascular aneurysm repair in nonagenarians is safe and effective. *J Vasc Surg.* 2010;52:1140-1146, Copyright 2010, with permission from the Society for Vascular Surgery.)

symptoms, patients over the age of 90 should be considered for EVAR (Figs 1 and 2).

▶ By the year 2050 (when I am set to turn 84), there will be an estimated 20.9 million Americans over the age of 85, representing 5% of the entire US population, up from just 1.5% in the year 2000.[1] With a current life expectancy of 6.4 years for 85-year-olds, it is projected that many octogenarians will live into their tenth decade.

This is the largest reported endovascular aneurysm repair (EVAR) series in nonagenarians. The Kaplan-Meier survival curves, as one might imagine, look like a steep cliff compared with those of other EVAR trials (Fig 1). The results are impressive, however, and shed some light on probably the most important aspect in caring for these patients—patient selection. Those patients with greater than 5 comorbidities fared poorly (Fig 2).

These authors can teach us all a few lessons in dealing with these elderly patients. They stress consideration of locoregional anesthetics when suitable and caution when treating elective patients who have greater than 5 comorbidities. Patients must be completely informed before embarking on a surgical approach that may take them from this earth before we expected them to go.

B. W. Starnes, MD

Reference

1. United States Census Bureau Population Estimates. [cited]. http://www.census.gov/popest/estimates.html. Accessed October 4, 2010.

Predicting the learning curve and failures of total percutaneous endovascular aortic aneurysm repair
Bechara CF, Barshes NR, Pisimisis G, et al (Baylor College of Medicine, Houston, TX; et al)
J Vasc Surg 57:72-76, 2013

Introduction.—Percutaneous endovascular aneurysm repair (PEVAR) has been shown to be feasible; however, technical success is variable, reported to be between 46.2% and 100%. The objective of this study was to quantify the learning curve of the PEVAR closure technique and identify predictors of closure failure.

Methods.—We reviewed patient- and procedure-related characteristics in 99 consecutive patients who underwent PEVAR over a 30-month period in a single academic institution. A suture-mediated closure device (Proglide or Prostar XL) was used. Forward stepwise logistic regression was used to investigate associations between the failure of the closure technique and a number of patient and operative characteristics. To ensure objective assessment of the learning curve, a time-dependent covariate measuring time in calendar quarters was introduced in the model. Poisson regression was

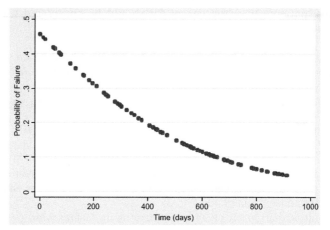

FIGURE 2.—Predicted probability of percutaneous failure over time. The curve is steepest during the first 18 months. (Reprinted from the Journal of Vascular Surgery. Bechara CF, Barshes NR, Pisimisis G, et al. Predicting the learning curve and failures of total percutaneous endovascular aortic aneurysm repair. *J Vasc Surg.* 2013;57:72-76, Copyright 2013, with permission from The Society for Vascular Surgery.)

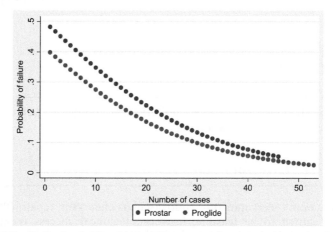

FIGURE 3.—Predicted probability of device failure over time (Prostar in the *blue curve* and Proglide in the *red curve*). Prior experience with Proglide use does not offer any advantage. For Interpretation of the references to color in this figure legend, the reader is referred to web version of this article. (Reprinted from the Journal of Vascular Surgery. Bechara CF, Barshes NR, Pisimisis G, et al. Predicting the learning curve and failures of total percutaneous endovascular aortic aneurysm repair. *J Vasc Surg.* 2013;57:72-76, Copyright 2013, with permission from The Society for Vascular Surgery.)

used to model the trend of observed failure events of the percutaneous technique over time.

Results.—Overall PEVAR technical success was 82%. Type of closure device ($P < .35$), patient's body mass index ($P < .86$), type of anesthesia ($P < .95$), femoral artery diameter ($P < .09$), femoral artery calcification ($P < .56$), and sheath size as measured in Fr ($P < .17$) did not correlate with closure failure rates. There was a strong trend for a decreasing number of failure events over time ($P < .007$). The average decrease in the odds of technical failure was 24% per calendar quarter. The predicted probability of closure failure decreased from 45% per patient at the time of the initiation of our PEVAR program to 5% per patient at the end of the 30-month period. There were two postoperative access-related complications that required surgical repair. Need for surgical cutdown in the event of closure failure prolonged the operative time by a mean of 45 minutes ($P < .001$). No groin infections were seen in the percutaneous group or the failed group.

Conclusions.—Technical failure can be reduced as the surgeon gains experience with the suture-mediated closure device utilized during PEVAR. Previous experience with the Proglide device does not seem to influence the learning curve (Figs 2 and 3).

▶ This topic has been near and dear to my heart for more than a decade. The pre-close technique was introduced in 1999 by Haas et al.[1] Benefits over standard surgical exposure and repair have been well documented and include less postoperative pain and fewer postoperative complications, such as infection, wound dehiscence, lymphatic complications, and femoral nerve injury. Suture-mediated closure devices were approved by the US Food and Drug Administration (FDA) and were available for closure of sheath sites up to and including 10F since 1996; yet, it has taken more than 15 years for this technique to be widely adopted. These authors (late adopters) began their percutaneous endovascular aneurysm repair (PEVAR) program in March 2009 and, in this report, detailed what they believed to be their learning curve with use of both the Prostar and Proglide devices (Abbott, Menlo Park, California). To ensure objective assessment of the learning curve, a time-dependent covariate measuring time in calendar quarters since the beginning of the PEVAR program was introduced into the model.

Type of closure, use of a hydrophilic sheath, type of anesthesia, femoral artery diameter, femoral artery calcification, and sheath size did not correlate with closure failure rates. The probability of failure over time decreased steadily (Figs 2 and 3). To achieve technical success of greater than 80%, they found that at least 15 cases were needed, and approximately 30 cases were needed to reach a technical success rate of 90%.

In 2007, I took a trip to the FDA in Rockville, Maryland to plead for approval of this technique without a randomized trial based on my own experience and the published literature. I was shot down. The results of the only randomized trial to date evaluating this method of access closure, the PEVAR trial, will be published this year. This technique should truly be the standard of care.

B. W. Starnes, MD

Reference

1. Haas PC, Krajcer Z, Diethrich EB. Closure of large percutaneous access sites using the Prostar XL Percutaneous Vascular Surgery device. *J Endovasc Surg.* 1999;6: 168-170.

Remodeling of proximal neck angulation after endovascular aneurysm repair

Ishibashi H, Ishiguchi T, Ohta T, et al (Aichi Med Univ Hosp, Nagakute, Japan)
J Vasc Surg 56:1201-1205, 2012

Objective.—This study investigated the remodeling of proximal neck (PN) angulations of abdominal aortic aneurysms (AAAs) after endovascular aneurysm repair (EVAR).

Methods.—A 64-row multidetector computed tomography scan of AAAs treated with EVAR was reviewed, and the PN angulation was measured on a volume-rendered three-dimensional image. The computed tomography scan was examined preoperatively, after EVAR at 1 week, 1 month, 6 months, 1 year, 1.5 years, 2 years, and then yearly. The study enrolled 78 patients, comprising 54 Zenith devices (Cook Medical, Bloomington, Ind) and 24 Excluder devices (W. L. Gore and Associates, Flagstaff, Ariz).

Results.—PN angulation was $50° \pm 20°$ preoperatively, and after EVAR was $36° \pm 14°$ at 1 week, $32° \pm 14°$ at 1 year, and $28° \pm 13°$ at 3 years. PN angulations $\leq 60°$ (n = 70, 77%) were $41° \pm 13°$ preoperatively, $31° \pm 12°$ 1 week after EVAR, $28° \pm 12°$ at 1 year, and $26° \pm 13°$ after 3 years. An angulation $>60°$ (n = 18, 23%) was $78° \pm 14°$ preoperatively, $51° \pm 11°$ 1 week after EVAR, $44° \pm 11°$ at 1 year, and $40° \pm 12°$ after 3 years. The greater the preoperative PN angulation, the greater its reduction immediately after EVAR ($r = .72$, $P < .001$). The diameter shrinkage of AAAs with a PN angulation $>60°$ was 3 ± 6 mm after 1 year; a significantly smaller shrinkage than with a PN angulation $\leq 60°$ (7 ± 7 mm, $P < .05$).

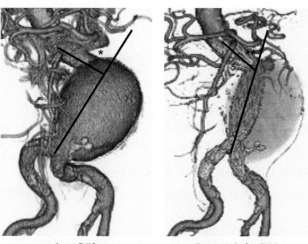

A: pre-EVAR   B: one week after EVAR

FIGURE 1.—**A,** Proximal neck (PN) angulation measurement before endovascular aneurysm repair (*EVAR*) was 95°(*). **B,** Proximal neck angulation was reduced to 65° (**) at 1 week after EVAR. (Reprinted from the Journal of Vascular Surgery. Ishibashi H, Ishiguchi T, Ohta T, et al. Remodeling of proximal neck angulation after endovascular aneurysm repair. *J Vasc Surg.* 2012;56:1201-1205, Copyright 2012, with permission from the Society for Vascular Surgery.)

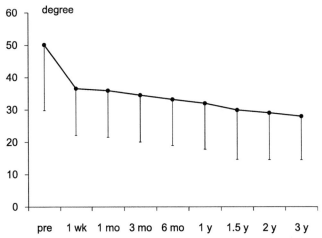

FIGURE 2.—Proximal neck (PN) angulation after endovascular aneurysm repair (EVAR) reduced greatly immediately after the procedure and subsequently reduced slowly and gradually long term. Mean data are shown with the standard deviation (*error bars*). Pre, Preoperative. (Reprinted from the Journal of Vascular Surgery. Ishibashi H, Ishiguchi T, Ohta T, et al. Remodeling of proximal neck angulation after endovascular aneurysm repair. *J Vasc Surg.* 2012;56:1201-1205, Copyright 2012, with permission from the Society for Vascular Surgery.)

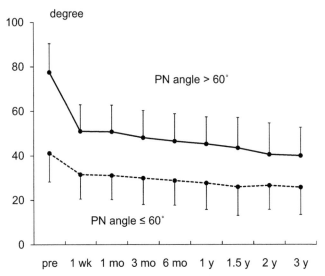

FIGURE 3.—Proximal neck (PN) angulation after endovascular aneurysm repair (EVAR) in PN angulation >60° (*dashed line*) and in angulation ≤60° (*solid line*). PN angulations in both groups reduced greatly immediately after the endovascular procedure, and PN angulation >60° had much greater reduction. Mean data are shown with the standard deviation (*error bars*). Pre, Preoperative. (Reprinted from the Journal of Vascular Surgery. Ishibashi H, Ishiguchi T, Ohta T, et al. Remodeling of proximal neck angulation after endovascular aneurysm repair. *J Vasc Surg.* 2012;56:1201-1205, Copyright 2012, with permission from the Society for Vascular Surgery.)

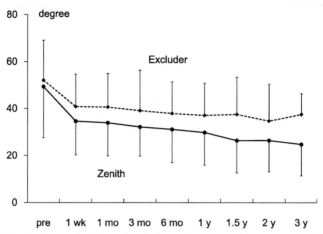

FIGURE 5.—Proximal neck (PN) angulation after endovascular aneurysm repair (EVAR) in Zenith (*solid line*) and Excluder (*dashed line*). PN angulation reduction after Zenith continued for a longer period at a slower pace after the endovascular procedure. Mean data are shown with the standard deviation (*error bars*). Pre, Preoperative. (Reprinted from the Journal of Vascular Surgery. Ishibashi H, Ishiguchi T, Ohta T, et al. Remodeling of proximal neck angulation after endovascular aneurysm repair. *J Vasc Surg.* 2012;56:1201-1205, Copyright 2012, with permission from the Society for Vascular Surgery.)

AAAs with a PN angulation >60° had a larger angulation reduction and a smaller diameter shrinkage after the EVAR procedure. The PN angulation of the 54 AAAs treated by Zenith was 49° ± 22° preoperatively, 34° ± 14° 1 week after EVAR, and 25° ± 13° after 3 years. The corresponding angulation of the 24 AAAs treated by Excluder devices was 52° ± 17°, 41° ± 14°, and 38° ± 9°, respectively. The PN angulation reduction of Zenith and Excluder was similar 1 week after the EVAR procedure. Unlike Excluder, however, the PN angulation in Zenith continued to reduce for a long period at a slow pace. There were no significant correlations between PN angulation reduction and diameter change and between PN length and diameter change ($P = .86$ and $.18$, respectively).

Conclusions.—Although the instructions for use of most commercially available stent grafts provide for a PN angulation of ≤60°, PN angulation was not a major issue in a midterm follow-up of AAAs with adequate PN length for patients in this series who received a Zenith or Excluder graft (Figs 1-3 and 5).

▶ Does proximal aortic neck angulation affect the durability of endovascular aneurysm repair? How does neck angulation change over time? Does it get worse or better? These are the questions that these authors set out to ask with this study. Seventy-eight patients underwent intensive follow-up after implantation of either a Zenith device (n = 54) or an Excluder device (n = 24). Proximal neck angulation was measured before surgery, at 1 week, 1 month, 6 months, 12 months, 18 months, 24 months, and then yearly out to 5 years.

The results were interesting and not what we would expect (Fig 1). Proximal neck angulation declined greatly in the first week and then continued to decline throughout the follow-up interval (Fig 2). Patients who had aortic neck angulation greater than 60° had a much greater reduction over time than those with angulation less than 60° (Fig 3). Interestingly, Zenith grafts exerted a greater reduction in neck angulation over a longer period (Fig 5). These findings go right to the heart of the Instructions for Use for these devices. After reading this report, you be the judge and answer the 3 questions that began this discussion above.

B. W. Starnes, MD

8 Thoracic Aorta

Late neurological recovery of paraplegia after endovascular repair of an infected thoracic aortic aneurysm

Mees BME, Bastos Gonçalves F, Koudstaal PJ, et al (Erasmus Univ Med Ctr, Rotterdam, The Netherlands)
J Vasc Surg 57:521-524, 2013

Spinal cord ischemia is a potentially devastating complication after thoracic endovascular aorta repair (TEVAR). Patients with spinal cord ischemia after TEVAR often develop paraplegia, which is considered irreversible, and have significant increased postoperative morbidity and mortality. We report the case of a patient with unusual late complete neurologic recovery of acute-onset paraplegia after TEVAR for an infected thoracic aortic aneurysm (Fig 2).

▶ Spinal cord ischemia (SCI) and resultant paraplegia are clearly the most feared complications after thoracic endovascular aneurysm repair (TEVAR). The current incidence is 3% to 4% in most series.[1] Risk factors for development of SCI after TEVAR include coverage of the left subclavian or hypogastric artery, embolization during intervention, renal failure, perioperative hypotension, prior abdominal aortic aneurysm repair, and greater proportion of aorta coverage (> 20 cm). We all know that when patients experience this complication, the outcome is nothing short of dismal.

These authors herein describe a 67-year-old patient with full paraplegia after TEVAR that had complete late neurologic recovery that began 1 month after TEVAR and continued for 1 year (Fig 2). I have seen this very situation in my own practice. Although not the norm, it certainly emphasizes that there is still so much that we do not know about spinal cord ischemia.

B. W. Starnes, MD

Reference

1. Rizvi AZ, Sullivan TM. Incidence, prevention, and management in spinal cord protection during TEVAR. *J Vasc Surg.* 2010;52:86S-90S.

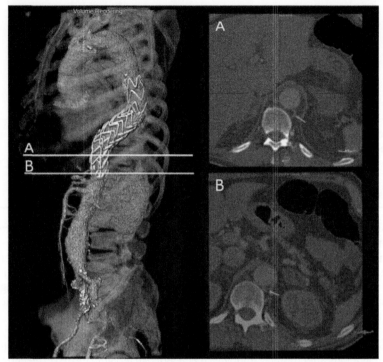

FIGURE 2.—Preoperative and postoperative computed tomographic (CT) angiograms showing the position of significant intercostal arteries at the T11-T12 level (*arrows*) covered by the stent graft. Five of seven pairs (on preoperative CT angiography) of intercostal arteries in the descending aorta were covered, including the large pair shown, which is the largest and located in the classic position of the artery of Adamkiewicz. One pair of lumbar arteries at the visceral aortic segment and four pairs at the infrarenal aorta were not covered and remained patent. The left subclavian and vertebral artery, the inferior mesenteric artery, and both hypogastric arteries with numerous collaterals all were patent. (Reprinted from the Journal of Vascular Surgery. Mees BME, Bastos Gonçalves F, Koudstaal PJ, et al. Late neurological recovery of paraplegia after endovascular repair of an infected thoracic aortic aneurysm. *J Vasc Surg.* 2013;57:521-524, Copyright 2013, with permission from the Society for Vascular Surgery.)

Staged total exclusion of the aorta for chronic type B aortic dissection

Perera AD, Willis AK, Fernandez JD, et al (Univ of Tennessee—Memphis)
J Vasc Surg 52:1339-1342, 2010

Hybrid techniques using extra-anatomic bypass of critical aortic branches to enable endovascular treatment of complex aortic pathology have been previously described. A staged endograft repair of a complex, chronic Stanford type B aortic dissection with aneurysmal degeneration is reported in a 50-year-old man. The aneurysmal portion of the dissection extended from the distal arch to both common iliac arteries and was covered with an endograft from the ascending aorta to both external iliac arteries. Aortic arch branches, visceral, and renal arteries were bypassed using open technique. The patient had no neurologic complications. This case report illustrates

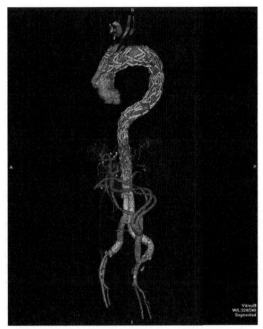

FIGURE 1.—Three-dimensional reconstruction shows the excluded aorta. (Reprinted from the Journal of Vascular Surgery. Perera AD, Willis AK, Fernandez JD, et al. Staged total exclusion of the aorta for chronic type B aortic dissection. *J Vasc Surg*. 2010;52:1339-1342, Copyright 2010, with permission from the Society for Vascular Surgery.)

the feasibility of the hybrid technique in selected high-risk patients when confronted with complex aortic pathology (Fig 1).

▶ This case report was of interest to me because it brings forth an interesting theory in treating patients with complex aortic pathology using endovascular techniques. Five separate operations were conducted on this 50-year-old male patient over a span of 99 days (Fig 1). Whether these authors were reacting to multiple inadequate initial procedures because of persistent endoleak is not known. What is very dramatic about this case is that the patient did not have a neurologic injury, despite coverage of so much of his aorta.

Which brings me to 2 questions: Does a staged procedure offer a period of enhanced collateralization of the spinal cord arterial circulation? Would this patient have had spinal cord injury if all of these procedures had been conducted at the same time? At the University of Washington, my colleague Dr Matthew Sweet is getting answers to this very question. He is staging his thoracic endovascular repairs separate from other portions of the aortic repair to allow for collateralization to occur. This case report lends some weight to our own bias.

B. W. Starnes, MD

Incidence of Descending Aortic Pathology and Evaluation of the Impact of Thoracic Endovascular Aortic Repair: A Population-based Study in England and Wales from 1999 to 2010

von Allmen RS, Anjum A, Powell JT, et al (Imperial College, London, UK)
Eur J Vasc Endovasc Surg 45:154-159, 2013

Objectives.—To investigate population trends in thoracic aortic disease (dissections and aneurysms) in England and Wales, with focus on the impact of thoracic endovascular aortic repair on procedure numbers and age at repair.

Materials and Methods.—Routine hospital statistics of England and Wales provided admission, procedure and mortality data from 1999 to 2010. All data were age-standardised, reported per 100,000 population, by age bands (>50 years or 50−74 years versus 75+ years) and gender. Only patients 50+ years were included, to focus on degenerative disease.

Results.—Between 1999 and 2010 hospital admissions for total (ascending and descending) have risen steadily for thoracic aortic dissection (TAD) from 7.2 to 8.8 and thoracic aortic aneurysm (TAA) from 4.4 to 9.0, principally attributable to increased admissions in those 75+ years. Total mortality declined steadily over the same period, for TAD from 4.4 to 3.2 and for TAA from 10.4 to 7.5. Procedure rates have risen sharply, driven

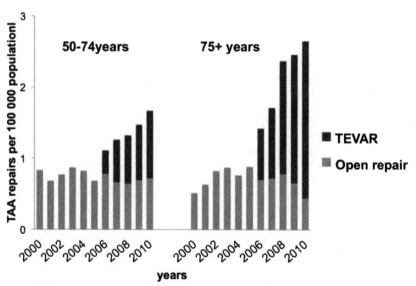

FIGURE 4.—Repairs for descending thoracic aortic aneurysm in England and Wales 1999−2010, by age. TAA open repairs (solid grey bars) and TEVARs (solid black bars); 50−74 years on the left hand side and 75+ years on the right hand side. Data were standardised by age group for procedural codes; L18.2, L19.2, L20.2, L21.2 (open repair), L27.3, L28.3 (TEVAR). (Reprinted from European Journal of Vascular and Endovascular Surgery. von Allmen RS, Anjum A, Powell JT. Incidence of descending aortic pathology and evaluation of the impact of thoracic endovascular aortic repair: a population-based study in england and wales from 1999 to 2010. *Eur J Vasc Endovasc Surg.* 2013;45:154-159, Copyright 2013, with permission from European Society for Vascular Surgery.)

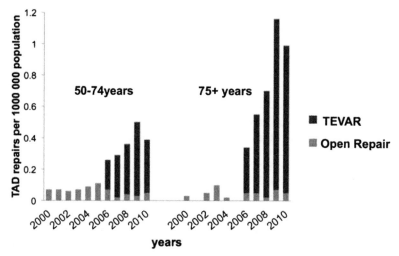

FIGURE 5.—Repairs for descending thoracic aortic dissection in England and Wales 1999–2010, by age. TAD open repairs (solid grey bars) and TEVARs (solid black bars); 50–74 years on the left hand side and 75+ years on the right hand side. Data were standardised by age group for procedural codes; L20.2, L21.2 (open repair), L27.4, L28.4 (TEVAR). (Reprinted from European Journal of Vascular and Endovascular Surgery. von Allmen RS, Anjum A, Powell JT. Incidence of descending aortic pathology and evaluation of the impact of thoracic endovascular aortic repair: a population-based study in england and wales from 1999 to 2010. *Eur J Vasc Endovasc Surg.* 2013;45:154-159, Copyright 2013, with permission from European Society for Vascular Surgery.)

by the implementation of TEVAR from 2006, for type B dissection from 0.06 to 0.53 and for descending TAA from 0.76 to 1.89. All figures are per 100,000 population with $P < 0.005$.

Conclusion.—Improvements in case ascertainment may have contributed to the increase in hospital admissions. The increased application of TEVAR, particularly for dissections, is mainly in those above 75 years and has not yet translated into an accelerated survival benefit (Figs 4 and 5).

▶ This is yet another interesting peripheral analysis of the value of health care in the United Kingdom from Janet Powell and her associates at Charing Cross in London.

Over the decade between 1999 and 2010, the number of thoracic endovascular aortic repair (TEVAR) procedures performed for thoracic aortic aneurysm (Fig 4) and thoracic aortic dissection (Fig 5) increased dramatically.

In this century, mortality from thoracic aortic disease has been on a downtrend, shadowing the trend of other cardiovascular diseases, such as myocardial infarction and abdominal aortic aneurysm.

Mortality for both thoracic aneurysm and thoracic dissection is decreasing steadily in the United Kingdom; however, the decrease started well ahead of the implementation of TEVAR and does not appear to have been accelerated by the increase of TEVAR procedures.

This study in England and Wales shows a meteoric increase in procedure rates for descending aortic disease, particularly for thoracic aortic dissection, driven by the use of TEVAR.

It is important to realize that TEVAR, unlike endovascular repair of abdominal aortic aneurysm, is still a practice without a solid evidence base. There are few randomized, controlled trials aimed at understanding the role of TEVAR for aortic dissection, but there are NONE for thoracic aortic aneurysms!

B. W. Starnes, MD

Reintervention for distal stent graft-induced new entry after endovascular repair with a stainless steel-based device in aortic dissection

Weng S-H, Weng C-F, Chen W-Y, et al (Taipei Veterans General Hosp, Taiwan; Natl Yang-Ming Univ School of Medicine, Taipei, Taiwan)
J Vasc Surg 57:64-71, 2013

Objective.—Stent graft-induced new entry (SINE) has been increasingly observed after thoracic endovascular aortic repair (TEVAR) for aortic dissection. We investigated the mechanism of late distal SINE, prevention strategies, proper size selection of the stent graft, and implantation sequence.

Methods.—From November 2006 to May 2011, 99 patients with aortic dissection underwent TEVAR with Zenith TX2 stent grafts (Cook, Bloomington, Ind) at our center. Among them, 27 distal SINEs were recognized. Eight of these patients with complicated distal SINE required intervention with new distal endografts, and all were enrolled for further analysis.

Results.—Eight of the 27 patients with distal SINE underwent a secondary endograft procedure from February 2011 to July 2011. All were successfully treated without any complications or deaths. A high taper ratio (35% ± 11%) and excessive oversizing of the true lumen area at the distal stent level (293% ± 76%) were noted among these patients.

Conclusions.—The incidence of distal SINE seemed to be high; however, there were also low rates of death and complications after TEVAR for aortic dissection using stainless steel-based stent grafts. Complicated distal SINE can successfully be resolved by distal endograft implantation. Excessive oversizing of the distal stent graft, as measured by the true lumen area, may be a significant factor causing delayed distal SINE. Precise size selection is crucial for the distal end of the stent, especially for high taper ratio dissection pathology in which the implantation sequence of a distal small-sized stent graft first might be considered to prevent future distal SINE (Fig 1).

▶ As stated elsewhere in this edition of VASCULAR YEAR BOOK, aortic dissection is a big problem in Asia. For this reason, many important studies are emerging from this region with important lessons from which we all can learn. Apparently, when chronic aortic dissections are managed with thoracic endovascular aortic repair (TEVAR) to seal the entry tear, over time there can be the development of stent graft—induced new entry (SINE) with the distal portion of the stent graft essentially rupturing into the false lumen (Fig 1). In this study, of 99 patients treated with TEVAR, 27 had SINE. The authors believe that this was related to excessive oversizing, but I would say that it probably is also related to extent of aortic coverage during the index procedure. It has been my practice to treat

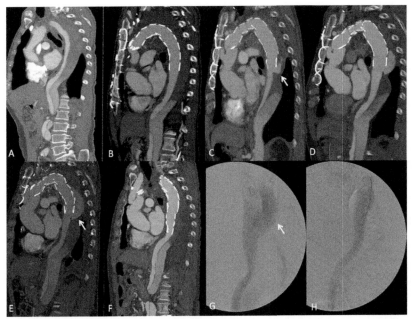

FIGURE 1.—Serial computed tomography imaging (sagittal view) of the index dissection, primary thoracic endovascular aortic repair (TEVAR), and follow-up period to reintervention for distal stent graft-induced new entry (SINE): (**A**) index dissection before primary TEVAR; (**B**) 2 weeks after primary TEVAR; (**C**) 8 months after primary TEVAR, first detection of distal SINE (*red arrow*); (**D**) 1 year after primary TEVAR; (**E**) 18 months after primary TEVAR, pseudoaneurysm formation with enlarged aortic aneurysm (*red arrow*); and (**F**) 1 week after reintervention. G, Digital subtraction angiography before distal endografting shows pseudoaneurysm formation (*red arrow*). **H**, Digital subtraction after distal endografting shows a new entry was covered successfully. For interpretation of the references to color in this figure legend, the reader is referred to web version of this article. (Reprinted from the Journal of Vascular Surgery. Weng S-H, Weng C-F, Chen W-Y, et al. Reintervention for distal stent graft-induced new entry after endovascular repair with a stainless steel-based device in aortic dissection. *J Vasc Surg.* 2013;57:64-71, Copyright 2013, with permission from the Society for Vascular Surgery.)

these patients all the way down to the celiac every time. This article also focused on the current limitations of available devices and materials. The goal in any of these chronic dissection cases is to treat the aneurysm to prevent death caused by aortic aneurysm rupture. This means the achievement of "favorable aortic remodeling" and complete false lumen thrombosis. Fortunately, all of the patients in this study were successfully treated with stent graft extension, which, as I stated before, is what should have been done in the first place.

B. W. Starnes, MD

Left subclavian artery coverage during thoracic endovascular aortic aneurysm repair does not mandate revascularization
Maldonado TS, Dexter D, Rockman CB, et al (NYU Langone Med Ctr; et al)
J Vasc Surg 57:116-124, 2013

Objective.—This study assessed the risk of left subclavian artery (LSA) coverage and the role of revascularization in a large population of patients undergoing thoracic endovascular aortic aneurysm repair.

Methods.—A retrospective multicenter review of 1189 patient records from 2000 to 2010 was performed. Major adverse events evaluated included cerebrovascular accident (CVA) and spinal cord ischemia (SCI). Subgroup analysis was performed for noncovered LSA (group A), covered LSA (group B), and covered/revascularized LSA (group C).

Results.—Of 1189 patients, 394 had LSA coverage (33.1%), and 180 of these patients (46%) underwent LSA revascularization. In all patients, emergency operations (9.5% vs 4.3%; $P =.001$), renal failure (12.7% vs 5.3%; $P =.001$), hypertension (7% vs 2.3%; $P =.01$), and number of stents placed (1 = 3.7%, 2 = 7.4%, $\geq$3 = 10%; $P =.005$) were predictors of SCI. History of cerebrovascular disease (9.6% vs 3.5%; $P =.002$), chronic obstructive pulmonary disease (9.5% vs 5.4%; $P =.01$), coronary artery disease (8.5% vs 5.3%; $P =.03$), smoking (8.9% vs 4.2%) and female gender (5.3% men vs 8.2% women; $P =.05$) were predictors of CVA. Subgroup analysis showed no significant difference between groups B and C (SCI, 6.3% vs 6.1%; CVA, 6.7% vs 6.1%). LSA revascularization was not protective for SCI (7.5% vs 4.1%; $P =.3$) or CVA (6.1% vs 6.4%; $P =.9$). Women who underwent revascularization had an increased incidence of CVA event compared with all other subgroups (group A: 5.6% men, 8.4% women, $P =.16$; group B: 6.6% men, 5.3% women, $P =.9$; group C: 2.8% men, 11.9% women, $P =.03$).

Conclusions.—LSA coverage does not appear to result in an increased incidence of SCI or CVA event when a strategy of selective revascularization is adopted. Selective LSA revascularization results in similar outcomes among the three cohorts studied. Revascularization in women carries an increased risk of a CVA event and should be reserved for select cases (Tables 3A—D and 8).

▶ Left subclavian artery coverage is required to obtain adequate proximal seal in up to 40% of patients undergoing thoracic endovascular aneurysm repair (TEVAR). Six high-volume aortic centers contributed to this analysis of the impact of left subclavian artery coverage during TEVAR on rates of cerebrovascular accident (CVA) and spinal cord injury (SCI) in the perioperative period. As reported in this article, 1189 patients were treated between 2000 and 2010, with 394 undergoing left subclavian artery coverage. Of these 394 patients, 180 underwent left subclavian revascularization.

The data are interesting. Not only do they describe major adverse event rates for a large cohort of patients (Table 3), they also go against conventional wisdom with regard to this practice. The authors essentially found that left subclavian

TABLE 3A.—Major adverse Events (*MAEs*), Including Paraplegia, Stroke, and Death, After Thoracic Endovascular Aortic Aneurysm Repair (TEVAR) (n = 1189) for All Pathologies (n = 1189)

Event	No. (%)
Paraplegia	74/1189 (6.2)
Stroke	77/1189 (6.5)
Mortality at 30 days	147/1189 (12.4)
Total MAEs	218/1189 (18.3)

TABLE 3B.—Major adverse Events (*MAEs*), Including Paraplegia, Stroke, and Death After Thoracic Endovascular Aortic Aneurysm Repair (TEVAR) for Thoracic Aortic Aneurysms (*TAA*)

Event	All Repairs	TAA Repair, No. (%) Elective	Emergency	P^a
Paraplegia	46/809 (5.6)	29/627 (4.6)	17/182 (9.3)	.016
Stroke	59/810 (7.2)	42/627 (6.7)	17/183 (9.3)	.235
Mortality at 30 days	97/822 (11.8)	55/627 (8.7)	42/183 (22.9)	<.001
Total MAEs	147/822 (17.9)	91/628 (14.5)	55/183 (30.1)	<.001

[a]Comparing elective vs emergency TAA.

TABLE 3C.—Major Adverse Events (*MAEs*), Including Paraplegia, Stroke, and Death After Thoracic Endovascular Aortic Aneurysm Repair (TEVAR) for All Thoracic Aortic Aneurysms (*TAA*) (n = 823) Comparing Group B (left subclavian artery [LSA] covered without revascularization) and C (LSA covered and revascularized)

Event	All TAA Repairs, No. (%) Group B	Group C	P
Paraplegia	5/111 (4.5)	6/136 (4.2)	.914
Stroke	5/106 (4.5)	11/132 (7.7)	.3
Mortality at 30 days	14/111 (12.6)	9/143 (6.3)	.08
Total MAEs	21/111 (18.9)	22/143 (15.3)	.456

TABLE 3D.—Major Adverse Events (*MAEs*), Including Paraplegia, Stroke, and Death Following Thoracic Endovascular Aortic Aneurysm Repair (TEVAR) for Elective Thoracic Aortic Aneurysms (*TAA*) (n = 628) Comparing Groups B (left subclavian artery [LSA] covered without revascularization) and C (LSA covered and revascularized)

Event	Elective Repair, No. (%) Group B	Group C	P
Paraplegia	2/74 (2.7)	5/119 (4.2)	.588
Stroke	4/74 (5.4)	7/119 (5.9)	.889
Mortality at 30 day	6/74 (8.1)	9/119 (7.6)	.549
Total MAEs	11/74 (14.9)	16/119 (13.4)	.782

TABLE 8.—Risk of Spinal Cord Ischemia (*SCI*), Cerebrovascular Accident (*CVA*), and Death at 30 Days in Patients Undergoing Thoracic Endovascular Aortic Aneurysm Repair (TEVAR) With Coverage of Left Subclavian Artery (LSA) With (group C) and Without Revascularization (group B)

Group	SCI No. (%)	CVA No. (%)	Death No. (%)
Group B	16/212 (7.5)	13/212 (6.1)	24/212 (11.3)
Group C	7/172 (4.1)	11/173 (6.4)	13/173 (7.5)
P	.2	.9	.5

artery revascularization was *not* protective for SCI and CVA (Table 8) when a strategy of selective revascularization was adopted. This selective approach was only applicable to patients with three conditions:

1. Patent left-internal mammary artery to coronary bypass
2. Dominant or isolated left vertebral artery
3. Functioning left upper extremity dialysis access fistula

Similar outcomes in terms of rates of SCI and CVA were reported for all 3 cohorts studied. The authors also found that revascularization in women carried an increased risk of CVA and should be reserved for select cases.

B. W. Starnes, MD

Triple-barrel Graft as a Novel Strategy to Preserve Supra-aortic Branches in Arch-TEVAR Procedures: Clinical Study and Systematic Review

Shahverdyan R, Gawenda M, Brunkwall J (Univ Hosp of Cologne, Germany)
Eur J Vasc Endovasc Surg 45:28-35, 2013

Objective.—To report our early experience with total endovascular repair of aortic-arch aneurysm using double chimney-grafts and present a literature overview.

Patients and Methods.—The double chimney-graft technique was performed in six male patients with contained ruptured aneurysm, dissecting aneurysm, pseudoaneurysm, penetrating aortic ulcer and proximal endoleak after TEVAR. Furthermore, a systematic electronic health database search of available articles was conducted according to PRISMA Guidelines.

Results.—In all cases, all supra-aortic vessels had to be covered with aortic stent-graft to receive a sufficient landing and sealing zone. Chimney-grafts were introduced to the ascending aorta slightly deeper than the thoracic stent-grafts through the cut-down exposure of the common carotid arteries. We deployed aortic stent-grafts and self-expandable chimney-grafts simultaneously and successfully. The patient with contained ruptured aneurysm died due to cardiopulmonary failure on day 19, the others survived. We detected two 'gutter' endoleaks. As a result of literature search, 12 articles met the inclusion criteria. Two articles described the double-chimney technique.

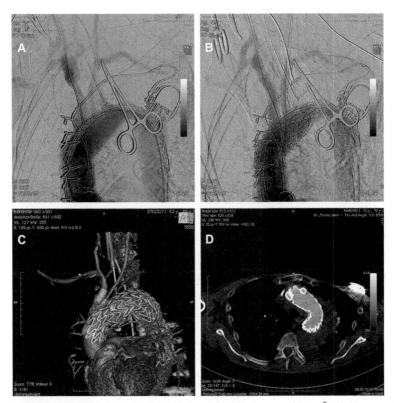

FIGURE 2.—(A) and (B): intraoperative angiogram showing deployment of CTAG® and chimney-grafts (C) and (D): postoperative 3- and 2- dimensional CTA-scan of excluded aneurysm. (Reprinted from European Journal of Vascular and Endovascular Surgery. Shahverdyan R, Gawenda M, Brunkwall J. Triple-barrel graft as a novel strategy to preserve supra-aortic branches in Arch-TEVAR procedures: clinical study and systematic review. *Eur J Vasc Endovasc Surg.* 2013;45:28-35, Copyright 2013, with permission from European Society for Vascular Surgery.)

Conclusions.—The use of double chimney-grafts is possible in high-risk patients where the proximal landing zone of endograft would be in zone 0. The available data is still limited. The long-term follow-up remains to be evaluated with the increased number of patients treated (Fig 2).

▶ Off-label use of commercially available devices has become rampant as more and more patients are approached with nontraditional innovative (but unproven) solutions. Very few published reports have assessed the use of some of these techniques because most experiences at this point are anecdotal.

Reported in this article is a single-institution experience of managing 6 patients with various aortic arch pathologies using a triple-barrel chimney technique (Fig 2). The only reason this case series and literature review is important is to give us a benchmark and at least an idea of how some of these devices and techniques perform. Even so, we must believe that the results published will be better than those in the real world as most interventionalists experimenting with these procedures do not write up their complications for publication.

Nonetheless, with chimney grafts placed within the aortic arch, we can expect *at least* a 6.5% 30-day mortality and *at least* a 19.7% endoleak rate. Furthermore, patients presenting urgently with severe comorbidities do not fare well in short-term follow-up.

Registries are desperately needed to compare these results with those of cervical debranchings, fenestrated techniques, and traditional open surgery.

B. W. Starnes, MD

Ex-vivo Haemodynamic Models for the Study of Stanford Type B Aortic Dissection in Isolated Porcine Aorta

Qing K-X, Chan YC, Lau SF, et al (The Univ of Hong Kong, Pokfulam Road)
Eur J Vasc Endovasc Surg 44:399-405, 2012

Objectives.—The aim of this study is to present novel ex-vivo models in the study of complex haemodynamical changes in Stanford type B aortic dissection (TBAD).

Materials and Methods.—Fifteen fresh porcine aortas were harvested and preserved with 4°C saline. Ex-vivo models were developed to simulate TBAD in three different situations: model A with patent false lumen, model

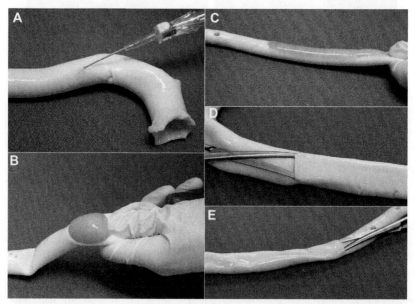

FIGURE 3.—Procedure of creating model A. A: using a 20-GA I.V. catheter puncture intima on a turned over aorta. B: creating a bleb with blood-stained saline. C: channelling the dissection flap. D: cutting the dissecting flap to create a primary entry in a proximal location with scissors. E: creating a re-entry on the distal portion of dissecting flap with scissors. (Reprinted from European Journal of Vascular and Endovascular Surgery. Qing K-X, Chan YC, Lau SF, et al. Ex-vivo haemodynamic models for the study of Stanford type B aortic dissection in isolated porcine aorta. *Eur J Vasc Endovasc Surg.* 2012;44:399-405, Copyright 2012, with permission from European Society for Vascular Surgery.)

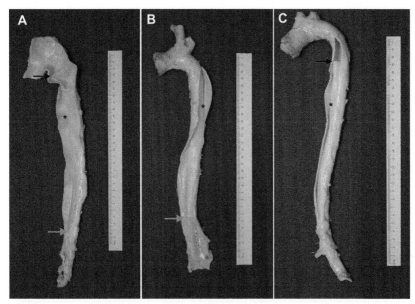

FIGURE 6.—Post-modelling gross examination of the three models. A: model A. B: model B. C: model C. *: false lumen. Black arrow: Proximal primary entry. Red arrow: Distal re-entry. For interpretation of the references to color in this figure legend, the reader is referred to web version of this article. (Reprinted from European Journal of Vascular and Endovascular Surgery. Qing K-X, Chan YC, Lau SF, et al. Ex-vivo haemodynamic models for the study of Stanford type B aortic dissection in isolated porcine aorta. *Eur J Vasc Endovasc Surg.* 2012;44:399-405, Copyright 2012, with permission from European Society for Vascular Surgery.)

B with distal re-entry only and model C with proximal primary entry only. These models were connected to standardised pulsatile pumps and the pressure waveforms were monitored and compared. The aortas were scanned with ultrasonography and subjected to post-experiment autopsy.

Results.—The three different models were successfully created ($n = 13$). Pulsatile flow testing was successful and the shapes of the pressure waveforms were similar to those taken from human aorta. Post-testing gross examination confirmed the success of modelling.

Conclusion.—Porcine aortas may prove to be useful ex-vivo models in the study of aortic dissection haemodynamics. These models are reproducible and may be used in the study of complex haemodynamic forces during the development and propagation of TBAD. Our three porcine models give a potential possibility in helping clinicians isolate and analyse complex haemodynamical factors in the development, propagation and prognosis of TBAD (Figs 3 and 6).

▶ Anyone who has conducted animal studies or computational fluid dynamics analysis related to acute aortic dissection realizes how truly difficult this can be. Dr Qing and colleagues, using porcine aortas, have created 3 different ex vivo models of acute type B aortic dissection (Fig 3). The first model simulates proximal and distal entry tears consistent with a patent true and false lumen. The second simulates a distal entry tear only (somewhat similar to a dissection treated with a stent graft) and the third a proximal entry tear only (similar to partial false lumen thrombosis).

Interestingly, consistent with prior findings,[1] partial false lumen thrombosis was associated with higher false lumen pressures and increased risk of rupture in these pressurized flow models (Fig 6).

Drawbacks and limitations of these models relate to the necessity to ligate branch intercostal vessels, thus likely altering pressure dynamics within the respective lumens. Nevertheless, these porcine ex vivo models of aortic dissection will hopefully help our understanding of this complex pathophysiologic process.

B. W. Starnes, MD

Reference

1. Tsai TT, Evangelista A, Nienaber CA, et al. Partial thrombosis of the false lumen in patients with acute type B aortic dissection. *N Engl J Med.* 2007;357:349-359.

Progress in Endovascular Management of Type A Dissection
Nordon IM, Hinchliffe RJ, Morgan R, et al (St George's Hosp, London, UK)
Eur J Vasc Endovasc Surg 44:406-410, 2012

Proximal acute aortic dissection [type A] remains a disease with a poor prognosis. High peri-operative open surgical mortality [up to 30%] and a significant turn-down rate [up to 40%] substantiate the bleak prospects for patients with this disease. Thoracic endovascular stent grafting has revolutionized the treatment of distal [type B] acute aortic dissection. Endovascular surgeons are now looking to improve the treatment of type A dissection by offering endovascular techniques to supplement conventional surgical therapy. Less invasive endovascular therapy, obviates the need for sternotomy and cardiopulmonary bypass, may reduce perioperative morbidity and offers a solution for those patients declined conventional intervention due to co-morbidity or severe complications of the disease. Thoracic stent grafting in the ascending aorta presents specific challenges due to proximity to the aortic valve, navigation over the steep aortic arch and pulsatile aortic movement. Endovascular surgeons have treated type A dissection off-license using aortic cuffs and stents designed for infra-renal aortic surgery. Now grafts specifically designed for treating type A dissection are being developed and deployed under trial [compassionate license] in patients deemed unfit for open surgery. This paper explores how endovascular solutions may fit into the future care of patients with acute type A dissection (Fig 2).

▶ Type A proximal aortic dissection represents nearly two-thirds of all dissection patients and technically is one of the most challenging operations that cardiac surgeons face.

This article nicely summarizes the early experience with a completely endovascular solution for managing type A dissections, including device requirements and current limitations. One thing is clear: endovascular solutions are coming and may one day replace open surgery in this challenging patient population (Fig 2).

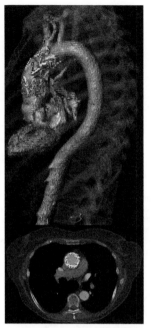

FIGURE 2.—Images demonstrating custom ascending aortic stent in-situ landing proximal to innominate artery [3 month follow-up scan]. Volume rendered 3D reconstruction and axial contrast-enhanced CT image. (Reprinted from European Journal of Vascular and Endovascular Surgery. Nordon IM, Hinchliffe RJ, Morgan R, et al. Progress in endovascular management of type a dissection. Eur J Vasc Endovasc Surg. 2012;44:406-410, Copyright 2012, with permission from the European Society for Vascular Surgery.)

The goals of surgical therapy are to resect the primary intimal tear, resect and repair the ascending aorta, achieve occlusion of the false lumen, restore aortic valve competence, and limit aortic dissection downstream. Most patients treated surgically do not require aortic valve replacement or coronary replant, although this is required in 10% to 20% of cases.

Increasing experience is being gained with short stent grafts in patients with suitable anatomy (see Fig 1 in the original article). We anxiously await good information from registries and case series on this exciting new development.

B. W. Starnes, MD

An in vitro phantom study on the influence of tear size and configuration on the hemodynamics of the lumina in chronic type B aortic dissections
Rudenick PA, Bijnens BH, García-Dorado D, et al (Univ Hosp and Res Inst Vall d'Hebron, Barcelona, Spain; ICREA-Universitat Pompeu Fabra, Barcelona, Spain)
J Vasc Surg 57:464-474.e5, 2013

Objective.—Management and follow-up of chronic aortic dissections continue to be a clinical challenge due to progressive dilatation and

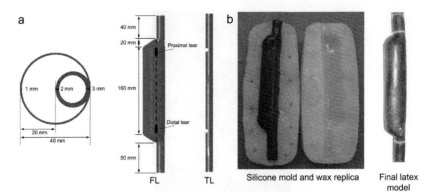

FIGURE 1.—a, Synthetic geometry of a type B aortic dissection. Schematic diagram of the dissected aortic section. b, Consecutive processing steps developed to make latex phantoms of type B aortic dissections. *FL*, False lumen; *TL*, true lumen. (Reprinted from the Journal of Vascular Surgery. Rudenick PA, Bijnens BH, García-Dorado D, et al. An in vitro phantom study on the influence of tear size and configuration on the hemodynamics of the lumina in chronic type B aortic dissections. *J Vasc Surg.* 2013;57:464-474.e5, Copyright 2013, with permission from The Society for Vascular Surgery.)

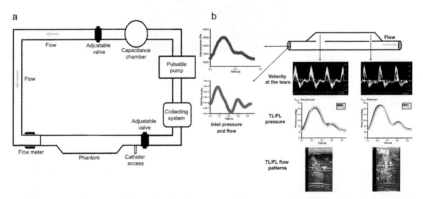

FIGURE 3.—a, Diagram of the pulsatile flow circuit. Valves are used to regulate the peripheral resistance, and a compliance chamber damps the pump outflow. b, Example of measurements performed in each model of dissection. *FL*, False lumen; *TL*, true lumen. (Reprinted from the Journal of Vascular Surgery. Rudenick PA, Bijnens BH, García-Dorado D, et al. An in vitro phantom study on the influence of tear size and configuration on the hemodynamics of the lumina in chronic type B aortic dissections. *J Vasc Surg.* 2013;57:464-474.e5, Copyright 2013, with permission from The Society for Vascular Surgery.)

subsequent rupture. To predict complications, guidelines suggest follow-up of aortic diameter. However, dilatation is triggered by hemodynamic parameters (pressures/wall shear stresses) and geometry of false (FL) and true lumen (TL), information not captured by diameter alone. Therefore, we aimed at better understanding the influence of dissection anatomy on TL and FL hemodynamics.

Methods.—In vitro studies were performed using pulsatile flow in realistic dissected latex/silicone geometries with varying tear number, size, and location. We assessed three different conformations: (1) proximal tear only; (2) distal tear only; (3) both proximal and distal tears. All possible combinations

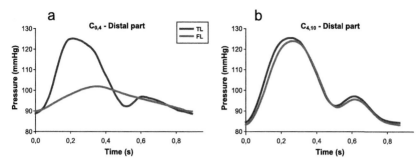

FIGURE 5.—Pressure profiles in the true lumen (*TL*) and false lumen (*FL*) (a) in the presence of only small tears and (b) in the presence of at least a big tear. C, Case. (Reprinted from the Journal of Vascular Surgery. Rudenick PA, Bijnens BH, García-Dorado D, et al. An in vitro phantom study on the influence of tear size and configuration on the hemodynamics of the lumina in chronic type B aortic dissections. *J Vasc Surg*. 2013;57:464-474.e5, Copyright 2013, with permission from The Society for Vascular Surgery.)

(n = 8) of small (10% of aortic diameter) and large (25% of aortic diameter) tears were considered. Pressure, velocity, and flow patterns were analyzed within the lumina (at proximal and distal sections) and at the tears. We also computed the FL mean pressure index (FPI$_{mean}$%) as a percentage of the TL mean pressure, to compare pressures among models.

Results.—The presence of large tears equalized FL/TL pressures compared with models with only small tears (proximal FPI$_{mean}$% 99.85 ± 0.45 vs 92.73 ± 3.63; distal FPI$_{mean}$% 99.51 ± 0.80 vs 96.35 ± 1.96; *P* <.001). Thus, large tears resulted in slower velocities through the tears (systolic velocity < 180 cm/s) and complex flows within the FL, whereas small tears resulted in lower FL pressures, higher tear velocities (systolic velocity > 290 cm/s), and a well-defined flow. Additionally, both proximal and distal tears act as entry and exit. During systole, flow enters the FL through all tears simultaneously, while during diastole, flow leaves through all communications. Flow through the FL, from proximal to distal tears or vice versa, is minimal.

Conclusions.—Our results suggest that FL hemodynamics heavily depends on cumulative tear size, and thus, it is an important parameter to take into account when clinically assessing chronic aortic dissections (Figs 1, 3, and 5).

▶ This is a fascinating study from a reputable group in Spain. These authors sought to have a better understanding of the influence of dissection anatomy on true lumen and false lumen hemodynamics. They created a latex, silicone model for assessing pressure, flow, and velocity of flow based on varying tear size (Figs 1 and 3). Recent findings have suggested an influence of tear size on chronic evolution to an aneurysm.

The authors' main findings were that pressures and, therefore, tear velocities mainly depend on the accumulated size of all tears. With large tears present, irrespective of location, true and false lumen pressures equalize, whereas with only small tears, false lumen pressures never reach true lumen levels.

In addition, during systole, flow enters the false lumen through all tears simultaneously, whereas during diastole, flow leaves through all communications. The false lumen pressure is dampened with damping inversely proportional to the cumulative size of connecting orifices (Fig 5). This is a start in helping us understand the complex fluid dynamics associated with this challenging disease process.

B. W. Starnes, MD

The results of stent graft versus medication therapy for chronic type B dissection
Jia X, Guo W, Li T-X, et al (Chinese PLA General Hosp, Beijing, China; Henan Provincial People's Hosp, Zhengzhou, China; The First Affiliated Hosp of Zhengzhou Univ, Zhengzhou, China; et al)
J Vasc Surg 57:406-414, 2013

Objective.—This prospective multicenter comparative study examined early and midterm results of medication and stent-graft therapies on chronic type B aortic dissection in China.

Methods.—The study consisted of 303 consecutive patients with chronic type B aortic dissection from four centers in China from January 2007 to December 2010 who were prospectively enrolled and treated by either optimal medical therapy (OMT) or thoracic endovascular aorta repair (TEVAR). Of the patients, 219 were male and 84 were female (average age, 53.6 ± 20.3 years; range, 29-81 years). Baseline diameter of the

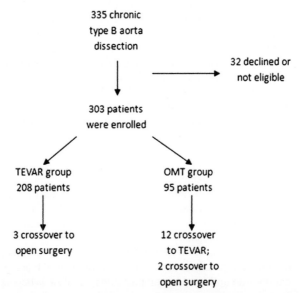

FIGURE 1.—Flowchart of the study. *OMT*, Optimal medical therapy; *TEVAR*, thoracic endovascular aorta repair. (Reprinted from the Journal of Vascular Surgery. Jia X, Guo W, Li T-X, et al. The results of stent graft versus medication therapy for chronic type B dissection. *J Vasc Surg.* 2013;57:406-414, Copyright 2013, with permission from the Society for Vascular Surgery.)

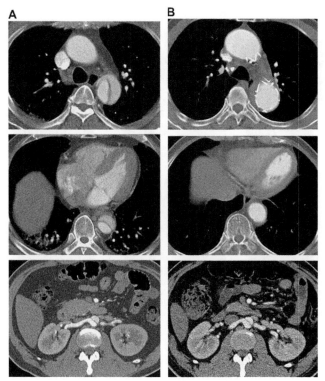

FIGURE 3.—Contrast-enhanced computed tomography (CT) of type B dissection (A) and comparable scans 12 months after thoracic endovascular aorta repair (TEVAR) (B) showing complete obliteration and progressive resolution of the false lumen in the thoracic aorta. (Reprinted from the Journal of Vascular Surgery. Jia X, Guo W, Li T-X, et al. The results of stent graft versus medication therapy for chronic type B dissection. *J Vasc Surg*. 2013;57:406-414, Copyright 2013, with permission from the Society for Vascular Surgery.)

thoracic aorta was 41.2 (19.1) mm (mean [standard deviation]), and dissection extended beyond the celiac axis in 87.1% of cases.

Results.—In total, there were 208 patients in the TEVAR group and 95 patients in the OMT group. Procedural success was 100%, and no deaths occurred during index hospitalization in the two groups. In the TEVAR group, two patients (0.9%) suffered from retrograde type A dissection, and two (0.9%) suffered from paraplegia or paraparesis. For in-hospital outcome, multivariate analysis revealed that age >75 years and American Society of Anesthesiologists class greater than III were independent predictors of major early adverse events. Average follow-up time for hospital survivors was 28.5 ± 16.3 months (range, 1.0-58 months). In the OMT group, five patients died from rupture of an enlarged false lumen, and six patients died suddenly of unknown reasons. Fourteen cases required crossover to TEVAR (n = 12) or surgical conversion (n = 2). In the TEVAR group, nine patients required reintervention or surgical conversion, and one died of postoperative multi-organ failure. One patient died of delayed retrograde type

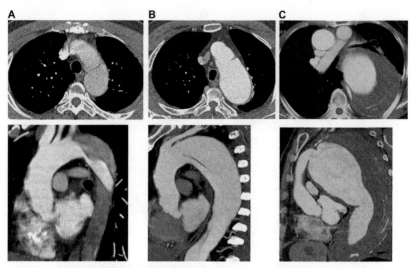

FIGURE 5.—Contrast-enhanced computed tomography (CT) of type B dissection (A) and comparable scans 24 months later (B) and 52 months later with emergent thoracic aorta rupture (C). (Reprinted from the Journal of Vascular Surgery. Jia X, Guo W, Li T-X, et al. The results of stent graft versus medication therapy for chronic type B dissection. *J Vasc Surg.* 2013;57:406-414, Copyright 2013, with permission from the Society for Vascular Surgery.)

A dissection, and four died suddenly of unknown reasons. The Kaplan-Meier analysis of survival probability at 2 and 4 years was 87.5% and 82.7% with TEVAR, respectively, and 77.5% and 69.1% with OMT, respectively ($P = .0678$, log-rank test). The estimated cumulative freedom from aorta-related death at 2 and 4 years was 91.6% and 88.1% with TEVAR, respectively, and 82.8% and 73.8% with OMT, respectively ($P = .0392$, log-rank test). The thoracic aorta diameter decreased from 42.4 (23.1) mm to 37.3 (12.8) mm in the TEVAR group and increased from 40.7 (18.6) mm to 48.1 (17.3) mm in the OMT group.

Conclusions.—This was the first prospective multicenter comparative study on the treatment of type B aortic dissection in China. TEVAR had a significantly lower aorta-related mortality compared with OMT but failed to improve overall survival rate or lower the aorta-related adverse event rate (Figs 1, 3, and 5).

▶ Aortic dissection is a catastrophic cardiovascular event that is associated with high morbidity and mortality rates. Dissection is a particularly vexing problem in China. Previous investigators have recognized that patients with type B aortic dissection in China are about 10 years younger than those in the Western world.[1] This is probably because of the high salt diet and high rates of undiagnosed and uncontrolled hypertension.

This prospective, multicenter, nonrandomized study evaluated the outcomes of patients with chronic aortic dissection treated with either thoracic endovascular aorta repair (TEVAR) or optimal medical therapy (OMT). The flowchart of the study is shown in Fig 1. Fig 3 displays the follow-up at 1 year of a patient successfully treated with TEVAR, whereas Fig 5 shows progression of a patient treated with OMT. In the TEVAR group, the risk of retrograde aortic dissection and paraplegia was less than 1% each, which is quite good for this patient population. Freedom from aortic-related death was significantly better in the TEVAR group, but overall, survival was no different between groups.

This study is important, as it gives us a partial glimpse into this promising therapy to manage chronic dissections. A randomized study is what will give us the real answer.

B. W. Starnes, MD

Reference

1. Xiong J, Jiang B, Guo W, Wang SM, Tong XY. Endovascular stent graft placement in patients with type B aortic dissection: a meta-analysis in China. *J Thorac Cardiovasc Surg*. 2009;138:865-872.

Acute type B aortic dissection in the absence of aortic dilatation
Trimarchi S, Jonker FHW, Froehlich JB, et al (Policlinico San Donato I.R.C.C.S, Milan, Italy; Yale Univ School of Medicine, New Haven, CT; Univ of Michigan Health System, Ann Arbor; et al)
J Vasc Surg 56:311-316, 2012

Background.—Increasing aortic diameter is thought to be an important risk factor for acute type B aortic dissection (ABAD). However, some patients develop ABAD in the absence of aortic dilatation. In this report, we sought to characterize ABAD patients who presented with a descending thoracic aortic diameter <3.5 cm.

Methods.—We categorized 613 ABAD patients enrolled in the International Registry of Acute Aortic Dissection from 1996 to 2009 according to the aortic diameter <3.5 cm (group 1) and ≥3.5 cm (group 2). Demographics, clinical presentation, management, and outcomes of the two groups were compared.

Results.—Overall, 21.2% (n = 130) had an aortic diameter <3.5 cm. Patients in group 1 were younger (60.5 vs 64.0 years; $P = .015$) and more frequently female (50.8% vs 28.6%; $P < .001$). They presented more often with diabetes (10.9% vs 5.9%; $P = .050$), history of catheterization (17.0% vs 6.7%; $P = .001$), and coronary artery bypass grafting (9.7% vs 3.4%; $P = .004$). Marfan syndrome was equally distributed in the two groups. The overall in-hospital mortality did not differ between groups 1 and 2 (7.6% vs 10.1%; $P = .39$).

Conclusions.—About one-fifth of patients with ABAD do not present with any aortic dilatation. These patients are more frequently females and younger, when compared with patients with aortic dilatation. This report is an initial investigation to clinically characterize this cohort, and further research is needed to identify risk factors for aortic dissection in the absence of aortic dilatation.

▶ Aortic dissections represent a challenging clinical entity. Despite the limitations of prospective randomized trials concerning alternative therapies, there is much to be gained from a well-maintained, prospectively gathered and validated registry such as the International Registry of Acute Aortic Dissection (IRAD). This article is this type of study, which adds to the current body of knowledge on the presentation and outcomes of aortic dissections, looking specifically at patients who develop the disease without antecedent aortic dilatation. The patient cohort identified at risk are younger women, a group that is generally not included in prospective randomized trials. Interestingly, more than 50% of those presenting with acute aortic dissection in the setting of normal aortic diameter were of the female gender in this cohort. The identification of those who may be at risk for acute aortic dissection is crucial in order to prevent potentially catastrophic complications. Of course, those patients identified with a dilated descending aorta may elicit concern in their provider, but what about those who have a normal aorta? Why would someone consider further examination in these patients? Perhaps younger women with malignant hypertension or a history of a collagen-vascular disease or other such inherited disorders in their family should undergo closer follow-up imaging of their thoracic aorta. I look forward to more studies and recommendations from the IRAD investigators concerning this unique group of patients.

R. L. Bush, MD, MPH

9 Aortoiliac Disease and Leg Ischemia

Midterm Outcomes of Embolisation of Internal Iliac Artery Aneurysms
Millon A, Paquet Y, Ben Ahmed S, et al (Univ Hosp of Lyon, France; Univ Hosp of Clermont Ferrand, France; et al)
Eur J Vasc Endovasc Surg 45:22-27, 2013

Objectives.—There is no standardised technique for internal iliac artery aneurysm (IIAA) embolisation and results of long-term prevention of rupture are unknown.

Design.—We retrospectively evaluated technical aspects and results of IIAA embolisation in a multicentre study.

Methods.—Aneurysm morphology and embolisation techniques were reviewed. Aneurysm-related death, rupture, diameter increase, endoleak, secondary procedure and complication related to the IIA occlusion were recorded.

Results.—Between 2001 and 2011, 53 patients with 57 IIAA were treated. Mean diameter of IIAA was 41 mm (range: 25−88 mm). Embolisation techniques were distal and proximal occlusion ($n = 24$), proximal occlusion $(n = 18)$ and sac packing $(n = 15)$. Cumulative overall survival rate was 92% at 1 year, 83% at 3 years and 59% at 5 years. No cause of deaths was related to aneurysm. Aneurysm diameter increased in five patients and endoleak was observed in 11 patients. One secondary open conversion and five secondary endovascular procedures were performed for increase of diameter or proximal endoleak. Two patients experienced a disabling buttock claudication.

Conclusions.—Embolisation of IIAA is safe in the short- and midterm. However, endoleak and aneurysm diameter increases are not rare. Yearly post-procedure computed tomography angiography seems appropriate (Table 3).

▶ Internal iliac artery aneurysms are rare but potentially associated with a fatal outcome. They represent 0.3% of all aortoiliac aneurysms and less than 20% of all isolated iliac artery aneurysms.[1] In addition, the natural history of these aneurysms is not well described. Historical data report a risk of rupture of up to 40% with a mortality rate of 80%, thus justifying treatment.

This five-institution report over 10 years describes the midterm outcomes of embolization as a therapy for managing these aneurysms.

TABLE 3.—Midterm Follow-up Results

	Total $n = 57$	Distal and Proximal Occlusion $n = 24$	Proximal Occlusion $n = 18$	Sac Packing $n = 15$	p
Mean Follow up (month)	30 (1–136)	25 (1–72)	40 (6–134)	30 (2–71)	0.376
Aneurysmal change n (%)					
Decrease	23 (40)	9 (38)	8 (44)	6 (40)	0.542
Stable	29 (51)	14 (54)	9 (50)	6 (40)	
Increase	5 (9)	1 (4)	1 (6)	3 (20)	
Endoleak n (%)	11 (19)	4 (17)	3 (17)	4 (27)	0.760
Proximal	5	0	1	4	
Distal	3	1	2	0	
Ilio-lumbar	3	3	0	0	
Secondary procedures n (%)	5 (9)	1 (4)	0	4 (27)	0.016
Buttock claudication n (%)	12 (21)	8 (38)	2 (11)	2 (13)	0.185

Fifty-three patients with 57 internal iliac artery aneurysms were treated with either distal and proximal occlusion, proximal occlusion alone, or aneurysm sac packing. No deaths during follow-up were attributed to the aneurysm. Five patients (9.4%) had aneurysm sac expansion requiring reintervention. Eleven patients (20.8%) had endoleak, and only 2 patients (3.7%) had disabling buttock claudication.

The midterm follow-up results were interesting (Table 3). The highest re-intervention rate was with aneurysm sac packing alone. The authors acknowledged that these procedures can be technically very difficult, especially with selection of the anterior and posterior divisions of the internal iliac artery off of a large aneurysm. Despite this, the authors recommend occlusion of the outflow vessels when possible.

B. W. Starnes, MD

Reference

1. Lucke B, Rea MH. Studies on aneurysm: I. General statistical data on aneurysms. *JAMA.* 1921;77:935-940.

Long-Term Follow-Up of Endovascular Treatment for Trans-Atlantic Inter-Society Consensus II Type B Iliac Lesions in Patients Aged <50 Years

Radak D, Babic S, Sagic D, et al (Inst for Cardiovascular Disease "Dedinje", Belgrade, Republic of Serbia; et al)
Ann Vasc Surg 26:1057-1063, 2012

Background.—To study the initial and long-term results of endovascular treatment in patients aged < 50 years with Trans-Atlantic Inter-Society Consensus-II type B unilateral iliac lesions and chronic limb ischemia.

Methods.—From January 2000 to February 2010, 60 consecutive endovascular interventions were performed on 23 women and 37 men aged ≤ 50 years. After successful treatment, all patients were followed up at 1, 3, 6, and 12 months after the procedure and every 6 months thereafter.

Results.—Successful percutaneous revascularization of the iliac artery was achieved in 56 patients (93.3%). The early vascular-related complication rate was 6.7%. The primary patency rates at 1, 3, and 5 years were 88%, 59%, and 49%, respectively. Cox univariate analysis revealed that an age range of 45 to 50 years (hazard ratio [HR]: 0.290; 95% confidence interval [CI]: 0.152−0.553; $P = 0.0001$), lower preprocedural ankle-brachial index (HR: 2.438; 95% CI: 1.04−5.715; $P = 0.047$), lesion length > 5 cm (HR: 0.838; 95% CI: 0.746−0.943; $P = 0.003$), and diabetes (HR: 2.005; 95% CI: 1.010−3.980; $P = 0.047$) had significant influence on decreasing primary patency.

Conclusions.—Endovascular treatment of TASC-II type B iliac lesions in patients aged < 50 years is a safe procedure with low procedural risk. Primary patency rates at 1, 3, and 5 years were 88%, 59%, and 49%, respectively.

▶ When a young patient presents with peripheral artery disease (PAD), we have to consider the cost-effectiveness of the chosen therapy. Most often the question of longevity becomes central, with the assumption that surgical therapy for iliac disease is synonymous with a one-and-done proposition for the patient vs an endovascular technique that will require expensive ongoing maintenance. These authors seek to examine the endovascular side of the argument. Ultimately, the series falls short on the longevity question, as the small series had very few patients who reached the 5-year to 10-year window (mean follow-up appears much less than the reported median follow-up). Primary patency is only 49% at 5 years, which is compared with several other single-center reports of young patients with aortobifemoral bypass who had highly variable outcomes. Perhaps the outcomes depicted herein seem acceptable, but with a prior study from Curi[1] regarding hypercoagulability in young patients with PAD strongly predicting poor survival, we do not have the data from this article to introduce that angle. Regardless, the study adds value to the proposition that endovascular techniques may have a cautious role in the very young patient with atherosclerotic iliac disease.

J. Black, MD

Reference

1. Curi MA, Skelly CL, Baldwin ZK, et al. Long-term outcome of infrainguinal bypass grafting in patients with serologically proven hypercoagulability. *J Vasc Surg.* 2003;37(2):301-306.

A systematic review of endovascular treatment of extensive aortoiliac occlusive disease

Jongkind V, Akkersdijk GJM, Yeung KK, et al (Spaarne Hosp, Hoofddorp, The Netherlands; VU Univ Med Ctr, Amsterdam, The Netherlands)
J Vasc Surg 52:1376-1383, 2010

Objectives.—Current multidisciplinary guidelines recommend to treat extensive aortoiliac occlusive disease (AIOD) by surgical revascularization. Surgery provides good long-term patency, but at the cost of substantial perioperative morbidity. Development of new technologies and techniques has led to increased use of endovascular therapy for extensive AIOD. We performed a systematic review of the literature to determine contemporary short- and long-term results of endovascular therapy for extensive AIOD.

Methods.—The Medline, Embase, and Cochrane databases were searched to identify all studies reporting endovascular treatment of extensive AIOD (TransAtlantic Inter-Society Consensus (TASC) type C and D) from January 2000 to June 2009. Two independent observers selected studies for inclusion, assessed the methodologic quality of the included studies, and performed the data extraction. Outcomes were technical success, clinical success, mortality, complications, long-term primary, and secondary patency rates.

Results.—Nineteen nonrandomized cohort studies reporting on 1711 patients were included. There was substantial clinical heterogeneity between the studies considering study population and interventional techniques. Technical success was achieved in 86% to 100% of the patients. Clinical symptoms improved in 83% to 100%. Mortality was described in seven studies and ranged from 1.2% to 6.7%. Complications were reported in 3% to 45% of the patients. Most common complications were distal embolization, access site hematomas, pseudoaneurysms, arterial ruptures, and arterial dissections. The majority of complications could be treated using percutaneous or noninvasive techniques. Four- or 5-year primary and secondary patency rates ranged from 60% to 86% and 80% to 98%, respectively.

Conclusions.—Endovascular treatment of extensive AIOD can be performed successfully by experienced interventionists in selected patients. Although primary patency rates are lower than those reported for surgical revascularization, reinterventions can often be performed percutaneously, with secondary patency comparable to surgical repair.

▶ The original Trans-Atlantic Inter-Society Consensus on the Management of Peripheral Arterial Disease (PAD; TASC) was published in 2000. The more complex lesion morphologies, the TASC C and D lesions, have open surgical reconstruction as the recommendation in the TASC guidelines. In 2007, the working group was expanded and an updated set of guidelines was published. According to the TASC website, the "TASC recommendations were updated with the aim of abbreviating the previous document and disseminating the information to primary care physicians who provide the day-to-day medical treatment for millions of patients affected by PAD across the world." Since 2000, there has been an explosion of new technology and technological advances in both implantable devices and auxiliary products used in the endovascular treatment of PAD. Furthermore, endovascular training is now taught in all vascular residencies and fellowships and broadly tested on in-training examinations as well as vascular certification and recertification tests. It only stands to reason that updated guidelines would include the technical advances and experience that has been gained in the past decade.

This systematic review emphasizes just these points. It summarizes 19 nonrandomized studies that include 1711 patients, all with TASC C or D lesions. Technical success rates are high, 86% to 100% symptomatic improvement in 83% to 100% of patients. There is wide variation in the types of complications reported, but only a 1.2% to 6.7% mortality rate. As stated in the authors' conclusion, "in the hands of experienced interventionalists," excellent outcomes can be obtained. The primary patency rates may not approach those of open revascularization; however, satisfactory percutaneous secondary patency rates may be obtained by reintervention. The practicing community of vascular surgeons and endovascular interventionalists has broadened the indications for endovascular treatment of extensive aortoiliac occlusive disease. Shouldn't the published guidelines reflect contemporary care?

R. L. Bush, MD, MPH

A contemporary experience of open aortic reconstruction in patients with chronic atherosclerotic occlusion of the abdominal aorta
West CA Jr, Johnson LW, Doucet L, et al (Louisiana State Univ Health Sciences Ctr, Shreveport; et al)
J Vasc Surg 52:1164-1172, 2010

Objective.—To examine and report surgical results from a contemporary experience of open abdominal aortic reconstruction in patients with chronic atherosclerotic abdominal aortic occlusion (CAAAO).

Methods.—Between January 1999 through May 2010, 54 patients with CAAAO were identified and retrospectively reviewed. CAAAOs were categorized into infrarenal aortic occlusions (IRAOs) and juxtarenal aortic occlusions (JRAOs) based on superior extension of thrombus and requirement for supra-renal aortic clamping to repair. Morbidity, mortality, hospital stay, and operative variables were assessed. The χ^2 or Fisher test and the Wilcoxon rank sum test were used to compare demographic and operative variables between two aortic occlusion groups (IRAO and JRAO). Univariate and multivariate analyses were performed to assess factors associated with surgical outcomes and hospital stay. The Kaplan-Meier method was used to calculate survival and patency rates.

Results.—Fifty patients underwent aortic reconstructions with aortobifemoral or iliac bypass, and three underwent a remote axillo-femoral bypass procedure. There were 35 (64.8%) males, and 19 (35.2%) females. Median age was 51.9 years (range, 32-72 years). Of the two CAAAO groups, there were 20 IRAOs and 33 JRAOs. Aorto-renal thromboendartectomy was performed in 26 (49.1%) patients; 26 (75.8%) among JRAOs versus 1 (5%) of IRAOs ($P < .01$). Proximal aortic clamps were required in 28 (85%) of JRAOs and 3 (15%) of IRAOs ($P < .01$). Thirty-day and in-hospital mortality was zero. Median length of hospital stay was 7 days (range, 4 to 66 days), and median intensive care unit length of stay was 3 days (range, 1-22 days). Complications included cardiopulmonary dysfunction in four (8%), postoperative renal insufficiency in 10 (18.9%), and other postoperative complications in 15 (28.3%). All 10 with renal insufficiency recovered renal function to baseline creatinine or a creatinine value < 1.1 mg/dL. Mean increases in right and left ankle-brachial indicess were 0.54 ± 0.25 and 0.59 ± 0.22, respectively. On univariate analysis, coronary artery disease and African American race were predictors of postoperative complications ($P = .048$). Age was significantly associated with total complications. Patients with postoperative complications and/or renal insufficiency were older than those without such complications ($P = .02$) Independent predictors of prolonged hospital stay were intraoperative blood replacement ($P = .003$), postoperative complications ($P < .01$), and postoperative renal insufficiency ($P < .01$). Prolonged intensive care unit stay was predicted by JRAO ($P = .04$), postoperative complications ($P = .02$), and postoperative renal insufficiency ($P = .013$). Survival at 3, 5, and 7 years were 86.6%, 76.5% and 50.9%, respectively. The reduced survival rates were predicted by previous myocardial infarction and existing coronary artery disease ($P < .01$).

Conclusion.—Abdominal aortic reconstruction is a safe method for treating CAAAO with low associated morbidity and mortality. Aorto-renal thromboendartectomy with supra-renal aortic clamping and aortic replacement remains an effective treatment for those with significant pararenal aortic disease, and can be performed without significant renal impairment.

▶ This is an excellent article that describes the modern outcomes that can be obtained with traditional open surgical reconstruction of the abdominal aorta for total aortic occlusion. Though most vascular surgeons have seen and treated this condition, it represents a rare disease entity. It is nice to be reminded in this era of "endovascular first" that conventional open surgery is truly indicated for aortic occlusion, with low complication rates and excellent patient results. Of note, renal insufficiency, though occurring in 18.9%, was temporary in this cohort. The authors describe exactly their protocol for intraoperative management of the renal arteries including renal protective medication administration.

Vascular surgical trainees need to be familiar with approaching the suprarenal aorta and for performing bilateral renal artery exclusion to prevent embolization during clamping. Furthermore, this series advocates a transperitoneal approach; however, one needs to be comfortable with this exposure as well as a retroperitoneal approach in patients who may have a hostile abdomen precluding a transperitoneal incision. Furthermore, alternatives such as axillobifemoral bypass and thoracobifemoral bypass need to be part of the surgeon's armamentarium for chronic aortic occlusion.

R. L. Bush, MD, MPH

Outcomes of angiosome and non-angiosome targeted revascularization in critical lower limb ischemia
Kabra A, Suresh KR, Vivekanand V, et al (Bhagwan Mahavir Jain Hosp, Bangalore, India)
J Vasc Surg 57:44-49, 2013

Objective.—Blood supply to the foot is from the posterior tibial, anterior tibial, and the peroneal arteries. Ischemic ulceration of the foot is the most common cause for major amputations in vascular surgical patients. It can be presumed that revascularization of the artery directly supplying the ischemic angiosome may be superior to indirect revascularization of the concerned ischemic angiosome.

Methods.—This was a prospective study of 64 patients with continuous single crural vessel runoff to the foot presenting with critical limb ischemia from January 2007 to September 2008. Direct revascularization (DR) of the ischemic angiosome was performed in 61% (n = 39), indirect revascularization (IR) in 39% (n = 25). Open surgery was performed in 60.9% and endovascular interventions in 39.1%. All patients were evaluated for the status of the wound and limb salvage at 1, 3, and 6 months. The study end points were major amputation or death, limb salvage, and wound epithelialization at 6 months.

Results.—In the study, 81.2% of patients had forefoot ischemia, 17.2% had ischemic heel, whereas 1.6% had midfoot nonhealing ischemic ulceration. The runoff involved the anterior tibial artery in 42.2% (27/64), posterior tibial artery in 34.4% (22/64), and the peroneal artery in 23.4% (15/64). All patients were followed at 1, 3, and 6 months postoperatively for ulcer healing, major amputation, or death. At the end of 6 months, nine patients expired, and six were lost to follow-up. Of 49 patients who completed 6 months, nine underwent major amputation, and 40 had limb salvage. Ulcer healing at 1, 3, and 6 months for DR vs IR were 7.9% vs 5%, 57.6% vs 12.5%, and 96.4% vs 83.3%, respectively. This difference in the rates of ulcer healing between the DR and IR groups was statistically significant ($P = .021$). The limb salvage in the DR group (84%) and IR group (75%) was not statistically significant ($P = .06$). The mortality was 10.2% for DR and 20% for IR at 6 months.

Conclusions.—To attain better ulcer healing rates combined with higher limb salvage, direct revascularization of the ischemic angiosome should be considered whenever possible. Revascularization should not be denied to patients with indirect perfusion of the ischemic angiosome as acceptable rates of limb salvage are obtained.

▶ In an effort to compare angiosome- and nonangiosome-targeted revascularization for critical limb ischemia (CLI), Kabra et al, after prospectively evaluating 64 patients presenting to their institution with CLI over a 21-month period, reported that direct revascularization (DR) to an angiosome resulted in faster healing rates than indirect revascularization (IR). Whereas the authors conclude that angiosome-targeted revascularization should be done whenever possible, this conclusion—certainly from this paper—is clearly an overreach given that there was no statistically significant difference in limb salvage rates between the DR and IR groups. This is particularly true given previously published, and larger, series confirming the efficacy of IR for limb salvage.[1] It would be more reasonable to recommend, as Neville et al have done, that among the multiple factors to be evaluated in choosing a target vessel for revascularization, consideration should also be given to the artery that directly feeds the ischemic angiosome.[2]

K. Hughes, MD

References

1. Berceli SA, Chan AK, Pomposelli FB Jr, et al. Efficacy of dorsal pedal artery bypass in limb salvage for ischemic heel ulcers. *J Vasc Surg.* 1999;30:499-508.
2. Neville RF, Attinger CE, Bulan EJ, Ducic I, Thomassen M, Sidawy AN. Revascularization of a specific angiosome for limb salvage: does the target artery matter? *Ann Vasc Surg.* 2009;23:367-373.

Subintimal Angioplasty of Long Chronic Total Femoropopliteal Occlusions: Long-Term Outcomes, Predictors of Angiographic Restenosis, and Role of Stenting
Siablis D, Diamantopoulos A, Katsanos K, et al (Patras Univ Hosp, Rion, Greece; et al)
Cardiovasc Intervent Radiol 35:483-490, 2012

Purpose.—The purpose of this article is to report the results of a prospective single-center study analyzing the longterm clinical and angiographic outcomes of subintimal angioplasty (SIA) for the treatment of chronic total occlusions (CTOs) of the femoropopliteal artery.

Materials and Methods.—Patients with severe intermittent claudication or critical limb ischemia (CLI) were enrolled in the study. All lesions were treated with SIA and provisional stenting. Primary end points were technical success, patient survival, limb salvage, lesion primary patency, angiographic binary restenosis (>50%), and target lesion revascularization (TLR). Regular clinical and angiographic follow-up was set at 6 and 12 months and yearly thereafter. Study end points were calculated with life-table survival analysis. Proportional-hazards regression analysis with a Cox-model was applied to adjust for confounding factors of heterogeneity.

Results.—Between May 2004 and July 2009, 98 patients (105 limbs, patient age 69.3 ± 9.9 years) were included in the study. Technical success rate was 91.4% with a lesion length of 121 ± 77 mm. Limb-salvage and survival rates were 88.7% and 84.1% at 3 years, respectively. After 12, 24, and 36 months, primary patency was 80.1%, 42.3%, and 29.0%, angiographic binary restenosis was 37.2%, 68.6%, and 80.0%, and TLR was 84.8%, 73.0%, and 64.5%, respectively. CLI was the only adverse predictor for decreased primary patency (hazard ratio [HR] 0.36; 95% confidence interval [CI] 0.16–0.80, $p = 0.012$), whereas significantly less restenosis was detected after spot stenting of the entry and/or re-entry site (HR 0.31;

95% CI 0.10−0.89, $p = 0.01$ and HR 0.20; 95% CI 0.07-0.56, $p = 0.002$, respectively).

Conclusions.—Subintimal angioplasty is a safe and effective revascularization technique for the treatment of CTOs of the femoropopliteal artery. Provisional stenting may have a role at the subintimal entry or true lumen re-entry site.

▶ This article describes an outstanding clinical outcome for subintimal angioplasty of long chronic femoral popliteal occlusions. One of the most interesting parts of the single-center study was the fact that all of the patients were premedicated for at least 3 days with aspirin and clopidogrel before the procedure. The majority of the procedures were performed with a 4F hydrophilic catheter and a hydrophilic guide wire. Only 7 cases (6.6%) required use of the reentry device. It was interesting to note that patients with claudication, that is, Rutherford categories 1 to 2, were excluded from the study as were patients with acute limb ischemia. The authors report a 91.4% technical success rate. They do report follow-up of as much as 3 years with evidence of primary patency of 80%, 43%, and 29%. The authors conclude that subintimal angioplasty is an effective revascularization technique. A complicating factor in this study was the fact that there was no mention of the specific Trans-Atlantic Inter-Society Consensus classification for the patients that were treated. It is important to know the extent of the runoff that could be associated with these lesions in the patients treated. Furthermore, they do mention that, based on their statistical analysis, they were able to predict that the full metal jacket lesion was a significant predictor of restenosis and, conversely, that stenting of the entry or reentry site was a predictor of less restenosis. It is interesting that these investigators were able to achieve a substantial technical success without the use of reentry devices. Although it is clear that these authors had considerable technical expertise, it is unclear what the anatomic characteristics of the patients treated were, particularly because their interventions were associated with limb salvage and survival rates of 88% and 84%, respectively.

M. T. Watkins, MD

A meta-analysis of endovascular versus surgical reconstruction of femoropopliteal arterial disease

Antoniou GA, Chalmers N, Georgiadis GS, et al (Central Manchester Univ Hosps, UK; Democritus Univ of Thrace, Alexandroupolis, Greece; et al)
J Vasc Surg 57:242-253, 2013

Background.—Controversy exists as to the relative merits of surgical and endovascular treatment of femoropoliteal arterial disease.

Methods.—A systematic review of the literature was undertaken to identify studies comparing open surgical and percutaneous transluminal methods for the treatment of femoropopliteal arterial disease. Outcome data were pooled and combined overall effect sizes were calculated using fixed or random effects models.

Results.—Four randomized controlled trials and six observational studies reporting on a total of 2817 patients (1387 open, 1430 endovascular) were included. Endovascular treatment was accompanied by lower 30-day morbidity (odds ratio [OR], 2.93; 95% confidence interval [CI], 1.34-6.41) and higher technical failure (OR, 0.10; 95% CI, 0.05-0.22) than bypass surgery, whereas no differences in 30-day mortality between the two groups were identified (OR, 0.92; 95% CI, 0.55-1.51). Higher primary patency in the surgical treatment arm was found at 1 (OR, 2.42; 95% CI, 1.37-4.28), 2 (OR, 2.03; 95% CI, 1.20-3.45), and 3 (OR, 1.48; 95% CI, 1.12-1.97) years of intervention. Progression to amputation was found to occur more commonly in the endovascular group at the end of the second (OR, 0.60; 95% CI, 0.42-0.86) and third (OR, 0.55; 95% CI, 0.39-0.77) year of intervention. Higher amputation-free and overall survival rates were found in the bypass group at 4 years (OR, 1.31; 95% CI, 1.07-1.61 and OR, 1.29; 95% CI, 1.04-1.61, respectively).

Conclusions.—High-level evidence demonstrating the superiority of one method over the other is lacking. An endovascular-first approach may be advisable in patients with significant comorbidity, whereas for fit patients with a longer-term perspective a bypass procedure may be offered as a first-line interventional treatment.

▶ This study is one of the most important review articles on the topic of open versus endovascular intervention for femoropopliteal arterial disease. It combines data from 4 randomized trials and 6 observational studies to determine the relative merits of these interventions. The strengths of this study are that it goes to great lengths to delineate the demographic and clinical characteristics of the study populations included in the review. The data are temporally reported over a 4-year period. It is amazing to learn that data on clinical improvement were provided in only 2 randomized trials. Predictably, lower 30-day morbidity was significantly favored in the endovascular group. Surprisingly, they report a transient benefit for surgical intervention versus endovascular interventions with respect to progression to amputation at years 2 and 3 following intervention, but not at year 4. Paradoxically, amputation-free survival became statistically favorable for open surgery only at 4 years following intervention. It is likely that the underlying medical condition for patients offered open versus endovascular intervention was significantly different, and this may account for the favorable amputation-free survival. The discussion part of this article is superb and balanced in the interpretation of the data. The limitations of the randomized and nonrandomized study data are presented with clarity and without prejudice. This article provides more than enough rationale to support the efforts of a number of groups to obtain funding for a multicenter prospective randomized trial comparing the outcome of these techniques for femoropopliteal occlusive disease.

M. T. Watkins, MD

A Randomized Prospective Multicenter Trial of a Novel Vascular Sealant
Stone WM, Cull DL, Money SR (Mayo Clinic, Scottsdale, AZ; Greenville
Memorial Hosp, SC)
Ann Vasc Surg 26:1077-1084, 2012

Background.—Increasing use of anticoagulant medications, particularly antiplatelet therapies, can increase the difficulty in obtaining adequate suture line hemostasis. Multiple vascular sealants have been used as adjuncts to surgical procedures, but none of them have been universally successful. The aim of this study was to evaluate the safety and effectiveness of a new prophylactic vascular sealant in arterial surgery.

Methods.—A randomized prospective multi-institutional trial was undertaken comparing ArterX Vascular Sealant (AVS) with Gelfoam Plus during open arterial reconstruction.

Results.—Three hundred thirty-one anastomotic sites in 217 patients were randomized. One hundred one of 167 (60.5%) anastomotic sites in the AVS group achieved immediate hemostasis compared with 65 of 164 (39.6%) in the control group ($P = 0.001$). In anastomoses with polytetrafluoroethylene grafts, 105 of 167 (62.5%) in the AVS group achieved immediate hemostasis compared with 56 of 164 (34.0%) in the control group ($P < 0.001$). No significant differences were noted in morbidity or mortality. Operative time was significantly less in the AVS group compared with the control group (3.2 vs. 3.8 hours, $P < 0.01$).

Conclusion.—Use of AVS results in superior hemostatic effectiveness compared with Gelfoam Plus, with no difference in safety. Although no cost analysis was performed, cost savings likely resulted from significantly decreased operative time.

▶ Suture line bleeding is an everyday problem for vascular surgeons seeking technical perfection after open arterial interventions. This well-designed trial compares the effectiveness of a novel sealant in managing suture line bleeding at 11 participating centers. The strength of the report is the fact that the data were obtained prospectively in a randomized fashion. Statistically significant differences in bleeding time and operating time were observed in the novel treatment group when compared with standard therapeutic intervention such as Gelfoam. The authors stratify control of suture line bleeding into immediate and a number of different time intervals. It was not clear that the amount of heparin administered to the patients and the level of anticoagulation were similar between the groups. This report attempts to provide additional information that may become more relevant and important in the setting of the need to decrease health care cost. Does the decrease in operating time observed in patients using the novel hemostatic agent offset the cost of the agent? The authors go to great lengths to discuss the potential side effects related to the use of the novel agent, as it contains bovine serum albumin. This report is included for this YEARBOOK because it is an important problem that has not been answered adequately. The authors are to be commended for their effort and excellent follow-up of this clinical problem. Without adequate comparison of the level of perioperative treatment with antiplatelet agents and the intraoperative use of heparin, a definitive answer to this problem will not be achieved.

M. T. Watkins, MD

A multicenter experience evaluating chronic total occlusion crossing with the Wildcat catheter (the CONNECT study)

Pigott JP, for the Connect Trial Investigators (Jobst Vascular Inst, Toledo, OH; et al)
J Vasc Surg 56:1615-1621, 2012

Objective.—Percutaneous techniques for crossing femoropopliteal chronic total occlusions (CTOs) offer an alternative to bypass surgery in patients deemed to be at increased risk due to advanced age or comorbidities. Recent reports document good success rates in catheters designed to reconstitute peripherally occluded arteries following failed guidewire passage. The Wildcat catheter (Avinger, Redwood City, Calif) is a novel device with a rotating distal tip and deployable wedges fashioned for channeling a passage through arterial occlusions. This report describes the results of a prospective, multicenter, nonrandomized trial evaluating the safety and efficacy of the Wildcat device when crossing de novo or restenotic femoropopliteal CTOs.

Methods.—Between August 2010 and April 2011, patients with peripheral arterial disease due to a femoropopliteal CTO >1 cm and ≤35 cm were evaluated for study enrollment at 15 U.S. sites. During treatment, the physician initially attempted to cross the CTO using conventional guidewires per protocol; if the guidewire successfully crossed, the patient was considered a screen failure and the Wildcat was not deployed. At 30 days, patients were reevaluated. The primary efficacy end point was successful crossing of the Wildcat into the distal true lumen as confirmed by angiography. Primary safety end points included no in-hospital or 30-day major adverse events, no clinically significant perforation or embolization, and no grade C or greater dissection. Additional data collected included lesion length, degree of calcification, and location.

Results.—Eighty-eight patients were enrolled in the trial. Of these, the Wildcat device was used in 84 patients (95%) per protocol. Successful CTO crossing was reported and confirmed by independent review in 89% (75/84) of cases with 5% (4/84) major adverse events as defined in the protocol (predominantly perforations sealed with balloon inflation). There were no clinically relevant events associated with any of the perforations. The mean CTO length was 174 ± 96 mm (range, 15-350 mm). Approximately 57% (n = 48) of all lesions were categorized as containing at least moderate calcification. Eighty-nine percent (n = 75) of vessels recanalized were superficial femoral arteries.

Conclusions.—In this multicenter study, the Wildcat catheter demonstrated an 89% crossing success rate with little associated morbidity. The

Wildcat catheter is a viable device for crossing moderately calcified femoropopliteal CTOs.

▶ These authors sought to evaluate the early results associated with using a Wildcat catheter to cross chronic total occlusions. In this trial, exclusion criteria included severe calcification on angiography or target lesions in a stent or bypass graft. By protocol, the investigators attempted to cross lesions that were less than 30 cm in length, and in all instances they were given at least 10 minutes to try to cross lesions using conventional techniques. In this study, the authors took great care to include the time involved in intent to treat, whether by usual catheter-based techniques or the Wildcat catheter. In this study, they found an 89% success rate treating lesions with the mean length of 174 mm. It is interesting to note that only 35% of the patients in the starting ankle-brachial indexes experienced intermittent claudication. For these studies, a reentry device was needed in 15 of the 88 interventions reported. The important components of this study are the fact that they were able to cross significantly challenging lesions in patients with significant symptomatology. Thus, this is a feasibility study, which seems to indicate that this device may be very useful in crossing complex chronic total occlusions. There are little long-term data available in this study. To determine whether this technology will be clinically useful, long-term results of this treatment will be important to put this device's efficacy in perspective.

M. T. Watkins, MD

One-year Clinical Outcome after Primary Stenting for Trans-Atlantic Inter-Society Consensus (TASC) C and D Femoropopliteal Lesions (The STELLA "STEnting Long de L'Artère fémorale superficielle" Cohort)
Davaine J-M, Azéma L, Guyomarch B, et al (CHU Nantes, France; et al)
Eur J Vasc Endovasc Surg 44:432-441, 2012

Objective.—The study aims to evaluate the safety and the efficacy of primary stenting for Trans-Atlantic Inter-Society Consensus Document II on Management of Peripheral Arterial Disease (TASC) C and D femoropopliteal lesions.

Design.—Prospective cohort study.

Methods.—Patients with TASC C and D *de novo* femoropopliteal lesions were treated with the same endovascular technique by implanting a primary nitinol self-expanding stent (LifeStent®, Bard Peripheral Vascular, Tempe, AZ, USA). Patients were included in a single-centre registry and prospectively followed up. The primary end point was primary sustained clinical improvement after 12 months. Secondary end points were secondary sustained clinical improvement, primary and secondary patency rates, freedom from target lesion revascularisation (TLR), freedom from target extremity revascularisation (TER) and stent fracture rate.

Results.—We enrolled 58 patients (62 limbs) suffering from either claudication (40.3%) or critical limb ischaemia (59.7%). Lesions were either TASC C (62.9%) or TASC D (37.1%). Median length of the treated segment was 220 ± 160 mm. The mean number of stents was 2.2. Mean follow-up was 17 months, with one patient lost to follow-up. At 1 year, the primary end point was 68.6% while secondary sustained clinical improvement was 82.6%. Freedom from TLR and TER rates were 81.1% and 96.3%. Primary and secondary patencies were 66% and 80.9%. One-year primary and secondary sustained clinical improvement rates were 76.7% ± 7.2 for TASC C and 46.3% ± 11.1 for TASC D ($p = 0.03$) and 87.6% ± 5.9 for TASC C and 67.3% ± 11.3 for TASC D ($p = 0.09$), respectively. The ankle–brachial pressure index increased from 0.58 to 0.94 ($p = 0.001$) at 1 year and the incidence of in-stent restenosis (ISR) was 19.3%. Stent fracture and disconnection rate was 17.7%.

Conclusions.—Primary stenting of TASC C and D lesions appears to be safe and efficient given the high-sustained clinical improvement and the low rate of ISR observed in our study. Endovascular treatment of such long and severe lesions exposes to high rate of stent fractures, which should not be a concern given their low clinical impact.

▶ This trial was formed as a prospective cohort study to determine the efficacy of primary stenting for long lesions (TASC II C and D) of the femoropopliteal segment. Notably, this was not sponsored by industry and the authors had no disclosures in reference to the LifeStents from Bard (Tempe, Arizona). Among the 58 treated patients, 60% were treated for rest pain (21%), ulceration (32%), or gangrene (7%). At 1 year, Rutherford class improvement of greater than 1 was appreciated in 68% of patients, with secondary target lesion revascularization yielding an improvement rate of 80%. Overall, the benefit of stenting in the authors' trial for such diffuse disease is slightly better than in prior studies, but their conclusions concerning stent fractures as benign entities are questionable. The average number of stents per patient was 2.2, and the contention has been made by others that stent fractures in overlap zones have more malignant potential. With so few patients in their trial, to conclude stent fractures are benign may represent a type II statistical error. In this regard, the best policy is likely to use appropriate length stents to avoid multiple implants.

J. Black, MD

Volume–Outcome Relationships in Lower Extremity Arterial Bypass Surgery
Moxey PW, Hofman D, Hinchliffe RJ, et al (St George's Vascular Inst, London, UK; St George's Univ of London, UK)
Ann Surg 256:1102-1107, 2012

Objective.—We sought to investigate whether a volume–outcome relationship exists for lower extremity arterial bypass (LEAB) surgery.

Methods.—All LEAB procedures performed in England between 2002 and 2006 were identified from Hospital Episode Statistics data. A Charlson-type risk profile, including operating hospital annual case volume, was identified per patient. Outcome measures of revision bypass, amputation, death and a composite measure were established during the index admission and at 1 year.

Quintile analysis and multilevel multivariate modeling were used to identify the existence of a volume—outcome relationship and allow adjustment of results for significant determinants of outcome.

Results.—A total of 27,660 femoropopliteal bypass and 4161 femorodistal bypass procedures were identified.

As volume increased, in-hospital mortality after popliteal bypass decreased from 6.5% to 4.9% ($P = 0.0045$), with a corresponding odds ratio of 0.980 [95% confidence interval (CI), 0.929—0.992; $P = 0.014$] for every increase of 50 patients per year. Major amputation decreased from 4.1% to 3.2% ($P = 0.006$) in high-volume hospitals, with a reduction in risk of 0.955 (95% CI, 0.928—0.983; $P = 0.002$) at 1 year.

For distal bypass, in-hospital mortality decreased from 9.8% to 5.5% ($P = 0.004$) and 1-year major amputation decreased from 25.4% to 18.2% ($P < 0.001$), with a corresponding odds ratio of 0.658 (95% CI, 0.517—0.838; $P < 0.0001$) as the volume increased.

An increase in the chance of revision surgery (10.6% vs 8.2%, $P < 0.001$) was seen with higher volume, with an increased odds ratio of 1.031 (95% CI, 1.005—1.057; $P = 0.018$).

Conclusions.—A positive volume—outcome relationship exists for LEAB procedures even after employing multilevel risk adjustment models. There are benefits in terms of mortality and limb salvage both in the short-term and at 1 year postsurgery.

▶ This article lends credence to the importance of volume in delivering better patient outcomes in lower extremity bypass surgery (LEAB). The authors identified all LEAB patients in England using a centralized government database and studied mortality, amputation, and revision procedure status for femoropopliteal (N = 27 660) and femorodistal bypass (N = 4161). Coding limitations do not allow separation of autogenous vs prosthetic bypass, thus missing a major area of resultant procedural improvement. Indeed, although hospital-level variables are assumed to be better in a high-volume setting, it is equally plausible that higher rates of autogenous bypasses could explain the better outcomes in the study. Nonetheless, the statistical comparisons across the volume quintiles reflect an important theme. Lower mortality, lower rates of amputation and, lastly, higher attempts at revision bypasses are seen at high-volume hospitals, but the latter item strikes to the heart of the matter. Higher-volume centers can likely mount efforts at rescuing an untoward outcome, more often from services that complement vascular surgeons, such as cardiology, nephrology, and hematology. Indeed, the failure to rescue, whether it be a clotted graft, impending gangrene, or evolving myocardial infarction, is appreciated in lower-volume hospitals and may reflect this phenomena, which underlies all volume—outcome studies. The authors take us to the brink of this step and highlight the next layer of complexity in the volume—outcome paradigm.

J. Black, MD

Effect on walking distance and atherosclerosis progression of a nitric oxide-donating agent in intermittent claudication

Gresele P, on behalf of the NCX 4016-X-208 Study Group (Univ of Perugia, Italy; et al)
J Vasc Surg 56:1622-1628, 2012

Background.—Peripheral arterial disease (PAD) is almost invariably associated with a generalized atherosclerotic involvement of the arterial tree and endothelial dysfunction. Previous short-term studies showed improvement of vascular reactivity and walking capacity in PAD patients by measures aimed at restoring nitric oxide (NO) production. NO is also known to prevent the progression of atherosclerosis. We wished to assess whether the prolonged administration of an NO-donating agent (NCX 4016) improves the functional capacity of PAD patients and affects the progression of atherosclerosis as assessed by carotid intima-media thickness (IMT).

Methods.—This prospective, double-blind, placebo-controlled study enrolled 442 patients with stable intermittent claudication who were randomized to NCX 4016 (800 mg, twice daily) or its placebo for 6 months. The primary study outcome was the absolute claudication distance on a constant treadmill test (10% incline, 3 km/h). The main secondary end point was the change of the mean far-wall right common carotid artery IMT.

Results.—The increase of absolute claudication distance at 6 months compared with baseline was 126 ± 140 meters in the placebo-treated group and 117 ± 137 meters in the NCX 4016-treated group, with no significant differences. Carotid IMT increased in the placebo-treated group ($+0.01 \pm 0.01$ mm; $P = .55$) and decreased in the NCX 4016-treated group (-0.03 ± 0.01 mm; $P = .0306$). Other secondary end points did not differ between the two treatments.

Conclusions.—Long-term NO donation does not improve the claudication distance but does reduce progression of atherosclerosis in patients with PAD. Further studies aimed at assessing whether long-term NO donation may prevent ischemic cardiovascular events are warranted.

▶ Medical therapy for peripheral arterial disease (PAD), in its current form, includes antiplatelet and statin and antihypertensive medications. β-blockers have been attacked by the POISE trial against general use, but they remain of benefit in PAD patients. This study examined a new oral medication to improve the nitric oxide dysfunction of PAD. The randomized and blinded trial was sponsored by the drug maker, but the authors had no financial interest and maintained editorial control. Although the drug did not translate into improvement in claudication distance, there was a difference in carotid intima-media thickness (IMT). Interestingly, the carotid IMT finding was not a reduction in carotid IMT with time from the baseline, but rather a reduction of progression of IMT vs the controls. IMT has many technical limitations and can be questioned on that level easily, and the prior reports of improving from baseline carotid IMT seen in statin trials is thus fundamentally different from what this trial purports as their benefit. However, the study indicates future trials to include IMT may benefit from a 6-month lead-in phase to determine the true IMT baseline before drug introduction.

J. Black, MD

Pilot Trial of Cryoplasty or Conventional Balloon Post-Dilation of Nitinol Stents for Revascularization of Peripheral Arterial Segments: The COBRA Trial

Banerjee S, Das TS, Abu-Fadel MS, et al (Univ of Texas Southwestern Med Ctr, Dallas; Presbyterian Hosp of Dallas, TX; Univ of Oklahoma Health Sciences Ctr, Oklahoma City; et al)

J Am Coll Cardiol 60:1352-1359, 2012

Objectives.—The purpose of this study is to compare post-dilation strategies of nitinol self-expanding stents implanted in the superficial femoral artery of diabetic patients with peripheral arterial disease.

Background.—Endovascular treatment of superficial femoral artery disease with nitinol self-expanding stents is associated with high rates of in-stent restenosis in patients with diabetes mellitus.

Methods.—We conducted a prospective, multicenter, randomized, controlled clinical trial of diabetic patients to investigate whether post-dilation of superficial femoral artery nitinol self-expanding stents using a cryoplasty balloon reduces restenosis compared to a conventional balloon. Inclusion criteria included diabetes mellitus, symptomatic peripheral arterial disease, and superficial femoral artery lesions requiring implantation of stents >5 mm in diameter and > 60 mm in length. Primary endpoint was binary restenosis at 12 months, defined as ≥ 2.5-fold increase in peak systolic velocity by duplex ultrasonography.

Results.—Seventy-four patients, with 90 stented superficial femoral artery lesions, were randomly assigned to post-dilation using cryoplasty (n = 45 lesions) or conventional balloons (n = 45 lesions). Mean lesion length was 148 ± 98 mm, mean stented length was 190 ± 116 mm, mean stent diameter was 6.1 ± 0.4 mm, and 50% of the lesions were total occlusions. Post-dilation balloon diameters were 5.23 ± 0.51 mm versus 5.51 ± 0.72 mm in the cryoplasty and conventional balloon angioplasty groups, respectively ($p = 0.02$). At 12 months, binary restenosis was significantly lower in the cryoplasty group (29.3% vs. 55.8%, $p = 0.01$; odds ratio: 0.36, 95% confidence interval: 0.15 to 0.89).

Conclusions.—Among diabetic patients undergoing implantation of nitinol self-expanding stents in the superficial femoral artery, post-dilation with cryoplasty balloon reduced binary restenosis compared to conventional balloon angioplasty. (Study Comparing Two Methods of Expanding Stents Placed in Legs of Diabetics With Peripheral Vascular Disease [COBRA]; NCT00827853).

▶ Enthusiasm for CryoPlasty in peripheral artery disease procedures has waned in recent years as trials have failed to demonstrate durable improvements in the femoropopliteal territory. The authors tried to define a role in diabetic patients in whom long segment disease would predict usage of stent and a concomitant risk of restenosis. After stent placement, the CryoPlasty balloon is applied, presumably to model the stent to the wall, vs a conventional balloon. The restenosis rate after CryoPlasty is greatly reduced, only 29% in the CryoPlasty group vs 55% in the regular percutaneous transluminal angioplasty. The results are compelling, but clearly cost is a major concern to invoke a routine policy of poststent CryoPlasty. I remain concerned that the stent and CryoPlasty group is still fading into restenosis at 1 year, so have we just kicked (or frozen) the can of restenosis farther down the street? The inevitable comparison to drug-eluting stents will come next, and indeed those vs the proposal of this study may be cost equivalent.

J. Black, MD

Micro-lightguide spectrophotometry for tissue perfusion in ischemic limbs
Jørgensen LP, Schroeder TV (Univ of Copenhagen, Denmark)
J Vasc Surg 56:746-752, 2012

Objective.—To validate micro-lightguide spectrophotometry (O2C) in patients with lower limb ischemia and to compare results with those obtained from toe blood pressure.

Methods.—We prospectively examined 59 patients, 24 of whom complained of claudication, 31 had critical ischemia, and four were asymptomatic. Diabetes was present in 19 (32%) patients. Saturation (SO_2) and flow measured with O2C were determined with the limb in the horizontal position followed by a 55-cm elevation. Toe pressures were determined in the horizontal position only. In addition, 13 patients were examined before and, on average, 3 days after revascularization.

Results.—Median SO_2 was 62% (25%-75% percentile: 37%-75%) with the limb in the horizontal position and 16% (3%-41%) with the limb elevated. Comparing the individual toe pressures with SO_2 values measured in the horizontal position and elevated position revealed a significant correlation ($r_s = 0.40$; $P < .01$ and $r_s = 0.56$; $P < .01$, respectively). A low SO_2 (ie, <40% in the horizontal position and <20% in the elevated position) was highly predictive of a toe pressure of 40 mm Hg or less. In the horizontal position, the positive predictive value was 100%, whereas the negative predictive value was 47%. The similar figures in the elevated position were a positive predictive value of 97% and a negative predictive value of 68%. Postoperatively, SO_2 increased significantly from 27% (P25%-75%: 11%-75%) to 79% (68%-87%) in the horizontal position ($P = .008$) and from 14% (P25%-75%: 2%-39%) to 55% (30%-73%) in the elevated position ($P = .011$), respectively. Looking at the individual 13 cases in which revascularization was performed, three patients had a partial reconstruction (ie, superficial femoral artery occlusion distal to a central reconstruction or reconstruction to a popliteal blind segment). These patients had significantly lower postoperative SO_2 as well as toe pressure compared with the 10 patients with unobstructed flow to the foot.

Conclusions.—O2C was easy to use, fast, and painless. The most useful finding was the high predictive value of a low saturation and the rise in O2C values after successful revascularization.

▶ The authors debut a new technology to assess limb perfusion using a probe that is attached to the target tissue to measure oxygen saturation. Notably, the authors have disclosed no financial interest in the company that manufactured the device. The device is small; however, the analysis unit is the size of a desktop computer. Thus, the unit is not likely to be useful outside of a vascular laboratory. This begs the question: in the vascular laboratory, what will it replace? The new device doesn't record a waveform, so it won't replace Doppler or the pulse volume recordings anytime soon. In its current iteration, the device is impractical.

J. Black, MD

Randomized controlled trial of remote endarterectomy versus endovascular intervention for TransAtlantic Inter-Society Consensus II D femoropopliteal lesions
Gabrielli R, Rosati MS, Vitale S, et al ("Policlinico Casilino", Rome, Italy; "Sapienza" Univ of Rome, Italy)
J Vasc Surg 56:1598-1605, 2012

Objective.—This study evaluated outcomes of remote endarterectomy (RE) vs endovascular (ENDO) interventions on TransAtlantic Inter-Societal Consensus (TASC)-II D femoropopliteal lesions and identified factors predictive of restenosis.

Methods.—From October 2004 to December 2008, 95 patients with TASC-II D lesions were randomized 1:1 to receive RE of the superficial femoral artery (SFA) with end point stenting (51 patients) or ENDO, consisting of subintimal angioplasty with stenting (44 patients). The groups were balanced for age, sex, atherosclerotic risk factors, and comorbidities. Categoric data were analyzed with χ^2 tests, and time to event provided two-sided *P* values with a level of significance at .05 and 95% confidence intervals (CIs). Survival curves for primary patency were plotted using the Kaplan-Meier method. Univariate analysis for diabetes, hypertension, dyslipidemia, smoking, and critical ischemia was performed according to the Cox proportional hazards model.

Results.—The mean follow-up was 52.5 months (range, 35-75 months). Five RE patients and four ENDO patients were lost to follow-up (censored). Primary patency was 76.5% (39 of 51) in RE and 56.8% (25 of 44) in ENDO (hazard ratio [HR], 2.6; 95% CI, 0.99-4.2; *P* =.05) at 24 months and was 62.7% (32 of 46) in RE and 47.7% (21 of 40) in ENDO (HR, 1.89; 95% CI, 0.94-3.78; *P* =.07) at 36 months. Assisted primary patency was 70.6% (36 of 51) in RE and 52.3% (23 of 44) in ENDO (HR, 2.45; 95% CI, 1.20-5.02; *P* =.01). Secondary patency overlapped the primary comparison data at 12 and 24 months; at 36 months, there was a slight but significative advantage for RE (HR, 2.26; 95% CI, 1.05-4.86;

$P=.03$). Univariate analysis demonstrated that hypercholesterolemia and critical limb ischemia (CLI) were significantly related to patency failure, whereas diabetes was significant only in ENDO. These factors (hypercholesterolemia and CLI) were independent predictors of patency on Cox multivariate analysis.

Conclusions.—RE is a safe, effective, and durable procedure for TASC-II D lesions. Our data demonstrate a significantly higher primary, assisted primary, and secondary patency of RE vs ENDO procedures. Furthermore, overall secondary patency rates remain within the standard limits, although preoperative CLI and dyslipidemia continue to be associated with worse outcomes. Taken together, these data suggest that RE should be considered better than an endovascular procedure in SFA long-segment occlusion treatment.

▶ Surgical revascularization via bypass grafting is suggested for TransAtlantic Inter-Societal Consensus (TASC) IID femoropopliteal lesions. Gabrielli et al present herein a prospective trial comparing the remote endarterectomy (RE) and end-point stenting technique with standard endovascular (ENDO) intervention using nitinol self-expanding stents. Approximately 60% of both groups included patients with rest pain or gangrene. In combining these groups as a single population, of which the rest pain comprised most, we are still left to contemplate where RE fits on the expected spectrum of intervention. The study recapitulates the horrible performance of ENDO for TASC IID with only a 26% primary patency at 3 years, yet the limb salvage success is statistically similar (96% vs 90%). Indeed, the authors conclude surgery should remain the mainstay in higher Rutherford classes but correctly offer RE as an option for those unfit for surgery. I look forward to seeing if a head-to-head comparison of RE and bypass surgery will best the results reflected in BASIL.

J. Black, MD

Effect of Supervised Exercise Therapy for Intermittent Claudication in Patients With Diabetes Mellitus
van Pul KM, Kruidenier LM, Nicolai SPA, et al (Atrium Med Ctr Parkstad, Heerlen, The Netherlands; Maxima Med Ctr, Veldhoven, The Netherlands; et al)
Ann Vasc Surg 26:957-963, 2012

Background.—Primary treatment for patients with intermittent claudication is exercise therapy. Diabetes mellitus (DM) is a frequently occurring comorbidity in patients with intermittent claudication, and in these patients, exercise tolerance is decreased. However, there is little literature about the increase in walking distance after supervised exercise therapy (SET) in patients with both intermittent claudication and DM. The objective of this study was to determine the effectiveness of SET for intermittent claudication in patients with DM.

Methods.—Consecutive patients with intermittent claudication who started SET were included. Exclusion criteria were Rutherford stage 4 to 6 and the inability to perform the standardized treadmill test. SET was administered according to the guidelines of the Royal Dutch Society for Physiotherapy. At baseline and at 1, 3, and 6 months of follow-up, a standardized treadmill exercise test was performed. The primary outcome measurement was the absolute claudication distance (ACD).

Results.—We included 775 patients, of whom 230 had DM (29.7%). At 6 months of follow-up, data of 440 patients were available. Both ACD at baseline and at 6 months of follow-up were significantly lower in patients with DM ($P < 0.001$). However, increase in ACD after 6 months of SET did not differ significantly ($P = 0.48$) between the DM group and the non-DM group (270 m and 400 m, respectively).

Conclusion.—In conclusion, SET for patients with intermittent claudication is equally effective in improving walking distance for both patients with and without DM, although ACD remains lower in patients with DM.

▶ Although practitioners and patients may assume that individuals with severe limitation of their daily activities are poor candidates for exercise therapy because of limited ability to participate, these results show that supervised exercise therapy (SET) should be pursued in all claudicants. The investigators hypothesized that metabolic changes associated with skeletal muscle and endothelial function might predispose diabetic patients to reduced benefits associated with SET, but similar increases in absolute claudication distance (ACD) were observed for both diabetic and nondiabetic patients at 6 months. Because diabetic patients had a lower baseline ACD, they potentially gained the most from SET in terms of functional status. The authors also provide a list of reasons for withdrawal from SET, which might be useful for individualizing treatment; it is interesting to note that sufficient result of SET was the reason provided by 7% of patients who withdrew. This study utilized community-based SET programs that allowed patients to participate within their neighborhoods; because such programs are not widely available in all countries, it would be interesting to compare these results with those from clinic- or hospital-based programs.

M. A. Corriere, MD, MS

Availability of Supervised Exercise Programs and the Role of Structured Home-based Exercise in Peripheral Arterial Disease
Makris GC, Lattimer CR, Lavida A, et al (Ealing Hosp, London, UK)
Eur J Vasc Endovasc Surg 44:569-575, 2012

Objectives.—The effectiveness of supervised exercise programs (SEPs) for the management of peripheral arterial disease (PAD) can be hampered by low accessibility and poor compliance. The current international availability and use of SEPs was evaluated and the evidence on alternative approaches such as structured, home-based exercise programs (HEPs) was reviewed.

Methods-Materials.—International survey on SEP availability among vascular surgeons using an online questionnaire. A systematic review on structured-HEPs effectiveness was also performed.

Results.—A total of 378 responses were collected from 43 countries, with the majority (95%) from Europe. Only 30.4% of the participants had access to SEPs and within this group there was significant heterogeneity on the way SEPs were implemented. This systematic review identified 12 studies on the effectiveness of HEPs. In 3 studies SEPs were superior to HEPs in improving functional capacity or equivalent in improving quality of life (QoL). HEPs significantly improved most of the functional capacity and QoL markers when compared to the "go home and walk" advice and baseline measurements.

Conclusions.—SEPs remain an underutilized tool despite recommendations. Structured HEPs may be effective and can be useful alternatives when SEPs are not available. Further research is warranted to establish cost-effectiveness.

▶ This report shows the importance of specificity and detail when counseling patients with intermittent claudication about exercise therapy. Although the supervised exercise program (SEP) has several advantages, which are detailed in the systematic review, the lack of widespread SEP access demonstrated by the survey results eliminates this option for most patients and providers. Even when available within the community, patients may not access SEPs because of lack of coverage or out-of-pocket costs.

The systematic review describes a number of useful alternatives that are more effective than the "go home and walk" advice (GHWA) that can be considered in environments in which SEPs are not an option. The more durable effect of home exercise programs (HEPs), attributed to incorporation of exercise into daily routine as opposed to within a specific environment, may be preferable in some ways to the more resource-intensive but less-sustainable SEP approach. Additional alternatives, including pedometers and online coaching, may impart structure where organized programs are unavailable but require patients to take on increasing personal responsibility for their treatment. Quoting the results of SEP- or HEP-based treatment to a patient embarking on a GHWA approach may have the unintended negative consequence of establishing patient expectations that are unrealistic outside of a more structured regimen.

M. A. Corriere, MD, MS

Comparison of initial hemodynamic response after endovascular therapy and open surgical bypass in patients with diabetes mellitus and critical limb ischemia
Zhan LX, Bharara M, White M, et al (Univ of Arizona, Tucson)
J Vasc Surg 56:380-386, 2012

Background.—While endovascular (ENDO) therapy has increasingly become the initial intervention of choice to treat lower extremity peripheral arterial disease, reported outcomes for ENDO in patients with critical limb ischemia (CLI) and diabetes have been reported to be inferior compared to open bypass surgery (OPEN). Objective data assessing the hemodynamic success of ENDO compared to the established benchmark of OPEN are sparse. We therefore evaluated and compared early hemodynamic outcomes of ENDO and OPEN in patients with diabetes with CLI at a single academic center.

Methods.—We studied 85 consecutive patients with diabetes and CLI who underwent 109 interventions, either ENDO (n = 78) or OPEN (n = 31). The mean patient age was 69 years; 62% were men. All patients presented with either rest pain and/or ulcer/gangrene. Per protocol, all were assessed using ankle brachial index (ABI) and toe pressure (TP) determinations before and early postintervention.

Results.—Both ENDO (ΔABI = 0.36 ± 0.24, $P < .0001$; ΔTP = 35.6 ± 24.1, $P < .0001$) and OPEN (ΔABI = 0.39 ± 0.17, $P < .0001$; ΔTP = 34.3 ± 24.0, $P < .0001$) resulted in significant hemodynamic improvement. There was no statistically significant initial difference between the two types of intervention (ABI, $P = .6$; TP, $P = .6$).

Conclusions.—These data suggest that with appropriate patient selection, each intervention is similarly efficacious in initially improving hemodynamics. If the intermediate or long-term results of ENDO for CLI in people with diabetes are inferior, the problem is not one of initial hemodynamic response, but more likely due to differing patient characteristics or durability of the intervention.

▶ This retrospective study compares postintervention changes in ankle brachial index (ABI) and toe pressures after surgical vs endovascular revascularization in a nonrandomized cohort of diabetic patients with critical limb ischemia. Similar degrees of improvement in both measures were observed for patients treated with surgical bypass vs endovascular intervention, and postintervention major amputation rates were also similar between treatments (11% for each group at a mean follow-up of 13—15 months). Two-thirds of the patients in the study received endovascular treatment as their initial intervention, suggesting a possible selection bias toward an endo-first approach, which is acknowledged in the discussion. Baseline Rutherford class, ABI, and toe pressures were similar between treatment groups, however, indicating that anatomic treatment selection criteria did not translate into huge differences in objective measures of disease severity. The authors concluded that long-term differences in outcomes between bypass and endovascular treatment may, therefore, be caused by durability of the interventions or patient factors. These results and conclusions are congruent with the findings of the randomized Bypass Versus Angioplasty in Severe Ischemia of the Leg (BASIL) trial, which reported similar early outcomes for surgery vs angioplasty-first intervention approaches,[1] although later outcomes from the treatment-received analysis also indicated a potential amputation-free survival advantage among participants surviving 2 years or longer who were treated with vein bypass.[2] These results indicate that endovascular treatment is a reasonable initial approach in many patients and may be preferred in situations in which limited life expectancy, significant comorbidities, or lack of a single segment of saphenous vein conduit potentially outweigh durability considerations.

M. A. Corriere, MD, MS

References

1. Bradbury AW, Adam DJ, Bell J, et al. Bypass versus Angioplasty in Severe Ischaemia of the Leg (BASIL) trial: An intention-to-treat analysis of amputation-free and overall survival in patients randomized to a bypass surgery-first or a balloon angioplasty-first revascularization strategy. *J Vasc Surg.* 2010;51(5 Suppl):5S-17S.
2. Bradbury AW, Adam DJ, Bell J, et al. Bypass versus Angioplasty in Severe Ischaemia of the Leg (BASIL) trial: Analysis of amputation free and overall survival by treatment received. *J Vasc Surg.* 2010;51(5 Suppl):18S-31S.

Outcomes of Open Operation for Aortoiliac Occlusive Disease After Failed Endovascular Therapy

Danczyk RC, Mitchell EL, Petersen BD, et al (Oregon Health and Science Univ, Portland)

Arch Surg 147:841-845, 2012

Objectives.—To compare patient outcomes of primary open operation for aortoiliac occlusive disease (AIOD) with those of secondary open operations for failed endovascular therapy (ET) of AIOD.

Design.—A retrospective cohort study was performed analyzing demographic characteristics, comorbidities, and outcomes.

Setting.—Affiliated Veterans Affairs Hospital from January 1, 1998, through March 31, 2010.

Patients.—Patients who underwent primary open operation for AIOD or secondary open operation for failed ET of AIOD.

Main Outcome Measures.—Overall survival and limb salvage.

Results.—Primary open operations (n = 153) were 67 aortobifemoral grafts (43.8%), 38 axillobifemoral grafts (24.8%), and 48 femoral-femoral grafts (31.4%). Secondary open operations (n = 35) were 28 aortobifemoral grafts (80.0%), 5 axillobifemoral grafts (14.3%), and 2 femoral-femoral grafts (5.7%). Mean (SD) 5-year survival was 48.2% (5.6%) and 66.8% (10.0%), respectively, for patients undergoing primary vs secondary open surgery for AIOD (P = .01). There were 7 amputations during a mean follow-up of 3 years, all in the primary open surgery group.

Conclusions.—Despite a higher proportion of coronary artery disease and a 20% conversion of claudication to critical limb ischemia after failed ET for AIOD, survival was longer in patients undergoing secondary vs primary open surgery. Patients who underwent open surgery after failed ET for AIOD did not require amputation. Failed ET for AIOD does not lead to worse outcomes for patients undergoing open surgery for AIOD.

▶ Surgical procedures for aortoiliac disease have been increasingly narrowed in indication with improvements in endovascular techniques. TASC II recommends aortobifemoral grafting for only the most diffuse and severe disease, so it comes as no surprise that Danczyk et al found higher amputation rates and less survival with the primary surgery group. Examination of their secondary surgical group, the majority of whom had surgery converted to aortobifemoral grafts (ABF), did far better with longer survival and fewer later events. In a retrospective review, such as this publication, it is very likely the secondary surgery group was more fit, and indeed the authors comment that among the primary group, only 43% had ABF vs the 80% in the secondary group in whom ABF was the procedure. They were also more likely to take clopidogrel, suggesting more aggressive medical management. Importantly, failure of endovascular therapy in the femoropopliteal region has been associated with a loss of the Society of Vascular Surgery tibial runoff score, yet the authors do not comment on runoff changes in their secondary group. Indeed, anatomic scoring of the runoff score in both groups would lend greatly to ensuring secondary aortoiliac surgery is as good as estimated.

J. Black, MD

Sirolimus-Eluting Stents for Treatment of Infrapopliteal Arteries Reduce Clinical Event Rate Compared to Bare-Metal Stents: Long-Term Results From a Randomized Trial
Rastan A, Brechtel K, Krankenberg H, et al (Herz-Zentrum Bad Krozingen, Germany; Eberhard-Karls-Universität, Tübingen, Germany; Universitäres Herz- und Gefäßzentrum Hamburg, Germany; et al)
J Am Coll Cardiol 60:587-591, 2012

Objectives.—The study investigated the long-term clinical impact of sirolimus-eluting stents (SES) in comparison with bare-metal stents (BMS) in treatment of focal infrapopliteal lesions.

Background.—There is evidence that SES reduce the risk of restenosis after percutaneous infrapopliteal artery revascularization. No data from randomized trials are available concerning the clinical impact of this finding during long-term follow-up.

Methods.—The study extended the follow-up period of a prospective, randomized, multicenter, double-blind trial comparing polymer-free SES with placebo-coated BMS in the treatment of focal infrapopliteal de novo lesions. The main study endpoint was the event-free survival rate defined as freedom from target limb amputation, target vessel revascularization, myocardial infarction, and death. Secondary endpoints include amputation rates, target vessel revascularization, and changes in Rutherford-Becker class.

Results.—The trial included 161 patients. The mean target lesion length was 31 ± 9 mm. Thirty-five (23.3%) patients died during a mean follow-up period of $1,016 \pm 132$ days. The event-free survival rate was 65.8% in the SES group and 44.6% in the BMS group (log-rank $p = 0.02$). Amputation rates were 2.6% and 12.2% ($p = 0.03$), and target vessel revascularization rates were 9.2% and 20% ($p = 0.06$), respectively. The median (interquartile range) improvement in Rutherford-Becker class was -2 (-3 to -1) in the SES group and -1 (-2 to 0) in the BMS group, respectively ($p = 0.006$).

Conclusions.—Long-term event-free survival, amputation rates, and changes in Rutherford-Becker class after treatment of focal infrapopliteal lesions are significantly improved with SES in comparison with BMS. (YUKON-Drug-Eluting Stent Below the Knee-Randomised Double-Blind Study [YUKON-BTX]; NCT00664963).

▶ This article follows up on the previous article[1] of a randomized, prospective, multicenter, double-blinded trial comparing sirolimus-eluting stents (SES) vs bare-metal stents (BMS). The previous trial, at 1-year follow-up, revealed higher patency and Rutherford class improvement in SES. Nonsignificant differences were noted in target vessel revascularization, limb salvage, and event-free survival. This study now takes follow-up to nearly 3 years, and as the SES matures, it shows more benefit. Target vessel revascularization is statistically better in SES than BMS, and amputation incidence drops from 12.2% in the BMS to 2.6% with SES. The favorable reductions in events, stenosis, and limb loss are impressive with SES, but the lesion characteristics are fairly atypical for most patients. The lesions are shorter, and surely most diabetic patients, for whom a preponderance of diffuse disease would be expected, would not fit the profile required to repeat these results. Furthermore, the absence of self-expanding stent scaffolds to deliver the drug to the vessel wall may reduce applicability of the current balloon-expandable SES designs. But what this study clearly reveals is that while the economics of SES has been a major consideration against wider use, the long-term improvements with SES for avoidance of amputation would pay for itself easily if one can be ensured that longer lesions follow up the nice results of this short-lesion study.

J. Black, MD

Reference

1. Rastan A, Tepe G, Krankenberg H, et al. Sirolimus-eluting stents vs. bare-metal stents for treatment of focal lesions in infrapopliteal arteries: a double-blind, multi-centre, randomized clinical trial. *Eur Heart J.* 2011;32:2274-2281.

Sex-based differences in the inflammatory profile of peripheral artery disease and the association with primary patency of lower extremity vein bypass grafts
Hiramoto JS, Owens CD, Kim JM, et al (Univ of California—San Francisco; et al)
J Vasc Surg 56:387-395, 2012

Objective.—This study was conducted to determine if there are sex-based differences in the inflammatory phenotype of patients undergoing lower extremity bypass (LEB) and if they correlate with clinical outcomes.

Methods.—This was a retrospective analysis of a prospective cohort of 225 patients (161 men and 64 women) who underwent autogenous vein LEB between February 2004 and May 2008. Fasting baseline blood samples were obtained before LEB, and the inflammatory biomarkers high-sensitivity C-reactive protein (CRP) and fibrinogen were assessed. All patients underwent ultrasound graft surveillance. CRP levels were dichoto-mized at 5 mg/L and fibrinogen levels at 600 mg/dL.

Results.—There were no significant differences in age, race, history of hypertension or diabetes mellitus, body mass index, or coronary artery disease between men and women. Men were more likely to be current smokers ($P =.02$), have a history of hypercholesterolemia ($P =.02$), and be taking sta-tins ($P =.02$). Women were more likely to present with critical limb ischemia ($P =.03$) and had higher median baseline CRP levels (5.15 mg/L; interquartile range [IQR], 1.51-18.62 mg/L) than men (2.70; IQR, 1.24-6.98 mg/L; $P =.02$). Median follow-up was 893 days (IQR, 539-1315 days). A multivar-iable Cox proportional hazards model for primary vein graft patency showed a significant interaction between sex and CRP ($P =.03$) and fibrin-ogen ($P =.02$). After adjustment for key covariates, primary vein graft patency was significantly less in women with CRP > 5 mg/L compared with women with CRP < 5 mg/L ($P =.02$). No such difference was seen in men ($P =.95$). Primary graft patency was also decreased in women with fibrino-gen > 600 mg/dL vs women with fibrinogen < 600 mg/dL ($P =.002$); again, this pattern was not evident in men ($P =.19$).

Conclusions.—Women undergoing LEB for advanced peripheral artery disease have a different inflammatory phenotype than men. Elevated base-line levels of CRP and fibrinogen are associated with inferior vein graft patency in women but not in men. These findings indicate an important interaction between sex and inflammation in the healing response of vein grafts for LEB. Women with elevated preoperative CRP and fibrinogen levels may benefit from more intensive postoperative graft surveillance protocols.

▶ Although women generally have lower rates of cardiovascular atherosclerotic occlusive disease than men, women who undergo lower extremity bypass have increased complications and lower graft patency. This prospective study demon-strated that elevated baseline C-reactive protein (CRP) levels and fibrinogen were each associated with autogenous vein graft failure in women, but not men. Chronic inflammation has been established as a strong risk factor for atheroscle-rosis and thrombotic events, and this study suggests a different underlying inflam-matory baseline profile in women compared with men who present with severe peripheral occlusive disease. It is the suggestion of this study that a predisposing underlying inflammatory phenotype may be associated with a disproportionate higher risk of subsequent graft failure in women. However, it is important to note that in this study only preoperative CRP and fibrinogen levels were measured without measurement at postoperative intervals or at time of graft failure. Further-more, the strength and generalizability of this association are also limited by the modest sample size, diverse study population, and focus on patients with advanced peripheral atherosclerosis undergoing autogenous vein graft. That said, these findings should provide enough interest to further extend the evalua-tion of the interaction of sex and inflammation on revascularization outcomes.

M. A. Passman, MD

Impact of Gender and Age on Outcomes of Tibial Artery Endovascular Interventions in Critical Limb Ischemia

Domenick N, Saqib NU, Marone LK, et al (Univ of Pittsburgh Med Ctr, PA)
Ann Vasc Surg 26:937-945, 2012

Background.—Female sex and older age are known risk factors for adverse outcomes in peripheral artery disease. This study reports on the outcomes of tibial artery endovascular intervention (TAEI) by age and gender in patients treated for critical limb ischemia.

Methods.—All TAEIs for tissue loss or rest pain (Rutherford classes 4, 5, and 6) from 2004 to 2010 were retrospectively reviewed. Patient demographics, comorbidities, intervention sites, complications, and outcome measurements, including limb salvage, wound healing, and patency, were recorded for each patient. Data were analyzed by gender and age using Fisher exact test, multivariate logistic regression, and Cox proportional hazards regression.

Results.—Two hundred twenty-one limbs (201 patients, 40% female) were treated for critical limb ischemia (74% with tissue loss, 26% with rest pain). Mean age of the patients was 73.3 years (39% were aged $\geq$ 80 - years). Comorbidities and indications for intervention were comparable. Isolated TAEI was performed in 46% of the limbs, whereas multilevel interventions were performed in 54%. Mean follow-up period was 8.7 ± 7.3 months. Complications were comparable between genders and ages (P = not significant [NS]). Limb salvage rate was 88% and was comparable by gender (P = NS). Major amputation was less frequent in octogenarians (6% vs. 16%, P = 0.03). Neither gender nor age was a predictor of limb loss (P = NS), but renal insufficiency was (hazard ratio = 2.81, 95% confidence interval = 1.14−6.90, P = 0.02). Age $\geq$ 80 years was a predictor of impaired wound healing (hazard ratio = 1.57, 95% confidence interval = 1.04−2.37, P = 0.03), but gender was not (P = NS). Overall primary patency rate was 62% at 1 year and was similar in women and octogenarians (P = NS). Overall reintervention rate was 53% at 1 year and was higher in women (65% vs. 46%, P = 0.03), but was not affected by age (P = NS).

Conclusions.—TAEI outcomes do not appear to be adversely affected by gender or age. Limb salvage appears equivalent in octogenarians, with amputations occurring less frequently. Women also appear to have outcomes similar to men after TAEIs, but may require repeat interventions to achieve equivalent limb salvage rates.

▶ The impact of female gender and advanced age on adverse outcomes after peripheral interventions has been mixed with some studies suggesting negative impact and others showing equivalence when compared with men and younger age groups. However, there are little data specific to endovascular interventions for critical limb ischemia from tibial-level occlusive disease. Although this study focuses on tibial interventions examining the effect of age and gender, the lack of difference here should be tempered by the small sample size, retrospective study design, inherent selection bias, and relatively short follow-up times.

Furthermore, lack of a standardized classification for tibial occlusive disease makes any comparisons difficult.

M. A. Passman, MD

Temporal Trends and Geographic Variation of Lower-Extremity Amputation in Patients With Peripheral Artery Disease: Results From U.S. Medicare 2000–2008
Jones WS, Patel MR, Dai D, et al (Duke Univ Med Ctr, Durham, NC)
J Am Coll Cardiol 60:2230-2236, 2012

Objectives.—This study sought to characterize temporal trends, patient-specific factors, and geographic variation associated with amputation in patients with lower-extremity peripheral artery disease (LE PAD) during the study period.

Background.—Amputation represents the end-stage failure for those with LE PAD, and little is known about the rates and geographic variation in the use of LE amputation.

Methods.—By using data from the Centers for Medicare & Medicaid Services (CMS) from January 1, 2000, to December 31, 2008, we examined national patterns of LE amputation among patients age 65 years or more with PAD. Multivariable logistic regression was used to adjust regional results for other patient demographic and clinical factors.

Results.—Among 2,730,742 older patients with identified PAD, the overall rate of LE amputation decreased from 7,258 per 100,000 patients with PAD to 5,790 per 100,000 ($p < 0.001$ for trend). Male sex, black race, diabetes mellitus, and renal disease were all independent predictors of LE amputation. The adjusted odds ratio of LE amputation per year between 2000 and 2008 was 0.95 (95% CI: 0.95-0.95, $p < 0.001$).

Conclusions.—From 2000 to 2008, LE amputation rates decreased significantly among patients with PAD. However, there remains significant patient and geographic variation in amputation rates across the United States.

▶ Using a large Medicare data set, this study shows a significant decrease in lower extremity amputation rates for patients with peripheral arterial disease (PAD) during the contemporary study period. Whether this reflects improved treatment strategies for patients with PAD, earlier detection, expanded revascularization options, or a combination thereof, is difficult to determine. However, the presence of geographic variation likely reflects an unmeasured effect of socioeconomic status, race, access to care, timing of presentation of patients with critical limb ischemia, and variable threshold to perform lower extremity amputation. Although there are limitations in this analysis reflecting a study design based on Medicare claims data, this study does identify an important need to standardize treatment of PAD across geographic boundaries.

M. A. Passman, MD

Impact of endovascular options on lower extremity revascularization in young patients

Chaar CIO, Makaroun MS, Marone LK, et al (Univ of Pittsburgh Med Ctr, PA)
J Vasc Surg 56:703-713.e3, 2012

Objective.—This study assessed outcomes of revascularization strategies in young patients with premature arterial disease.

Methods.—Lower extremity revascularization outcomes from 2000 to 2008 were retrospectively compared among consecutive patients with comparable indications and procedures: age <50 years (group A) at the time of revascularization, 51 to 60 years (group B), and >60 years (control group C). Patency, limb salvage, and survival by limb or patient level were assessed by Kaplan-Meier and Cox proportional hazards analyses.

Results.—A total of 409 limbs in 298 patients were treated: 44% for claudication and 56% for critical limb ischemia (CLI). Group A patients were more likely to be smokers and have a hypercoagulable state but less likely to have diabetes and renal failure. Treatment indications were comparable among groups, and procedures were equally distributed between open surgical and endovascular interventions. Two perioperative deaths occurred in group C (2%). Mean follow-up was 29 months, and 16% of claudicant patients in group A progressed to CLI (B, 3%; C, 2%; $P < .001$). Overall, 2-year primary, primary assisted, and secondary patency were significantly lower in group A (50.5%, 65.2%, 68.2%; $P = .045$) vs B (65.7%, 81.4%, 86.8%; $P = .01$) and C (57.9%, 78.9%, 83.9%; $P < .001$). Claudicant patients in group A had an unexpectedly low 2-year freedom from major amputation after intervention of only 90%. Results were more comparable across groups for CLI. The 2-year freedom from reintervention was similar (A, 81.0%; B, 78.9%; C, 83.5%), irrespective of the indication for intervention ($P = .60$). Younger patients had a significantly higher 3-year survival (A, 89.5%; B, 85.3%) compared with patients aged >60 years (C, 71.4%; $P = .005$). The 2-year freedom from major amputation rate was significantly lower in claudicant patients in group A vs C undergoing endovascular revascularization ($P = .002$), but not in patients treated with open revascularization ($P = .40$). Predictors of loss of primary patency included age <50 years ($P = .003$), endovascular revascularization ($P = .005$), and progression from claudication to CLI ($P < .001$). Age <50 years was also an independent predictor of limb loss vs age >60 years ($P = .05$).

Conclusions.—Endovascular options are commonly being used in young patients, especially those with claudication, but patency rates and outcomes remain very poor (Fig 3).

▶ These authors present an exhaustive examination of lower extremity revascularization, stratified by age. Following upon the prior YEAR BOOK's review of Radak, we now see the thematic issues of the young vasculopath crystallize. First, the younger patients were far more likely to be smokers and have hypercoagulability disorders. This is evidenced by higher rates of deep vein thrombosis and pulmonary embolism and history of warfarin use—events not seen in any of

Two-year primary patency rates by age groups – endovascular procedures

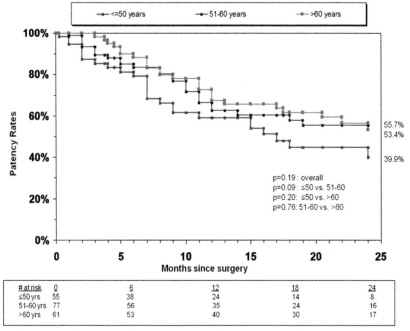

FIGURE 3.—Kaplan-Meier curves show 2-year primary patency for patients in groups A (*blue line*), B (*black line*), and C (*red line*) treated with an endovascular procedure. For interpretation of the references to color in this figure legend, the reader is referred to web version of this article. (Reprinted from the Journal of Vascular Surgery. Chaar CIO, Makaroun MS, Marone LK, et al. Impact of endovascular options on lower extremity revascularization in young patients. *J Vasc Surg.* 2012;56:703-713.e3, Copyright 2012, with permission from The Society for Vascular Surgery.)

the patients above 50 years of age. Second, primary patency of endovascular interventions is poor at 39% at 24 months (Fig 3) and also the amputation-free survival is lower. This should reflect that younger patients are truly biologically different from older patients. On the other hand, the outcomes of open surgery in the over 50-year-old category were also examined, but the amputation-free survival was not similarly reduced. The study undoubtedly suggests that the younger patient may be better served with surgical revascularization, but I was stymied by the short follow-up. I look forward to seeing the long-term survival considerations in the young vasculopath solidified.

J. Black, MD

A multicenter experience evaluating chronic total occlusion crossing with the Wildcat catheter (the CONNECT study)

Pigott JP, for the Connect Trial Investigators (Jobst Vascular Inst, Toledo, OH; et al)
J Vasc Surg 56:1615-1621, 2012

Objective.—Percutaneous techniques for crossing femoropopliteal chronic total occlusions (CTOs) offer an alternative to bypass surgery in patients deemed to be at increased risk due to advanced age or comorbidities. Recent reports document good success rates in catheters designed to reconstitute peripherally occluded arteries following failed guidewire passage. The Wildcat catheter (Avinger, Redwood City, Calif) is a novel device with a rotating distal tip and deployable wedges fashioned for channeling a passage through arterial occlusions. This report describes the results of a prospective, multicenter, nonrandomized trial evaluating the safety and efficacy of the Wildcat device when crossing de novo or restenotic femoropopliteal CTOs.

Methods.—Between August 2010 and April 2011, patients with peripheral arterial disease due to a femoropopliteal CTO > 1 cm and ≤35 cm were evaluated for study enrollment at 15 U.S. sites. During treatment, the physician initially attempted to cross the CTO using conventional guidewires per protocol; if the guidewire successfully crossed, the patient was considered a screen failure and the Wildcat was not deployed. At 30 days, patients were reevaluated. The primary efficacy end point was successful crossing of the Wildcat into the distal true lumen as confirmed by angiography. Primary safety end points included no in-hospital or 30-day major adverse events, no clinically significant perforation or embolization, and no grade C or greater dissection. Additional data collected included lesion length, degree of calcification, and location.

Results.—Eighty-eight patients were enrolled in the trial. Of these, the Wildcat device was used in 84 patients (95%) per protocol. Successful CTO crossing was reported and confirmed by independent review in 89% (75/84) of cases with 5% (4/84) major adverse events as defined in the protocol (predominantly perforations sealed with balloon inflation). There were no clinically relevant events associated with any of the perforations. The mean CTO length was 174 ± 96 mm (range, 15-350 mm). Approximately 57% (n = 48) of all lesions were categorized as containing at least moderate calcification. Eighty-nine percent (n = 75) of vessels recanalized were superficial femoral arteries.

Conclusions.—In this multicenter study, the Wildcat catheter demonstrated an 89% crossing success rate with little associated morbidity. The Wildcat catheter is a viable device for crossing moderately calcified femoropopliteal CTOs.

▶ The growing array of devices available for management of chronic total occlusion (CTO) in the setting of lower extremity peripheral arterial disease (PAD) continues to expand the proportion of patients who are candidates for endovascular treatment. This study characterizes one such device, the Wildcat catheter, in a nonrandomized, multicenter study in which a variety of definitive revascularization techniques (including atherectomy, angioplasty, stent placement, and laser ablation) were used after crossing the lesion. With the exception of one patient treated for asymptomatic disease (no explanation was provided for intervention in this scenario), two-thirds of the study cohort were claudicants, whereas the remainder had either rest pain or tissue loss. Consistent with most safety studies characterizing novel devices for endovascular PAD management, this study achieved primary safety and efficacy performance goals in the setting of strictly defined anatomic inclusion criteria without a comparison or control group. In the introduction, the authors allude to the need for crossing devices in the setting of a long, fibrotic, and calcified CTO in which an intraluminal crossing attempt with a conventional guide wire may be impossible; severe target lesion calcification and lesion length greater than 30 cm, however, were both exclusion criteria. The safety and efficacy data provided in this article are useful but must be interpreted within the restrictions of the study design.

In the current era of resource-restricted health care environments, a minimalist approach is often the best means of controlling the equipment costs associated with endovascular interventions. From that perspective, it is interesting to note that the mean time spent attempting to cross the lesion with a guide wire was 4.6 minutes, which was significantly less than the 10-minute time limit specified in the protocol and much less than the mean time of 22.1 minutes spent with the Wildcat device. It is, therefore, possible that more vigorous or persistent attempts at wire crossing may have achieved success, avoiding the need for a CTO device as well as the need for a reentry device required in 17% of these interventions. It is, therefore, unclear how many of these procedures would have truly required the Wildcat for technical success, and direct comparisons are needed to determine the utility of the Wildcat vs other CTO devices or subintimal approaches when guide wire passage fails.

M. A. Corriere, MD, MS

Calf muscle oxygen saturation and the effects of supervised exercise training for intermittent claudication
Beckitt TA, Day J, Morgan M, et al (Bristol Royal Infirmary, UK)
J Vasc Surg 56:470-475, 2012

Objective.—The mechanisms underlying the symptomatic improvement witnessed as a result of exercise training in intermittent claudication remain unclear. There is no reproducible evidence to support increased limb blood flow resulting from neovascularization. Changes in oxygenation of active muscles as a result of blood redistribution are hypothesized but unproven. This study sought evidence of improved gastrocnemius oxygenation resulting from exercise training.

Methods.—The study recruited 42 individuals with claudication. After an initial control period of exercise advice, participants undertook a 3-month supervised exercise program. Spatially resolved near-infrared spectroscopy monitored calf muscle oxygen saturation (Sto_2) during exercise and after a period of cuff-induced ischemia. Comparison was made with 14 individuals undergoing angioplasty for calf claudication. Clinical outcomes of claudication distance and maximum walking distance were measured by treadmill assessment.

Results.—Significant increases occurred in mean [interquartile range] claudication disease (57 [38-78] to 119 [97-142] meters; $P = .01$) and maximum walking distance (124 [102-147] to 241 [193-265] meters; $P = .02$) after supervised exercise but not after the control period. No change occurred in resting Sto_2 at any interval. Angioplasty (27% [21-34] to 19% [13-29]; $P = .02$) but not exercise training (26% [21-32] vs 23% [20-31]; $P > .20$) resulted in a reduced Sto_2 desaturation in response to submaximal exercise and an increased hyperemic hemoglobin oxygen recovery rate after ischemia (0.48 [0.39-0.55] to 0.63 [0.52-0.69] s^{-1}; $P = .01$). However supervised exercise reduced the Sto_2 recovery half-time by 17% (82 [64-101] to 68 [55-89] seconds; $P = .02$).

Conclusions.—Supervised exercise training is not associated with increased gastrocnemius muscle oxygenation during exercise or increased hyperemic hemoglobin flow after a model of ischemia. This suggests that the symptomatic improvement witnessed is not the result of increased oxygen delivery to the active muscle. The enhanced recovery after exercise training therefore reflects a combination of enhanced metabolic economy and increased oxidative capacity, suggesting that exercise training helps reverse an acquired metabolic myopathy (Table 3).

▶ This study provides us with insight into the contrast between mechanisms of action for angioplasty vs supervised exercise training (SET) for intermittent claudication. The authors observed increases in both initial claudication distance and maximum walking distance in both study groups, whereas only the angioplasty group had significant reduction in exercise-induced calf muscle oxygen desaturation measured by near-infrared spectroscopy (Table 3). The results suggest that symptomatic improvement through SET is the result of enhanced metabolic activity, rather than enhanced oxygen delivery through collaterals as previously hypothesized. Although consensus recommendations direct practitioners to consider these treatment interventions from a hierarchical perspective

TABLE 3.—Oxygen Saturation (Sto_2) Responses at the Conclusion of the Study

Outcome	Exercise Group (n = 42)			Angioplasty Group (n = 14)		
	Recruitment	Completion	P^a	Recruitment	Completion	P^a
Resting Sto_2, %	56 (48-63)	56 (49-63)	>.50	55 (48-63)	57 (47-65)	>.30
Peak Sto_2 desaturation						
Maximal, %	38 (33-44)	40 (33-45)	>.30	38 (32-44)	33 (26-36)	>.10
Submaximal, %	26 (21-32)	23 (20-31)	>.20	27 (21-34)	19 (13-29)	.02
Recovery T_{50} submaximal, sec	79 (61-97)	68 (55-89)	.02	75 (59-94)	53 (38-67)	<.01

T_{50}, Half-time.
$^a P$ values < .05 are statistically significant.

(proceeding with angioplasty only in the setting of a suboptimal result with exercise therapy), the different mechanisms for improvement with each of these therapeutic interventions raise the question of whether an even greater and perhaps synergistic effect would occur in patients treated with both angioplasty and SET. These findings suggest that considering SET and revascularization therapy from an either/or perspective may not achieve the maximum benefit in terms of functional outcomes. The authors appear to have a pessimistic attitude toward pharmacotherapy, as cilostazol was not included as part of the therapeutic approach in either treatment group or as an alternative control.

M. A. Corriere, MD, MS

Anatomical Predictors of Major Adverse Limb Events after Infrapopliteal Angioplasty for Patients with Critical Limb Ischaemia due to Pure Isolated Infrapopliteal Lesions

Iida O, Soga Y, Yamauchi Y, et al (Kansai Rosai Hosp, Amagasaki, Hyogo, Japan; Kokura Memorial Hosp, Kitakyushu, Fukuoka, Japan; Kikuna Memorial Hosp, Yokohama, Japan; et al)
Eur J Vasc Endovasc Surg 44:318-324, 2012

Objective.—To identify anatomical factors associated with major adverse limb events (MALE) after angioplasty as the basis for a novel morphology-driven classification of infrapopliteal lesions.

Design.—Retrospective-multicenter study.

Materials and Methods.—Between March 2004 and October 2010, 1057 limbs from 884 patients with CLI due to isolated infrapopliteal lesions were studied. Freedom-from MALE, defined as major amputation or any reintervention, was assessed out to 2 years by the Kaplan—Meier methods. Anatomical predictors and risk stratification for MALE were analyzed by multivariate analysis.

Results.—Freedom-from MALE was 47 ± 1% at 2 years. Lesion calcification, target vessel diameter <3.0 mm, lesion length >300 mm and no below-the-ankle (BA) run-off were positively associated with MALE by multivariate-analysis. The total number of risk factors was used to calculate the risk score for each limbs for subsequent categorization into 3 groups with 0 or 1 (low-risk), 2 (moderate-risk) and 3 or 4 (high-risk) factors. Freedom-from MALE at 2 year-rates was 59% in low-risk, 46% in moderate-risk, and 29% in high-risk, respectively.

Conclusion.—Target vessel diameter <3.0 mm, lesion calcification, lesion length >300 mm and no-BA run-off were associated with MALE after infrapopliteal angioplasty. Risk stratification based on these predictors allows estimation of future incidence of MALE in CLI with isolated infrapopliteal lesions (Tables 2 and 3).

▶ This retrospective analysis of a large multicenter cohort takes on the formidable task of identifying a novel set of anatomic predictors of major adverse limb events (MALE), defined as revascularization or major amputation, among patients with

TABLE 2.—Baseline Lesion Characteristics Before Below-the-Knee Angioplasty

Variables	Overall, $n = 1057$
TASC 2000 classification (A/B/C), (%)	3%/1%/7%
TASC 2000 D	89% (945)
Lesion calcification	65% (682)
Target lesion length (mm)	190 ± 96
Lesion length >100 mm	81% (855)
Target lesion % diameter stenosis before angioplasty	98 ± 5
Below-the-knee Chronic total occlusion	62% (651)
Below-the-ankle Chronic total occlusion	62% (659)
Target lesion reference vessel diameter (mm)	2.5 ± 0.5
Anterior tibial artery (ATA)	
Vessel diameter (mm)	2.5 ± 0.4
Intact/diseased	8% (85)/92% (972)
Occlusion	70% (737)
Posterior tibial artery	
Vessel diameter (mm)	2.4 ± 0.4
Intact/diseased	9% (98)/91% (959)
Occlusion	72% (760)
Peroneal artery	
Vessel diameter (mm)	2.2 ± 0.4
Intact/diseased	32% (340)/68% (717)
Occlusion	43% (457)
Number of below the knee run-offs	0.50 ± 0.68
Three-vessel disease	60% (634)
Dorsalis pedis artery	
Intact/diseased	62% (659)/38% (398)
Plantar artery	
Intact/diseased	58% (617)/42% (440)
Presence of below-the-ankle disease	59% (627)
Number of below-the-ankle (BA) run-offs	1.2 ± 0.8

TABLE 3.—Uni and Multivariable Analysis for MALE

Lesion Characteristics	Unadjusted HR [95% CI]	Adjusted HR [95% CI]
TASC 2000 class D	1.16 [0.84, 1.60]	1.03 [0.71, 1.50]
Lesion calcification	1.42 [1.16, 1.73]**	1.38 [1.12, 1.69]**
Target lesion length ≥300 mm	1.47 [1.20, 1.81]**	1.47 [1.18, 1.82]**
Chronic total occlusion in BTK	1.28 [1.04, 1.58]*	1.22 [0.98, 1.53]
Lesion reference diameter <3 mm	1.37 [1.10, 1.71]**	1.26 [1.01, 1.58]*
Number of BTK run-offs (vs. 3 run-offs)	1.00 (Ref)	1.00 (Ref)
2 run-offs	0.94 [0.58, 1.53]	0.85 [0.52, 1.39]
1 run-off	0.90 [0.58, 1.40]	0.71 [0.45, 1.15]
No run-off	0.95 [0.62, 1.46]	0.65 [0.41, 1.05]
Number of BA run-offs (vs. 2 run-offs)	1.00 (Ref)	1.00 (Ref)
1 run-off	1.04 [0.84, 1.29]	1.15 [0.92, 1.44]
No run-off	1.62 [1.23, 2.05]**	1.75 [1.36, 2.25]**
Diseased calcaneal branch	0.98 [0.81, 1.18]	0.98 [0.80, 1.19]

$*p < 0.05$, $**p < 0.01$.
TASC: Trans-Atlantic Inter-Society Consensus.
BTK: below the knee, BA: below the ankle.

critical limb ischemia (CLI) treated with angioplasty for isolated infrapopliteal disease. The authors assert the need for a new anatomic classification system given the lack of concordance between the Trans-Atlantic Inter-Society Consensus (TASC) guidelines and current clinical practice trends in procedural utilization. With the exception of target vessel diameter, however, the variables identified as predictors of MALE (Table 3) are also used in some fashion to determine TASC classification (lesion length, calcification, and runoff).[1] Although the presented anatomic classification has many of the same predictors included by other risk stratification systems, this analysis still provides useful information that may facilitate decision making and patient information from a lesion-based perspective. Because most patients with CLI do not have isolated infrapopliteal disease (as evidenced by the database utilized, where 1198 of 2519 patients were excluded because of treatment of other anatomic locations), these results cannot be generalized beyond the described disease distribution. Although baseline patient disease characteristics are provided among the descriptive statistics, they are conspicuously absent from the list of variables considered for modeling MALE; beyond lesion-specific considerations, some of these factors (including lesion calcification and poor runoff) may additionally reflect systemic effects of diabetes, end-stage renal disease, smoking, and other predictive patient-level factors. The high prevalence of anatomically challenging lesion characteristics (including TASC D disease, long and calcified lesions, and small vessel diameters in most patients; Table 2) would be expected to negatively impact outcomes associated with any treatment. A more realistic perspective might, therefore, be to consider postangioplasty repeat revascularization as an anticipated and necessary part of limb salvage, rather than an adverse event.

M. A. Corriere, MD, MS

Reference

1. Norgren L, Hiatt WR, Dormandy JA, et al. Inter-Society Consensus for the Management of Peripheral Arterial Disease (TASC II). *J Vasc Surg.* 2007;45: S5-S67.

Long-term limb salvage and survival after endovascular and open revascularization for critical limb ischemia after adoption of endovascular-first approach by vascular surgeons
Dosluoglu HH, Lall P, Harris LM, et al (VA Western NY Healthcare System, Buffalo; State Univ of New York at Buffalo)
J Vasc Surg 56:361-371.e3, 2012

Objective.—The adoption of endovascular interventions has been reported to lower amputation rates, but patients who undergo endovascular and open revascularization are not directly comparable. We have adopted an endovascular-first approach but individualize the revascularization technique according to patient characteristics. This study compared characteristics of patients who had endovascular and open procedures and assessed the long-term outcomes.

Methods.—From December 2002 to September 2010, 433 patients underwent infrainguinal revascularization for critical limb ischemia (CLI; Rutherford IV-VI) of 514 limbs (endovascular: 295 patients, 363 limbs; open: 138 patients, 151 limbs). Patency rates, limb salvage (LS), and survival, as also their predictors, were calculated using Kaplan-Meier and multivariate analysis.

Results.—The endovascular group was older, with more diabetes, renal insufficiency, and tissue loss. More reconstructions were multilevel (72% vs 39%; $P < .001$) and the most distal level of intervention was infrapopliteal in the open group (64% vs 49%; $P = .001$). The 30-day mortality was 2.8% in the endovascular and 6.0% in the open group ($P = .079$). Mean follow-up was 28.4 ± 23.1 months (0-100). In the endovascular vs open groups, 7% needed open, and 24% needed inflow/runoff endovascular reinterventions with or without thrombolysis vs 6% and 17%. In the endovascular vs open group, 5-year LS was 78% ± 3% vs 78% ± 4% ($P = .992$), amputation-free survival was 30% ± 3% vs 39% ± 5% ($P = .227$), and survival was 36% ± 4% vs 46% ± 5% ($P = .146$). Five-year primary patency (PP), assisted-primary patency (APP), and secondary patency (SP) rates were 50 ± 5%, 70 ± 5% and 73 ± 6% in endovascular, and 48 ± 6%, 59 ± 6% and 64 ± 6% in the open group, respectively ($P = .800$ for PP, 0.037 for APP, 0.022 for SP). Multivariate analysis identified poor functional capacity (hazard ratio, 3.5 [95% confidence interval, 1.9-6.5]; $P < .001$), dialysis dependence (2.2 [1.3-3.8]; $P = .003$), gangrene (2.2 [1.4-3.4]; $P < .001$), need for infrapopliteal intervention (2.0 [1.2-3.1]; $P = .004$), and diabetes (1.8 [1.1-3.1]; $P = .031$) as predictors of limb loss. Poor functional capacity (3.3 [2.4-4.6]; $P < .001$), coronary artery disease (1.5 [1.1-2.1]; $P = .006$), and gangrene (1.4 [1.1-1.9]; $P = .007$) predicted poorer survival. Statin use predicted improved survival (0.6 [0.5-0.8]; $P = .001$). Need for infrapopliteal interventions predicted poorer PP (0.6 [0.5-0.9-2.2]; $P = .007$), whereas use of autologous vein predicted better PP (1.8 [1.1-2.9]; $P = .017$).

Conclusions.—Patients who undergo endovascular revascularization for CLI are medically higher-risk patients. Those who have bypass have more complex disease and are more likely to require multilevel reconstruction and infrapopliteal intervention. Individualizing revascularization results in optimization of early and late outcomes with acceptable LS, although survival remains low in those with poor health status.

▶ This study is truly exhaustive in its scope to examine the outcomes of endovascular and open operations to manage critical limb ischemia (CLI). Although the BASIL (Bypass vs Angioplasty in Severe Ischaemia of the Leg) trial has assumed the mantle of CLI outcomes because of its randomized design, it is appropriate to challenge and reconsider the BASIL trial in the era wherein vascular surgeons become the primary operators for all aspects of the open and endovascular paradigm. In this regard, this study takes the lead and demonstrates several important changes that have leveled the playing field.

First, this study includes a substantial number of multilevel and infrapopliteal interventions that are absent from BASIL. Second, the study includes modern endovascular techniques, whereas BASIL comprised only angioplasty procedures, which are proven to be associated with failure in TransAtlantic Inter-Society Consensus II B, C, and D anatomy typical of CLI. Lastly, the study refutes that an endovascular-first approach failure may compromise a subsequent surgical intervention, with their groups all having similar amputation-free survival. This latter insight is critically important to understand; it is highly unlikely we will see a randomized controlled trial reemerge to answer the debate, but this study provides the best estimate that an endovascular-first approach does not burn any bridges with our current armamentarium of techniques.

J. Black, MD

A Prospective Randomized Multicenter Comparison of Balloon Angioplasty and Infrapopliteal Stenting With the Sirolimus-Eluting Stent in Patients With Ischemic Peripheral Arterial Disease: 1-Year Results From the ACHILLES Trial
Scheinert D, on behalf of the ACHILLES Investigators (Park-Krankenhaus Leipzig-Südost GmbH, Germany; et al)
J Am Coll Cardiol 60:2290-2295, 2012

Objectives.—The study investigated the efficacy and safety of a balloon expandable, sirolimus-eluting stent (SES) in patients with symptomatic infrapopliteal arterial disease.

Background.—Results of infrapopliteal interventions using balloon angioplasty and/or bare stents are limited by a relatively high restenosis rate, which could be potentially improved by stabilizing the lesion with a SES.

Methods.—Two hundred patients (total lesion length 27 ± 21 mm) were randomized to infrapopliteal SES stenting or percutaneous transluminal balloon angioplasty (PTA). The primary endpoint was 1-year in-segment binary restenosis by quantitative angiography.

Results.—Ninety-nine and 101 patients (mean age 73.4 years; 64% diabetics) were randomized to SES and PTA, respectively (8 crossover bailout cases to SES). At 1 year, there were lower angiographic restenosis rates (22.4% vs. 41.9%, $p = 0.019$), greater vessel patency (75.0% vs. 57.1%, $p = 0.025$), and similar death, repeat revascularization, index-limb amputation rates, and proportions of patients with improved Rutherford class for SES versus PTA.

Conclusions.—SES implantation may offer a promising therapeutic alternative to PTA for treatment of infrapopliteal peripheral arterial disease (Figs 2 and 3).

▶ In this randomized trial of balloon-expandable sirolimus-eluting stents (SES) vs balloon angioplasty for infrapopliteal peripheral arterial disease (PAD), patients randomized to SES had significantly lower rates of angiographic

A   B   C

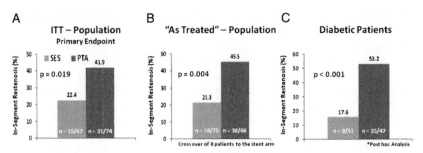

FIGURE 2.—Angiographic results at 12-month follow-up. Primary endpoints for the intention-to-treat (ITT) population (**A**), the as-treated population (**B**), and the diabetic subpopulation (**C**). Abbreviations as in Figure 1. (Reprinted from Scheinert D, on behalf of the ACHILLES Investigators. A prospective randomized multicenter comparison of balloon angioplasty and infrapopliteal stenting with the sirolimus-eluting stent in patients with ischemic peripheral arterial disease: 1-year results from the ACHILLES trial. *J Am Coll Cardiol.* 2012;60:2290-2295, Copyright 2012, with permission from the American College of Cardiology.)

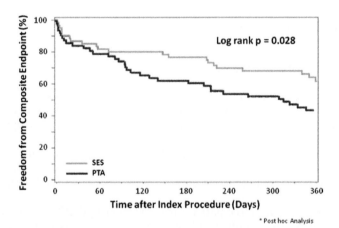

FIGURE 3.—Freedom from death, target lesion revascularization, bypass, amputation, and rutherford class ≥4. The SES group had significantly greater freedom from the composite endpoint relative to the balloon angioplasty group. Abbreviations as in Figure 1. (Reprinted from Scheinert D, on behalf of the ACHILLES Investigators. A prospective randomized multicenter comparison of balloon angioplasty and infrapopliteal stenting with the sirolimus-eluting stent in patients with ischemic peripheral arterial disease: 1-year results from the ACHILLES trial. *J Am Coll Cardiol.* 2012;60:2290-2295, Copyright 2012, with permission from the American College of Cardiology.)

restenosis (22.4% vs 41.9%), greater patency (75.0% vs 57.4%), and greater freedom from the composite endpoint at 1 year (Fig 3). Identification of a specific benefit associated with SES versus angioplasty in diabetic patients (Fig 2) is a particularly encouraging finding, given the predisposition for tibial disease in this patient population. Interestingly, the device success rate of PTA (defined by achievement of a final residual diameter stenosis of less than 30% using the assigned device only) was only 58.2%, while the lesion success rate (defined by less than 50% residual in-stent or balloon diameter stenosis using any percutaneous method) was 96.9%. The adjunctive techniques used to convert device failure to lesion success, however, were not described or accounted for in the results. Because patients undergoing PTA received low-dose aspirin alone post-procedure, while those in the SES treatment arm were also treated with either clopidogrel or ticlopidine for 6 months, it is possible that some of the benefit observed in the SES randomization arm may have resulted from more aggressive antiplatelet therapy (especially if bare metal stents were frequently used to achieve lesion success in the PTA arm). Because clinical outcomes of repeat revascularization, amputation, or improvement in symptomatic status were not statistically different between randomization groups, whether these impressive patency advantages translate into clinical results that justify the higher cost of drug-eluting stents remains to be determined.

M. A. Corriere, MD, MS

Combination therapy with warfarin plus clopidogrel improves outcomes in femoropopliteal bypass surgery patients
Monaco M, Di Tommaso L, Pinna GB, et al (Istituto Clinico Pineta Grande, Castel Volturno (CE), Italy; Univ "Federico II", Naples, Italy)
J Vasc Surg 56:96-105, 2012

Background.—Patients having undergone femoropopliteal bypass surgery remain at significant risk of graft failure. Although antithrombotic therapy is of paramount importance in these patients, the effect of oral anti-coagulation therapy (OAT) on outcomes remains unresolved. We performed a randomized, prospective study to assess the impact of OAT plus clopidogrel vs dual antiplatelet therapy on peripheral vascular and systemic cardiovascular outcomes in patients who had undergone femoropopliteal bypass surgery.

Methods.—Three hundred forty-one patients who had undergone femo-ropopliteal surgery were enrolled and randomized: 173 patients received clopidogrel 75 mg/d plus OAT with warfarin (C + OAT), and 168 patients received dual antiplatelet therapy with clopidogrel 75 mg/d plus aspirin 100 mg/d (C + acetylsalicylic acid [ASA]). Study end points were graft patency and the occurrence of severe peripheral arterial ischemia, and the incidence of bleeding episodes.

Results.—Follow-up ranged from 4 to 9 years. The graft patency rate and the freedom from severe peripheral arterial ischemia was significantly higher in C + OAT group than in C + ASA group ($P = .026$ and $.044$, respectively, Cox-Mantel test). The linearized incidence of minor bleeding complications was significantly higher in C + OAT group than in C + ASA group (2.85% patient-years vs 1.37% patient-years; $P = .03$). The incidence of major adverse cardiovascular events, including mortality, was found to be similar ($P = .34$) for both study groups.

Conclusions.—In patients who have undergone femoropopliteal vascular surgery, combination therapy with clopidogrel plus warfarin is more effective than dual antiplatelet therapy in increasing graft patency and in reducing severe peripheral ischemia. These improvements are obtained at

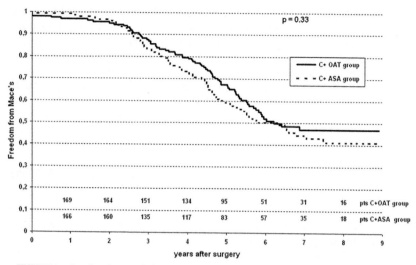

FIGURE 2.—Freedom from graft failure for the two study groups. C + ASA, Clopidogrel plus acetyl-salicylic acid therapy patients; C + OAT, clopidogrel plus oral anticoagulation therapy patients. (Reprinted from the Journal of Vascular Surgery. Monaco M, Di Tommaso L, Pinna GB, et al. Combination therapy with warfarin plus clopidogrel improves outcomes in femoropopliteal bypass surgery patients. *J Vasc Surg.* 2012;56:96-105, Copyright 2012, with permission from The Society for Vascular Surgery.)

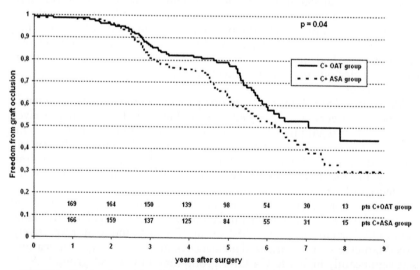

FIGURE 3.—Freedom from major adverse cardiovascular events, including mortality, for the two study groups. C + ASA, Clopidogrel plus acetylsalicylic acid therapy patients; C + OAT, clopidogrel plus anti-coagulation therapy patients. (Reprinted from the Journal of Vascular Surgery. Monaco M, Di Tommaso L, Pinna GB, et al. Combination therapy with warfarin plus clopidogrel improves outcomes in femoropopliteal bypass surgery patients. *J Vasc Surg.* 2012;56:96-105, Copyright 2012, with permission from The Society for Vascular Surgery.)

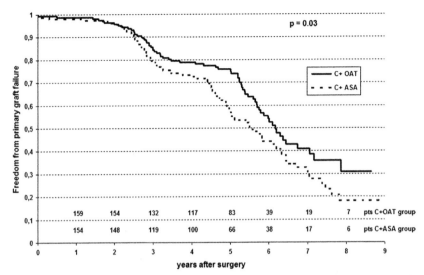

FIGURE 4.—Freedom from primary graft failure for the two study groups. C + ASA, Clopidogrel plus acetylsalicylic acid therapy patients; C + OAT, clopidogrel plus oral anticoagulation therapy patients. (Reprinted from the Journal of Vascular Surgery. Monaco M, Di Tommaso L, Pinna GB, et al. Combination therapy with warfarin plus clopidogrel improves outcomes in femoropopliteal bypass surgery patients. *J Vasc Surg.* 2012;56:96-105, Copyright 2012, with permission from The Society for Vascular Surgery.)

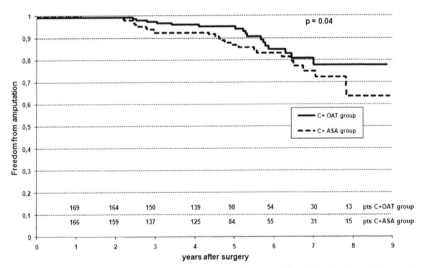

FIGURE 5.—Freedom from amputation for the two study groups. C + ASA, Clopidogrel plus acetylsalicylic acid therapy patients; C + OAT, clopidogrel plus oral anticoagulation therapy patients. (Reprinted from the Journal of Vascular Surgery. Monaco M, Di Tommaso L, Pinna GB, et al. Combination therapy with warfarin plus clopidogrel improves outcomes in femoropopliteal bypass surgery patients. *J Vasc Surg.* 2012;56:96-105, Copyright 2012, with permission from The Society for Vascular Surgery.)

TABLE 4.—Cox Hazards Regression: Independent Predictors of Long-Term Graft Failure and of Bleeding Rate

Predictors	P Value	Graft Failure Exp (B)	95% CI	P Value	Bleeding Rate Exp (B)	95% CI
Age	.001	0.59	0.44-0.79	.02	0.61	0.40-0.92
Age^2	.0006	0.35	0.23-0.68	.001	2.98	1.68-5.27
Urgent operation	.0001	2.87	1.81-4.55	.005	0.09	0.01-0.58
Preoperative ABPI	.0001	3.25	2.15-4.87	.15	1.43	0.88-2.33
Diabetes	.0001	2.42	1.58-3.78	.01	1.65	1.11-2.64
Poor arterial run-off	.0001	1.08	1.04-1.12	.22	0.84	0.68-1.10

ABPI, Ankle-brachial pressure index.
All tested variables are listed in the text.

the expenses of an increase in the rate of minor anticoagulation-related complications (Figs 2-5, Table 4).

▶ This randomized study provides long-term outcomes related to postoperative anticoagulation after femoropopliteal bypass (above-knee bypasses with synthetic conduit and below-knee bypasses with saphenous vein). With a median follow-up of 6.6 years, the results showed no difference in graft failure between the 2 study groups, whereas those treated with clopidogrel plus warfarin had greater risk of minor bleeding complications but significant advantages in freedom from major adverse cardiovascular events, primary graft failure, and amputation (Figs 2-5). Although these outcomes suggest an overall advantage favoring treatment with clopidogrel plus warfarin over dual antiplatelet therapy, it is a bit surprising to note that the treatment randomization was noninfluential in the multivariable Cox proportional hazards models of graft failure and bleeding (Table 4). Several factors that have been shown to influence patency, amputation-free survival, and overall survival after lower extremity bypass (including presence of critical limb ischemia and vein graft diameter) were not included among the descriptive statistics or accounted for in the randomization strategy but may have affected the results. Because patients across the entire spectrum of symptomatic peripheral artery disease (including intermittent claudication, rest pain, ulcers, gangrene, and blue toe syndrome) included in the study would be expected to have distinct levels of risk for the outcomes evaluated, inability to stratify the results by symptomatic status makes it challenging to determine which individuals are most likely to benefit from more aggressive anticoagulation.

M. A. Corriere, MD, MS

A phase II dose-ranging study of the phosphodiesterase inhibitor K-134 in patients with peripheral artery disease and claudication

Brass EP, Cooper LT, Morgan RE, et al (Harbor-UCLA Ctr for Clinical Pharmacology, Torrance; Mayo Clinic, Rochester, MN; Kowa Res Inst, Morrisville, NC; et al)

J Vasc Surg 55:381-389.e1, 2012

Background.—Phosphodiesterase inhibitors have been shown to improve claudication-limited exercise performance in patients with peripheral artery disease. K-134, a novel phosphodiesterase inhibitor, was evaluated in a phase II trial incorporating an adaptive design to assess its safety, tolerability, and effect on treadmill walking time.

Design.—Patients with peripheral artery disease were randomized to receive placebo (n = 87), K-134 at a dose of 25 mg (n = 42), 50 mg (n = 85), or 100 mg (n = 84), or cilostazol at a dose of 100 mg (n = 89), each twice daily for 26 weeks. Peak walking time (PWT) was assessed using a graded treadmill protocol at baseline and after 14 and 26 weeks of treatment. A Data and Safety Monitoring Board-implemented adaptive design was used that allowed early discontinuation of unsafe or minimally informative K-134 arms.

Results.—As determined by the prospectively defined adaptive criteria, the 25-mg K-134 arm was discontinued after 42 individuals had been randomized to the arm. During the 26-week treatment period, PWT increased by 23%, 33%, 37%, and 46% in the placebo, 50-mg K-134, 100-mg K-134, and cilostazol arms, respectively (primary analysis placebo vs 100-mg K-134 arm not statistically significant, $P = .089$). Secondary analyses showed that cilostazol significantly increased PWT after 14 weeks of treatment and that the 100-mg K-134 dose and cilostazol both increased PWT vs placebo after 14 and 26 weeks in those individuals who completed the 26-week trial and were compliant with the study drug, or when the data were analyzed using a mixed-effects model incorporating all time points. K-134 had tolerability and adverse effect profiles similar to that of cilostazol. Both drugs were associated with an increase in withdrawals before study completion due to adverse events compared with placebo.

Conclusions.—K-134 was generally well tolerated. K-134 at a dose of 100 mg twice daily did not affect PWT according to the primary analysis, but K-134 and cilostazol both increased PWT when analyzed using a mixed-effects model and in the per-protocol population (Tables 1-4).

▶ In the United States, there are few medical treatments that are effective in the treatment of intermittent claudication. Currently, cilostazol is the only US Food and Drug Administration—indicated drug for treating claudication secondary to arterial occlusive disease. In this randomized, controlled, placebo-controlled, double-blind study that included 25 sites in the United States and 23 sites in Russia, a new phosphodiesterase inhibitor type III (K-134) was tested for efficacy on a standardized treadmill test for tolerability and safety. This was a 5-arm study that analyzed 3 different K-134 doses (25 mg, 50 mg, and 100 mg), cilostazol

TABLE 1.—Demographics of Study Patients[a]

Variable	Placebo (n = 78)	K-134 arm				P[b]	All subjects at sites		P[c]
		25 mg (n = 42)	50 mg (n = 76)	100 mg (n = 75)	Cilostazol (n = 74)		Russia (n = 271)	USA (n = 74)	
Age, y	62.9 (44-82)	63.3 (41-88)	63.8 (45-90)	62.8 (42-84)	64.5 (50-84)	.732	62.0 (41-81)	68.6 (51-90)	<.001
Male sex, %	89.7	83.3	86.8	82.3	94.6	.187	92.6	70.3	<.001
Race, %						.750			<.001
White	97.4	100	97.4	97.3	97.3		100	89.2	
Black	2.6	0.0	2.6	1.3	2.7		0.0	9.5	
Asian	0.0	0.0	0.0	0.0	0.0		0.0	0.0	
Other	0.0	0.0	0.0	1.3	0.0		0.0	1.4	
Diabetic, %	15.4	11.9	13.2	12.0	14.9	.964	8.1	33.8	<.001
Cigarette use, %						.943			<.001
Never	9.0	4.8	13.2	12.0	9.5		10.3	9.5	
Former	29.5	40.5	40.8	34.7	39.2		31.0	56.8	
Current	61.5	54.8	46.1	53.3	51.4		58.7	33.8	
Medications, %									
Statin	44.9	47.6	51.3	49.3	47.3	.950	38.0	85.1	<.001
Antiplatelet	74.4	81.0	86.8	85.3	87.8	.158	84.1	79.7	.369
Baseline									
ABI	0.58 ± 15	0.61 ± 0.16	0.65 ± 0.14	0.64 ± 0.15	0.62 ± 0.15	.063	0.61 ± 0.15	0.66 ± 0.14	.029
PWT, sec	318 ± 156	314 ± 141	303 ± 160	291 ± 154	265 ± 142	.241	283 ± 152	349 ± 144	.001
COT, sec	141 ± 93	132 ± 65	135 ± 102	127 ± 90	116 ± 60	.458	127 ± 86	141 ± 83	.239

ABI, Ankle-brachial index; *COT*, claudication onset time; *PWT*, peak walking time.
[a]Mean data are shown with the range or standard deviation. Data are for the modified intention-to-treat population, except for the 25-mg K-134 arm, for which data are from all randomized subjects. Data by country includes the modified intention-to-treat population and the 42 subjects randomized to 25 mg of K-134. P values for continuous variables were calculated from a one-way analysis of variance, and the χ^2 test was used for categoric variables.
[b]For differences between treatment arms.
[c]For differences between countries.

TABLE 2.—Change in Treadmill Performance with Treatment[a]

Variable	Placebo (n)	Placebo (sec)	50 mg K-134 (n)	50 mg K-134 (sec)	100 mg K-134 (n)	100 mg K-134 (sec)	Cilostazol (n)	Cilostazol (sec)
Change in peak walking time								
Baseline to week 14	78	39 ± 136	76	71 ± 171	74	94 ± 156	73	83 ± 118
Baseline to week 26	78	72 ± 196	76	100 ± 221	75	108 ± 160	74	122 ± 190
Change in claudication onset time								
Baseline to week 14	78	26 ± 83	75	40 ± 129	75	60 ± 108	74	35 ± 70
Baseline to week 26	78	44 ± 102	75	50 ± 114	75	66 ± 117	74	60 ± 95

Note that one patient in the cilostazol arm withdrew and had an exit visit that was tabulated as a week 26 visit. Two patients in the 100-mg K-134 arm had week 14 visits with COT assessments, but no valid PWT determination (treadmill test stopped early).
[a]Data are from the modified intention-to-treat population and presented as arithmetic means ± standard deviation. Baseline values are presented in Table I.

TABLE 3.—Secondary Analyses of Treatment Effects on Peak Walking Time[a]

Variable	Placebo	50 mg K-134	100 mg K-134	Cilostazol
ANCOVA mITT				
ln (week 14 PWT)/(baseline PWT)	0.077 ± 0.349	0.118 ± 0.392	0.221 ± 0.385	0.235 ± 0.333[b]
No.	78	76	73	73
P		.486	.067	.011
ln (week 26 PWT)/(baseline PWT)	0.146 ± 0.402	0.182 ± 0.427	0.259 ± 0.411	0.266 ± 0.438
No.	78	76	75	74
P		.411	.224	.079
Per-protocol population				
ln (week 14 PWT)/(baseline PWT)	0.064 ± 0.374	0.141 ± 0.375	0.259 ± 0.389[a,b]	
No.	63	66	60	63
P		.506	.015	.003
ln (week 26 PWT)/(baseline PWT)	0.146 ± 0.426	0.181 ± 0.425	0.307 ± 0.413[a,b]	
No.	63	66	62	64
P		.755	.048	.034
Mixed-effects model mITT				
Baseline ln PWT	5.64 ± 0.50	5.56 ± 0.58	5.53 ± 0.56	5.44 ± 0.56
No.	78	76	75	74
Week 14 ln PWT	5.72 ± 0.57	5.69 ± 0.75	5.73 ± 0.68	5.70 ± 0.63
No.	78	74	68	70
Week 26 ln PWT	5.80 ± 0.62	5.73 ± 0.75	5.84 ± 0.65	5.71 ± 0.75
No.	75	75	71	72
P vs placebo		.515	.029	.020

ANCOVA, Analysis of covariance; ln, natural log; mITT, modified intention to treat; PWT, peak walking time.
[a]ANCOVA was done using treatment, site, and baseline PWT as effects. The per-protocol population included only those subjects who completed 26 weeks of study drug treatment and had a week 26 treadmill assessment. The mixed-effects model included treatment, time point, and treatment-by-time point interaction as fixed categoric effects, site and patient as random effects, and baseline PWT as a covariate. Differences in PWT are expressed as ln (PWT/PWT at baseline) to correct for non-normality and are in mean seconds ± SD. ANCOVA P values shown are in contrast to placebo.
[b]P < .05 vs placebo.

100 mg, and placebo, all prescribed twice a day, with the intention to discontinue the 25-mg arm once tolerability was established and increase recruitment in the study arms using the higher doses of K-134. Of interest is that the groups were well matched, but most (78%) patients were enrolled in Russia, and there were significant differences between patients enrolled from Russia vs those enrolled

TABLE 4.—Effect of 100 mg of K-134 on Peak Walking Time by Country Site of Randomization[a]

Country	(n)	Placebo Mean ± SD	(n)	Cilostazol Mean ± SD	(n)	100 mg K-134 Mean ± SD
Russia	59	0.167 ± 0.431	61	0.299 ± 0.460	61	0.310 ± 0.402
USA	19	0.079 ± 0.029	13	0.115 ± 0.272	14	0.036 ± 0.390
P (between countries)		.410		.065		.024

SD, Standard deviation.
[a]Data are peak walking time expressed as natural log (week 26 PWT)/(baseline PWT). Data are from the modified intention-to-treat population. P values were calculated using a two-sample t test.

in the US with respect to age, race, diabetes, smoking history, statin and antiplatelet therapy, and baseline ankle-brachial index and peak walking time (PWT) (Table 1). The primary outcome measure of change in PWT (defined as the time between initiation of treadmill walking and the time at which the patient could walk no further due to maximally tolerated claudication symptoms) increased from baseline for both doses of K-134 and placebo and was highest for cilostazol at the 26-week treatment time point. However, there was no difference in percent change of PWT between placebo and K-134 at the 50- or 100-mg dose or cilostazol (Table 2). In the secondary efficacy analysis, there was an improvement in the change of PWT from baseline for both K-134 at 100-mg dose and cilostazol vs placebo at 14 weeks in the modified intention-to-treat population, and at 14 and 26 weeks in the per-protocol population (Table 3). Interestingly, the change in PWT was significantly better in patients treated in Russia with K-134 than those treated in the US (Table 4), which, after looking at the baseline characteristics, may be related to a younger population with less diabetes, but further work will be required to confirm these findings because the sample size in each group was not large. Important learning points from this study and the value in performing randomized trials is the sound methodology, the meticulous inclusion and exclusion criteria, the critical and timely follow-up periods, the attention to safety and tolerability of drug, assessment of biomarkers and inflammatory markers, potential of drug-drug interactions with K-134, and the meticulous statistical analysis performed. Future studies are required to assess the effectiveness of drugs in the treatment of patients with intermittent claudication during normal daily activities and with particular attention to whether the drug improves the quality of life as measured by disease-specific questionnaires.

J. D. Raffetto, MD

Anatomical Predictors of Major Adverse Limb Events after Infrapopliteal Angioplasty for Patients with Critical Limb Ischaemia due to Pure Isolated Infrapopliteal Lesions

Iida O, Soga Y, Yamauchi Y, et al (Kansai Rosai Hosp, Amagasaki, Hyogo, Japan; Kokura Memorial Hosp, Kitakyushu, Fukuoka, Japan; Kikuna Memorial Hosp, Yokohama, Japan; et al)
Eur J Vasc Endovasc Surg 44:318-324, 2012

Objective.—To identify anatomical factors associated with major adverse limb events (MALE) after angioplasty as the basis for a novel morphology-driven classification of infrapopliteal lesions.

Design.—Retrospective-multicenter study.

Materials and Methods.—Between March 2004 and October 2010, 1057 limbs from 884 patients with CLI due to isolated infrapopliteal lesions were studied. Freedom-from MALE, defined as major amputation or any reintervention, was assessed out to 2 years by the Kaplan—Meier methods. Anatomical predictors and risk stratification for MALE were analyzed by multivariate analysis.

Results.—Freedom-from MALE was 47 ± 1% at 2 years. Lesion calcification, target vessel diameter < 3.0 mm, lesion length > 300 mm and no below-the-ankle (BA) run-off were positively associated with MALE by multivariate-analysis. The total number of risk factors was used to calculate the risk score for each limbs for subsequent categorization into 3 groups with 0 or 1 (low-risk), 2 (moderate-risk) and 3 or 4 (high-risk) factors. Freedom-from MALE at 2 year-rates was 59% in low-risk, 46% in moderate-risk, and 29% in high-risk, respectively.

Conclusion.—Target vessel diameter < 3.0 mm, lesion calcification, lesion length > 300 mm and no-BA run-off were associated with MALE after infrapopliteal angioplasty. Risk stratification based on these predictors allows estimation of future incidence of MALE in CLI with isolated infrapopliteal lesions.

▶ It is difficult, if not impossible, to identify patients who may be at risk for a less than ideal outcome. This multicenter retrospective study was performed to define anatomical predictors for major adverse limb events after endovascular intervention performed on infrapopliteal lesions for critical limb ischemia. The authors concluded that small vessels (< 3 mm), long lesions (> 300 mm), calcification, and absence of below ankle runoff were predictors of poorer outcomes. They used these anatomical features to categorize patients into low-risk, moderate-risk, and high-risk levels for adverse limb outcomes based on a simple scoring system.

Traditionally, classification of these lesions has been based on the Trans-Atlantic Inter-Society Consensus (TASC) for management of peripheral arterial disease. TASC has been used to classify lesions for intervention decision making and analysis of database-derived cohorts to ensure comparison of equivalent lesions. Since TASC originally was described in 2000, the classification for infrapopliteal lesions has not been revised to reflect and include the most current intervention data that reflect the latest endovascular technology. Of note, the TASC guidelines for iliofemoral lesions were modified in the second iteration of this document. The armamentarium of balloons and stents, re-entry devices and atherectomy catheters, as well as the interventionalist's skill, have rapidly evolved in the past decade. Thus, it only seems logical that classification schemes and treatment guidelines should change in parallel with technology, outcomes, and new contributions to the literature.

R. L. Bush, MD, MPH

10 Upper Extremity Ischemia/Dialysis Access

Angiotensin receptor blockers and antiplatelet agents are associated with improved primary patency after arteriovenous hemodialysis access placement

Jackson RS, Sidawy AN, Amdur RL, et al (Veterans Affairs Med Ctr, Washington, DC)

J Vasc Surg 54:1706-1712, 2011

Objective.—Dialysis access failure is a major cause of morbidity, mortality, and cost in end-stage renal disease. We undertook a study to determine the influence of medication use on dialysis access failure.

Methods.—After institutional review board approval, we performed a retrospective analysis of all upper extremity hemodialysis accesses placed from 2005 to 2009 at the Washington DC Veterans Affairs Medical Center. For each access, the date of failure was recorded. For patients who died or were lost to follow-up, the date of the last documented functional patency (censoring) was recorded. The primary exposures were 12 medication classes. Patient demographics, behaviors, comorbidities, and access characteristics were used as covariates. Patency rates were calculated using Kaplan-Meier methods. Cox proportional hazard models controlling for patient characteristics and all medication classes, with procedures clustered within patients, were used to determine the influence of medication class on primary patency.

Results.—Two hundred sixty autogenous and 126 prosthetic newly placed accesses were identified. Of these, three lower extremity accesses and six accesses with unknown thrombosis date were excluded. Forty-five (18%) of the remaining 257 autogenous accesses were excluded for primary nonfunctionality (patent, but with inadequate venous dilatation for initial hemodialysis), because the primary outcome was long-term functional patency. The remaining 212 autogenous and 120 prosthetic accesses were analyzed. Primary patency rates at 1 and 2 years were 55.2% and 49.1% for autogenous accesses, and 50.2% and 29.7% for prosthetic accesses, respectively. On multivariable analysis, angiotensin receptor blockers (ARBs) were associated with reduced hazard of both autogenous (hazard

173

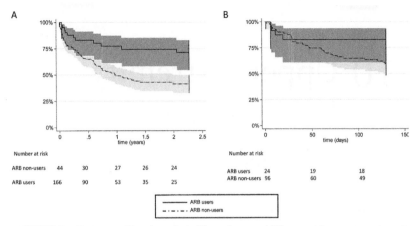

FIGURE 2.—Autogenous (**A**) and prosthetic (**B**) arteriovenous (AV) access primary patency, in angiotensin receptor blocker (*ARB*) users and nonusers. Shaded areas indicate 95% confidence interval (CI). (Reprinted from the Journal of Vascular Surgery. Jackson RS, Sidawy AN, Amdur RL, et al. Angiotensin receptor blockers and antiplatelet agents are associated with improved primary patency after arteriovenous hemodialysis access placement. *J Vasc Surg.* 2011;54:1706-1712, Copyright 2011, with permission from The Society for Vascular Surgery.)

ratio [HR], 0.35; 95% confidence interval [CI], 0.16-0.76; $P = .008$) and prosthetic (HR, 0.41; 95% CI, 0.18-0.95; $P = .039$) access failure. On subgroup analysis, ARBs prolonged autogenous access primary patency among patients receiving antiplatelet medication (aspirin, clopidogrel; HR, 0.16; 95% CI, 0.05-0.52; $P = .002$) but had no demonstrable benefit among patients not receiving antiplatelets (HR, 1.35; 95% CI, 0.34-5.31; $P = .670$). There were no significant drug–drug interactions in the analysis of prosthetic accesses. Weighted regression models demonstrated low multicollinearity among the model variables.

Conclusion.—Our data suggest that therapy with an ARB plus antiplatelet agent is associated with prolonged autogenous access primary patency, and therapy with an ARB with or without antiplatelet agents is associated with prolonged prosthetic access primary patency. Randomized studies are needed to confirm the causal role of ARBs and to determine the optimal therapeutic regimen (dose, timing, and duration) to promote access patency (Fig 2).

▶ One of the primary concerns in hemodialysis access is the patency and function of the arteriovenous fistula (AVF). Significant improvements have been made by the Disease Outcomes Quality Initiative guidelines in a fistula-first campaign, having at least 50% of fistula be constructed from autogenous vein. Constructing the fistula is not the problem, but what remains is the ability of the fistula to remain patent and mature for use. In this retrospective study spanning 5 years, patients with autogenous AVF and prosthetic AVF were evaluated for primary fistula functional patency and the influence of 12 medication classes on primary functional patency. After excluding nonfunctional, lower extremity, and unknown AVF, the remaining 212 autogenous and 120 prosthetic accesses were analyzed. The utilization of angiotensin receptor blockers (ARBs) reduced both the autogenous and prosthetic hazard of access failure at 2 years (Fig 2). On multivariable analysis, ARBs reduced the risk of autogenous access failure by 65% (hazard ratio [HR], 0.35; 95% confidence interval [CI], 0.16—0.76; $P = .008$). There was a statistically significant interaction between ARBs and antiplatelets on autogenous access primary patency ($P = .022$). On subgroup analysis, ARBs prolonged autogenous access primary patency by 84% among patients receiving antiplatelet agents (HR, 0.16; 95% CI, 0.05—0.52; $P = .002$) but interestingly had no demonstrable benefit among patients not receiving antiplatelet agents (HR, 1.35; 95% CI, 0.34—5.31; $P = .670$). This may be caused by the multimechanistic modality required (vasodilation, inhibition of neointimal hyperplasia, and platelet inhibition) by both ARBs and antiplatelet medications. On multivariable analysis, ARBs reduced the risk of prosthetic access failure by 59% (HR, 0.41; 95% CI, 0.18—0.95; $P = .039$). ARBs did not have significant interaction with any other medication class in the analysis of prosthetic access patency. Future research will need to assess the utilization of ARBs in conjunction with antiplatelets in randomized clinical trials that are double blinded and placebo controlled and assess functional patency, safety, and cost analysis in this at-risk group of patients with chronic renal failure on dialysis. In addition, this study raises important mechanistic questions that will need basic science research to fully understand the role of ARBs in reducing AVF failure and potentially develop new adjunctive treatment modalities to preserve the functioning and precious autogenous AVF.

J. D. Raffetto, MD

Cost-effectiveness of Vascular Access for Haemodialysis: Arteriovenous Fistulas Versus Arteriovenous Grafts

Leermakers JJPM, Bode AS, Vaidya A, et al (Maastricht Univ Med Ctr (MUMC), The Netherlands; Maastricht Univ, The Netherlands)
Eur J Vasc Endovasc Surg 45:84-92, 2013

Background.—The use of an arteriovenous fistula (AVF) for haemodialysis treatment may be associated with a high early failure rate, but usually good long-term patency, while using an arteriovenous graft (AVG) yields a lower early failure rate with worse long-term patency. The aim of this study was to calculate and compare the costs and outcome of AVF and AVG surgery in terms of early and long-term patencies.

Methods.—A decision tree and a Markov model were constructed to calculate costs and performance of AVFs and AVGs. The model was populated with a retrospective cohort of HD patients receiving their first VA. The outcomes were determined probabilistically with a 5-year follow-up.

Results.—AVFs were usable for a mean (95% CI) of 28.5 months (24.6—32.5 months), while AVGs showed a patency of 25.5 months (20.0—31.2 months). The use of AVFs was the dominant type of VA and €631 could be saved per patient/per month patency compared to AVG use. Regardless of the willingness to pay, the use of AVFs yielded a higher probability of being cost-effective compared to AVGs.

Conclusions.—AVFs are more cost-effective than AVGs. Nonetheless, early failure rates significantly influence AVF performance and initiatives to reduce early failure can improve its cost-effectiveness.

▶ Comparative effectiveness studies necessitate concomitant analyses of cost-effectiveness if not already included within the meaning of the term cost-effectiveness. As we move forward with attempts to reform the health care system in the United States and create a sustainable structure, looking at costs along with efficacy is paramount to progress and success.

This article addresses both of these issues nicely in a study of dialysis access procedures. Because patients are living longer and surviving on dialysis for years, even decades, maintaining functional lasting access is vital. Autologous access creation has been recommended in guidelines and by advocacy groups because of the longer patency rates and lower complication rates. However, this enthusiasm for outcomes must be tempered with the known rate of maturation failures and need for secondary procedures. Patients and providers do not ignore the high early failure rates of autogenous arteriovenous fistulas (AVFs); however, the guidelines may only account for those accesses that actually went on to functional maturation.

This article is a must read for surgeons and interventionalists who operate on AVFs and grafts. There are data on costs of initial access creation and myriad interventions. AVFs do indeed fall within the statistical modeling method used herein; they have lower overall costs, even for failed AVFs. Thus, there needs to be better predictive methods and techniques for increasing maturation of AVFs. Many have tried venous and arterial ultrasound mapping, balloon-assisted maturation, and other modalities. There may be a combination of tips and tricks to increase maturation rates, and as stated in this article, this is perhaps where the next research focus should be.

R. L. Bush, MD, MPH

Evaluation of Immature Hemodialysis Arteriovenous Fistulas Based on 3-French Retrograde Micropuncture of Brachial Artery

Yan Y, Soulen MC, Shlansky-Goldberg RD, et al (Univ of Pennsylvania Med Ctr, Philadelphia)
AJR Am J Roentgenol 199:683-690, 2012

Objective.—The objective of our study was to assess outcomes after evaluation of immature hemodialysis arteriovenous fistulas (AVFs) via 3-French brachial artery access and to identify the incidence of arterial and venous puncture site spasm.

Materials and Methods.—One hundred twenty-three outpatients (82 men, 41 women; mean age, 58 years; age range, 20—90 years) with immature AVF were identified retrospectively in whom diagnostic fistulography was performed via 3-French retrograde brachial artery puncture. Percutaneous transluminal angioplasty was performed via a separate venous puncture during the same visit in 95 patients. Patient age and sex, fistula age and type, and technical success and complications were recorded. Images were reviewed for lesion location, potentially competing vessels, and arterial and venous puncture—related spasms.

Results.—The mean fistula age was 99 days (range, 21—639 days). There were 49 AVFs in the left forearm; 30 in the left upper arm; 26 in the right forearm; and 18 in the right upper arm. Twenty-eight AVFs were transposed. Angioplasty was technically successful in 81 of 95 patients (85%; mean diameter, 7 mm; range, 4—10 mm). Brachial artery puncture caused no major complication. Arterial spasm occurred in 19 patients (15%) and was severe in one patient. There were two hematomas (1.6%). Venous spasm, ranging from mild (four patients) to occlusive (8 patients), occurred in 38 patients (40%) at the site of venipuncture for intervention. Nitroglycerin (mean, 325 mcg; range, 100—600 mcg) was used in 26 procedures (21%). Venous spasm was more common with forearm (50%) than upper arm (24%) fistulas ($p = 0.02$) and with decreasing vein diameter ($p = 0.02$).

Conclusion.—Evaluation of immature AVFs based on 3-French micropuncture of the brachial artery can be safely performed on an outpatient basis. Spasm is more common in forearm AVFs and in smaller veins.

▶ The practice of surgical placement of autogenous hemodialysis fistulae (AVF) has increased in the past several years as a result of Fistula First initiatives and revised guidelines. Along with this increase in AVF effort, there has also been a corresponding increase in the number of fistulae that fail to mature as marginal veins may be used. As an alternative to venous fistulography, this study describes a different method for assessing immature AVFs. This group studies the AVFs using a retrograde brachial artery approach with a 3 Fr catheter. With this technique, the group avoids unnecessary spasm that can occur by directly accessing the vein itself. Such spasm could potentially be misinterpreted as a stenosis and, furthermore, avoiding a fragile immature vein may be beneficial. Once an arterial or venous cause for the failure to mature is found, a separate puncture is used to perform endovascular interventions.

As someone who performs quite a few AVFs, particularly in an older population, I am aware of the difficulty with maturation that can occur. I often use marginal veins in attempts to create an autogenous access. Having ability to image AVFs, discover anatomic reasons for the failure, and correct in the same setting will hopefully increase the success and usability rate. The difficulty will arise in patients not yet on hemodialysis and in whom even a small amount of contrast is contraindicated. Using diluted contrast in very small amounts combined with subtraction angiography and gentle hydration should avoid or alleviate this issue. This is a technique that will be added to our armamentarium for assessment of immature AVFs.

R. L. Bush, MD, MPH

Long-term results of femoral vein transposition for autogenous arteriovenous hemodialysis access

Bourquelot P, Rawa M, Van Laere O, et al (Clinique Jouvenet, Paris, France; Polyclinique Cornette de St Cyr, Meknés, Morocco; CMC Ambroise Paré, Neuilly sur Seine, France; et al)
J Vasc Surg 56:440-445, 2012

Introduction.—When all access options in the upper limbs have been exhausted, an autogenous access in lower limb is a valuable alternative to arteriovenous grafts. We report our experience of transposition of the femoral vein (tFV).

Methods.—From June 1984 to June 2011, 70 patients underwent 72 tFV in two centers (Paris and Meknès) with the same technique. All patients had exhausted upper arm veins or had central vein obstructions. Patients were followed by serial duplex scanning. All complications were recorded and statistical analysis of patency was performed according to intention to treat using the life-table method.

Results.—The mean interval between initiation of dialysis and creation of the tFV was 10 years. The sex ratio was even (one female/one male). Mean age was 48 years (range, 1-84 years), and there were no postoperative infections. Duplex measurements in 33 patients indicated high-flow: mean = 1529 ± 429 mL/min; range, 700-3000 mL/min. Two immediate failures were observed and four patients were lost to follow-up soon after the access creation. Ten patients (14%) experienced minor complications (hematoma, five; lymphocele, one; delayed wound healing, two; distal edema, two) and 30 patients (42%) experienced mild complications (femoral vein and outflow stenosis, 16 [treated by percutaneous transluminal angioplasty, 13, or polytetrafluoroethylene patch, three]; puncture site complications, three [ischemia, two; infection, one]; reversible thrombosis, three [two surgical and one percutaneous thrombectomy]; abandoned thrombosis, eight [11%] after a mean patency of 8.1 years). Thirteen patients (18%) experienced major complications necessitating fistula ligation (ischemic complications, five diabetic patients with peripheral arterial occlusive disease [one major amputation included]; lower leg compartment syndrome, one; acute venous hypertension, two; secondary major edema, two; high-output cardiac failure, one; bleeding, two). All the patent accesses (59/72) were utilized for dialysis after a mean interval of 2 ± 1 months (range, 1-7 months) resulting in an 82% success rate. According to life-table analysis, the primary patency rates at 1 and 9 years were 91% ± 4% and 45% ± 11%, respectively. The secondary patency rates at 1 and 9 years were 84% ± 5% and 56% ± 9%, respectively.

Conclusions.—Femoral vein transposition in the lower limb is a valuable alternative to arteriovenous grafts in terms of infection and long-term patency. Secondary venous percutaneous angioplasties may be necessary.

High flow rates are frequently observed and patient selection is essential to avoid ischemic complications.

▶ For those of us that perform procedures for hemodialysis access, running out of upper extremity options is a known dilemma. Because of improvements in medical care, medications, and a more thorough understanding of the pathophysiology of chronic kidney disease, the life expectancy of patients on hemodialysis has lengthened. Thus, it is prudent to be resourceful, as well as creative, with autogenous fistula (AVF) creation in order to avoid prosthetic grafts and central venous catheters as long-term dialysis solutions. This being said, earlier reports on lower extremity autogenous fistulae have demonstrated mixed results, with infection and lower extremity ischemia being feared complications. Some authors have even reported the need for lower extremity amputation resulting from a femoral vein transposition.

These authors from France describe their experience with 72 transposed femoral veins in 70 patients as well as the necessity for proper patient selection to optimize outcomes. The article follows their experience and changes that they made in the procedure and patient selection as they encountered difficulties. Their experience has led to the exclusion of diabetic patients and those with significant distal peripheral vascular disease. The study also emphasizes the need for surveillance for congestive heart failure because of the high-flow nature of lower extremity transposition AVFs. In addition, there may be an increased incidence of outflow stenoses because of this high flow. I commend these authors for an excellent and informational series of patients. The article is a must read for those doing a reasonable volume dialysis access as we will all need to rely on other forms of AVFs in order to maintain an autogenous access.

R. L. Bush, MD, MPH

Ethnic differences in arm vein diameter and arteriovenous fistula creation rates in men undergoing hemodialysis access
Ishaque B, Zayed MA, Miller J, et al (Univ of California, Los Angeles (UCLA); Stanford Univ Med Ctr, CA; et al)
J Vasc Surg 56:424-432, 2012

Objective.—The National Kidney Foundation recommends that arteriovenous fistulas (AVFs) be placed in at least 65% of hemodialysis patients. Some studies suggest that African American patients are less likely to receive a first-time AVF than patients of other ethnicities, although the reason for this disparity is unclear. The purpose of our study is to determine (1) whether there are ethnic differences in AVF creation, (2) whether this may be related to differences in vein diameters, and (3) whether AVF patency rates are similar between African American and non-African American male patients.

Methods.—Consecutive male patients undergoing first-time hemodialysis access from 2006 to 2010 at two institutions were retrospectively reviewed. Data collected included age, ethnicity, weight, height, body mass index, diabetes, hypertension, congestive heart failure, smoking history, intravenous drug abuse, need for temporary access placement, and preoperative venous ultrasound measurements. Categoric variables were compared using χ^2 analysis, and the Wilcoxon rank-sum test was used to compare continuous variables.

Results.—Of 249 male patients identified, 95 were African American. Median age in African American and non-African American patients was 63 years. Hypertension and hyperlipidemia were statistically significantly greater in African American patients. The need for temporary access before hemoaccess was similar between the cohorts. African American patients demonstrated significantly smaller median basilic and cephalic vein diameters at most measured sites. Overall, 221 of 249 (88.8%) underwent AVF first. An AV graft was created in 17.9% of African American patients vs in only 7.1% of non-African Americans (odds ratio, 2.8; 95% confidence interval, 1.3-6.4; $P = .009$). The difference between median vein diameters used for autologous fistula creation in African American and non-African American patients was not significant. There was no significant difference in the primary patency (80.8% vs 76.2%; $P = .4$), primary functional patency (73.1% vs 69.2%; $P = .5$), or secondary functional patency rates (91.0% vs 96.5%; $P = .1$). Average primary fistula survival time was 257 days in African American and 256 in non-African American patients ($P = .2$).

Conclusions.—African American patients are less likely than non-African American patients to undergo AVF during first-time hemodialysis access surgery. This ethnic discrepancy appears to be due to smaller arm vein diameters in African American patients. In African American patients with appropriate vein diameters who do undergo AVF, primary and functional patencies are equivalent to non-African American patients.

▶ Vascular surgeons strive to increase arteriovenous fistula (AVF) creation in patients with chronic kidney disease to match national guidelines and ensure better long-term outcomes for the access site than that of prosthetic grafts or tunneled catheters. There have been data suggesting racial disparities in AVF percentages with African-Americans (AA) receiving less first-time AVFs. This is an interesting single-center study looking at whether or not there are anatomical reasons, which may account for these racial differences in AVF creation between AA and non-AA male patients.

Many reasons for racial disparities in access to care and actual care delivered exist. Data support a multifactorial rationale including transportation, family support, socioeconomic status, geographic location, and presentation at advanced stages of disease. This is the first study that I have seen looking at anatomical variations that may exist among racial and ethnic groups. Though the cohort is small (< 300), the authors did find that AAs had smaller vein diameters than non-AA patients. Furthermore, those AA patients that had AVFs had equivalent primary and functional patency rates to non-AA patients. The message to be gleaned from this study is to take an aggressive approach to first-time AVF creation in patients with chronic kidney disease regardless of time of presentation as long as there is a suitable vein preferably determined by preoperative vein mapping by ultrasound. Too many surgeons rely on physical examination alone, which may identify a vein of adequate size, but may overlook intraluminal irregularities, wall thickening, or important accessory veins that need ligation for fistula maturation. This reviewer recommends accepting a higher personal AVF failure rate with the expectation of achieving a first-time AVF.

R. L. Bush, MD, MPH

11 Carotid and Cerebrovascular Disease

Carotid Artery Surgery: High-Risk Patients or High-Risk Centers?
Bouziane Z, Nourissat G, Duprey A, et al (St Etienne Univ Hosp, France)
Ann Vasc Surg 26:790-796, 2012

Background.—Carotid angioplasty and stenting has been proposed as an alternative to carotid endarterectomy (CEA) in patients deemed as at high risk for this surgical procedure. To date, definitely accepted criteria to identify "high-risk" patients for CEA do not exist. Our objective was to assess the relevance of numerous supposed high-risk factors in our experience, as well as their possible effect on our early postoperative results.

Methods.—A retrospective review of 1,033 consecutive CEAs performed during a 5.6-year period at a single institution was conducted (Vascular Surgery Department, St. Etienne University Hospital, France). Early results in terms of mortality and neurologic events were recorded. Univariate and multivariate analyses for early risk of stroke, myocardial infarction, and death were performed, considering the influence of age, sex, comorbidities, clinical symptoms, and anatomic features.

Results.—The cumulative 30-day stroke and death rate was 1.2%. A total of 10 strokes occurred and resulted in three deaths. The postoperative stroke risk was significantly higher in the subgroup of patients treated for symptomatic carotid artery disease: 2,6% ($P = 0,004$). Univariate analysis and logistic regression did not show statistical significance for 30-day results in any of the considered variables.

Conclusion.—Patients with significant medical comorbidities, contralateral carotid occlusion, and high carotid lesions can undergo surgery without increased complications. Those parameters should not be used as exclusion criteria for CEA.

▶ Bouziane et al reported their series of 1033 consecutive carotid endarterectomies (CEA) performed over 5.6 years with an associated 30-day stroke/death rate of 1.2% and opine if there is, indeed, such a condition as "high operative risk" for undergoing carotid endarterectomy. Their analysis found no significant correlation of stroke with the variables typically considered as high operative risk. As cited by the authors, there are indeed many outstanding groups of vascular surgeons performing CEA who routinely achieve excellent results even for these high operative risk groups. These surgeons need not feel any pressure to perform—or refer their patients for—carotid stenting. Attention to these designated high operative risk groups will perhaps be of more benefit to the average vascular surgeon. I suspect, however, that the practicing vascular/endovascular surgeon today who is equally facile with performing both CEA and carotid artery stenting (CAS) will likely choose CAS for these high operative risk groups.

K. Hughes, MD

No Benefit from Carotid Intervention in Fatal Stroke Prevention for >80-Year-old Patients

De Rango P, Lenti M, Simonte G, et al (Hosp S.M. Misericordia, Perugia, Italy; et al)

Eur J Vasc Endovasc Surg 44:252-259, 2012

Background.—Invasive management of patients ≥80 years of age with carotid stenosis may be questionable. The higher likelihood of stroke needs to be balanced with the increased perioperative risk and the reduced life expectancy of this ageing population. The purpose of this study was to evaluate the clinical relevance of carotid stenosis revascularisation in octogenarians.

Methods.—All patients ≥80 years of age who received carotid revascularisation in 2001-2010 were reviewed for perioperative and 5-year outcomes. The experience was comprehensive of carotid endarterectomy (CEA) and carotid stenting (CAS) performed during the training frame when age was not a contraindication for this procedure. Mortality rates were compared to those of octogenarians of the same geographical territory according to all-cause and stroke-related mortality national statistics datasets.

Results.—A total of 348 procedures performed in ≥80-year-old patients (272 males) were reviewed: 162 (46.6%) were by CAS and 169 (48.6%) were for symptomatic disease. Perioperative stroke/death rate was 5.5% and was non-significantly higher for symptomatic disease (7.1% vs. 3.9% asymptomatic; $p = 0.24$), after CAS (6.2% vs. 4.8% CEA; $p = 0.64$) and in females (6.6% vs. 5.1% males; $p = 0.57$). At median follow-up of 36.18 months, 95 deaths and 21 new ischaemic strokes (12 fatal) occurred with 5-year Kaplan-Meier freedom from stroke of 84.8% (78.7%, symptomatic vs. 90.3% asymptomatic; $p = 0.003$). According to national datasets, in 80-85-year-old resident population 5-year mortality was 29.9% (23.4% females, 40.6% males) and ischaemic stroke-related mortality was 14.9% (16.8% females, 13.0% males). Corresponding figures from treated population showed a 5-year mortality of 49.4%, higher in males (39.5% females, 52.5% males) and ischaemic stroke-related mortality of 20.2%, higher in females (40.0% females, 15.6% males). Comparing data from the study population with residents' figures, ischaemic stroke-related mortality hazard was significantly higher in the study females: odds ratio

(OR) 3.2, 95% confidence interval (CI) 1.16-9.17; $p = 0.029$ (for males: OR 0.97, 95% CI 0.89-1.10; $p = 0.99$).

Conclusions.—Despite perioperative stroke/death risks being lower compared with CAS, the benefit of surgical carotid revascularisation in old patients remains controversial due to limited life expectancy and high fatality of stroke in this ageing population. Invasive treatment of carotid stenosis may not be warranted in most patients ≥ 80 years of age with carotid stenosis, especially when female and asymptomatic.

▶ Although the stroke-risk reduction benefit of carotid endarterectomy (CEA) and carotid artery stenting (CAS) is evident in relatively younger patients with carotid artery disease, much controversy exists when considering carotid interventions on elderly patients with carotid artery disease. This population-based study calls into question the true benefit, or lack thereof, of carotid interventions in octogenarians.

Comparing a group of patients 80 to 85 years of age who underwent either CEA or CAS for well-established indications with age-matched individuals with unknown carotid artery disease status from the same region in Italy, this study fails to demonstrate a mortality benefit or stroke reduction in the carotid intervention group. Further analysis shows that women and asymptomatic patients with carotid artery disease were even less likely to benefit from CEA or CAS.

Although this study cannot definitely show that carotid interventions are not indicated in the elderly, especially individuals with asymptomatic carotid artery disease, it does bring to our attention the need for a well-designed, randomized, controlled trial comparing best medical management with carotid artery interventions in octogenarians.

B. G. Peterson, MD

Prospective neurocognitive evaluation of patients undergoing carotid interventions
Zhou W, Hitchner E, Gillis K, et al (VA Palo Alto Health Care System, CA; et al)
J Vasc Surg 56:1571-1578, 2012

Objective.—Distal cerebral embolization is a known complication of carotid interventions. We prospectively investigated whether subclinical microembolization seen on postoperative magnetic resonance imaging (MRI) leads to cognitive deficits in patients undergoing carotid revascularization procedures.

Methods.—Patients undergoing carotid interventions and eligible for MRI scanning were recruited. Among 247 patients who received preoperative and postoperative MRI evaluations, 51 also completed neuropsychologic testing before and at 1 month after their procedure. Cognitive evaluation included the Rey Auditory Verbal Learning Test (RAVLT) for memory evaluation and the Mini-Mental State Examination (MMSE) for general cognitive impairment screening.

Results.—The 51 patients (all men), comprising 16 with carotid artery stenting (CAS) and 35 with carotid endarterectomy (CEA), were a mean age of 71 years (range, 54-89 years). Among them, 27 patients (53%) were symptomatic preoperatively, including 11 who had prior stroke and 16 who had prior preoperative transient ischemic attack symptoms. Most patients had significant medical comorbidities, including hypertension (96%), diabetes (31.3%), coronary artery disease (47%), and chronic obstructive pulmonary disease (15.7%). Two patients (4%) had prior ipsilateral CEA and eight had contralateral carotid occlusion (15.7%). Memory decline evident on RAVLT was identified in eight CAS patients and 13 CEA patients. Eleven patients had evidence of procedure-related microemboli. Although there was no significant difference in baseline cognitive function or memory change between the CEA and CAS cohorts, the CAS cohort had a significantly higher incidence of microembolic lesions. Multivariate regression analysis showed that procedure-related microembolization was associated with memory decline ($P = .016$) as evident by change in RAVLT. A history of neurologic symptoms was significantly associated with poor baseline cognitive function (MMSE; $P = .03$) and overall cognitive deterioration (change in MMSE; $P = .026$), as determined by Wilcoxon rank sum test and linear regression analysis, respectively.

Conclusions.—Although CEA and CAS are effective in stroke prevention, with minimal neurologic complication, neurocognitive effects remain uncertain. Procedure-associated microembolization and pre-existing neurologic symptoms are associated with poor baseline cognitive function and memory decline after the procedures. Further comprehensive cognitive evaluation to determine the benefit of carotid interventions is warranted.

▶ Zhou et al, in seeking to evaluate the cognitive effects of microemboli associated with carotid revascularization in a prospective clinical trial, used pre- and postoperative diffusion-weighted magnetic resonance imaging as well as a battery of neurocognitive testing. As has been previously reported, this study also found a significantly higher rate of microembolization among carotid angioplasty and stenting (CAS) patients (50%) compared with that of carotid endarterectomy patients (8.6%). Although this study—perhaps hindered by its small sample size of only 51 patients—failed to establish an association between microembolization and overall cognitive decline, the identification that microembolization was an independent predictor of memory decline after carotid revascularization is significant. Given that the cardiac surgical literature has established a convincing association between postoperative cognitive dysfunction and long-term cognitive decline, those of us who perform CAS (author included) would do well to temper our enthusiasm for this procedure. Indeed, attention to Dr LoGerfo's commentary[1] may serve us well if we seek assistance in modulating this enthusiasm.

K. Hughes, MD

Reference

1. LoGerfo FW. Carotid stents: unleashed, unproven. *Circulation.* 2007;116: 1596-1601.

Variability in Carotid Endarterectomy Practice Patterns Within a Metropolitan Area
Kansara A, Miller D, Damani R, et al (Wayne State Univ, Detroit, MI; Henry Ford Hosp, Detroit, MI; et al)
Stroke 43:3105-3107, 2012

Background and Purpose.—Previous clinical studies have suggested that patients with carotid stenosis with high surgical risk features may fare better with carotid artery stenting or aggressive medical therapy. The extent to which carotid endarterectomy is still being performed in this group of patients is unclear.

Methods.—A retrospective audit was performed among 4 hospitals over a 2-year period. The proportion of high surgical risk patients was compared and the in-hospital stroke, myocardial infarction, and death rates were compared among conventional and high surgical risk patients.

Results.—Three hundred thirty-five carotid endarterectomy operations were performed (63% asymptomatic) with 37.9% being high surgical risk subjects. The stroke, myocardial infarction, and death rate was 4.6% in conventional risk subjects and 10.2% in high surgical risk patients ($P < 0.05$). The only hospital with multidisciplinary carotid conferences had the lowest proportion of carotid endarterectomy operations in asymptomatic patients.

Conclusions.—A substantial proportion of carotid endarterectomy operations are performed in patients with high surgical risk features. These patients experienced a 2-fold increase in major in-hospital complications, raising doubts about whether they benefit from carotid surgery. The use of preintervention multidisciplinary conferences may improve patient safety.

▶ Naturally, composite endpoints of stroke, myocardial infarction, and death are higher with carotid endarterectomy (CEA) being performed in high-risk patients (10.2% in this study) compared with conventional risk patients (4.6%). Comparing 4 hospitals within a 30-mile radius of each other and using one of these hospitals as the reference hospital, because it had in place a multidisciplinary case conference, this group found that a large number of CEAs are still being performed in high-risk individuals. The main value of this article is that it suggests that surgeons remain skeptical about the value of aggressive medical management or carotid artery stenting in high-risk patients with carotid artery disease.

The authors suggest that the use of a multidisciplinary case conference to determine which patients will benefit from CEA may put fewer patients at risk, change practice patterns, and perhaps improve outcomes. I tend to agree and believe that this is most important when considering the type of intervention, be it medical management, carotid artery stenting, or CEA, in high-risk individuals. Too many carotid interventions are being performed for various reasons, but perhaps putting more thought into which patients are truly going to benefit and live long enough to realize that benefit may lead to a better understanding of carotid artery disease. Thankfully, the authors bring this to light in this report.

B. G. Peterson, MD

Stroke After Carotid Stenting and Endarterectomy in the Carotid Revascularization Endarterectomy Versus Stenting Trial (CREST)

Hill MD, for the CREST Investigators (Univ of Calgary, Alberta, Canada; et al)
Circulation 126:3054-3061, 2012

Background.—Stroke occurs more commonly after carotid artery stenting than after carotid endarterectomy. Details regarding stroke type, severity, and characteristics have not been reported previously. We describe the strokes that have occurred in the Carotid Revascularization Endarterectomy versus Stenting Trial (CREST).

Methods and Results.—CREST is a randomized, open-allocation, controlled trial with blinded end-point adjudication. Stroke was a component of the primary composite outcome. Patients who received their assigned treatment within 30 days of randomization were included. Stroke was adjudicated by a panel of board-certified vascular neurologists with secondary central review of clinically obtained brain images. Stroke type, laterality, timing, and outcome were reported. A periprocedural stroke occurred among 81 of the 2502 patients randomized and among 69 of the 2272 in the present analysis. Strokes were predominantly minor (81%, n = 56), ischemic (90%, n = 62), in the anterior circulation (94%, n = 65), and ipsilateral to the treated artery (88%, n = 61). There were 7 hemorrhages, which occurred 3 to 21 days after the procedure, and 5 were fatal. Major stroke occurred in 13 (0.6%) of the 2272 patients. The estimated 4-year mortality after stroke was 21.1% compared with 11.6% for those without stroke. The adjusted risk of death at 4 years was higher after periprocedural stroke (hazard ratio, 2.78; 95% confidence interval, 1.63–4.76).

Conclusions.—Stroke, particularly severe stroke, was uncommon after carotid intervention in CREST, but stroke was associated with significant morbidity and was independently associated with a nearly 3-fold increased future mortality. The delayed timing of major and hemorrhagic stroke after revascularization suggests that these strokes may be preventable.

▶ Hill et al re-examined CREST (Carotid Revascularization Endarterectomy versus Stenting Trial) findings to elucidate details regarding stroke type and severity. The authors determined that strokes occurred twice as frequently in the carotid angioplasty and stenting (CAS) arm compared with the carotid endarterectomy (CEA) arm. Most strokes were minor, which is encouraging. The finding, however, that these strokes were associated with a nearly 3-fold (hazard ratio, 2.78) higher risk of death in the long term is significant. Whereas the greater risk of stroke in the CAS arm combined with this nearly 3-fold risk of death would lead one to question the overall benefit of CAS, it is important to note that this relative increase in death was very similar to that associated with perioperative myocardial infarction (hazard ratio, 3.67)—primarily a complication of CEA.

Significant attention should be paid to the discovery that major strokes, diagnosed in only 0.6% of patients, occurred at a median time of 3 days postoperatively. As indicated by the authors, this suggests that there may be substantial opportunity to prevent these strokes, perhaps with optimization of medical management.

K. Hughes, MD

The impact of race and ethnicity on the outcome of carotid interventions in the United States
Schneider EB, Black JH III, Hambridge HL, et al (The Johns Hopkins Hosp, Baltimore, MD)
J Surg Res 177:172-177, 2012

Objective.—Previous studies have demonstrated an adverse impact of African American race and Hispanic ethnicity on the outcomes of carotid endarterectomy (CEA), although little is known about the influence of race and ethnicity on the outcome of carotid angioplasty and stenting (CAS). The present study was undertaken to examine the influence of race and ethnicity on the outcomes of CEA and CAS in contemporary practice.

Methods.—The nationwide inpatient sample (2005–2008) was queried using International Classification of Diseases-9 codes for CEA and CAS in patients with carotid artery stenosis. The primary outcomes were postoperative death or stroke. Multivariate analysis was performed adjusting for age, gender, race, comorbidities, high-risk status, procedure type, symptomatic status, year, insurance type, and hospital characteristics.

Results.—Overall, there were 347,450 CEAs and 47,385 CASs performed in the United States over the study period. After CEA, Hispanics had the greatest risk of mortality ($P < 0.001$), whereas black patients had the greatest risk of stroke ($P = 0.02$) compared with white patients on univariate analysis. On multivariable analysis, Hispanic ethnicity remained an independent risk factor for mortality after CEA (relative risk 2.40; $P < 0.001$), whereas the increased risk of stroke in black patients was no longer significant. After CAS, there were no racial or ethnic differences in mortality. On univariate analysis, the risk of stroke was greatest in black patients after CAS ($P = 0.03$). However, this was not significant on multivariable analysis.

Conclusion.—Hispanic ethnicity is an independent risk factor for mortality after CEA. While black patients had an increased risk of stroke after CEA and CAS, this was explained by factors other than race. Further studies are warranted to determine if Hispanic ethnicity remains an independent risk factor for mortality after discharge.

▶ Utilizing the Nationwide Inpatient Sample (NIS) database, Schneider et al examined the impact of race and ethnicity on the outcomes of carotid revascularization. Consistent with other studies such as CREST (Carotid Revascularization Endarterectomy vs Stenting Trial),[1] the authors showed that there is an increased stroke/death risk after carotid angioplasty and stenting (CAS) compared with carotid endarterectomy (CEA). It is notable that blacks undergoing both CEA and CAS were noted to have an increased rate of stroke, although this difference disappeared on multivariate analysis, suggesting that this was attributable to other variables. One such variable may be the significant finding that blacks were more likely to present with symptomatic disease. Perhaps the key finding of this study is that Hispanic race was determined to be independently associated with an increased risk of mortality after CEA (relative risk, 2.4). Unfortunately, the limitations of the NIS do not allow for a specific causal relationship to be established. It is imperative that additional investigation into these outcomes disparities be conducted.

K. Hughes, MD

Reference

1. Brott TG, Hobson RW II, Howard G, et al. Stenting versus endarterectomy for treatment of carotid-artery stenosis. *N Engl J Med.* 2010;363:11-23.

Visual outcomes after carotid reconstructive surgery for ocular ischemia
Neroev VV, Kiseleva TN, Vlasov SK, et al (The Helmholtz Moscow Res Inst of Eye Diseases, Moscow, Russia; Russian Academy of Med Science, Moscow, Russia)
Eye 26:1281-1287, 2012

Aims.—This study aimed to determine the influence of carotid artery surgery on ocular functions and ocular blood flow in patients with ocular ischaemic syndrome (OIS) in the late postoperative period.

Methods.—One hundred and eighty patients with OIS were operated on; 104 of them suffered from acute forms of the ischaemic disease and 76 patients had chronic forms of ocular ischaemia. Before surgery and in the course of 6 months and 12 months afterwards, all the patients were examined. Visual acuity, electrophysiological investigations (the threshold of electrical sensitivity (TES) and the level of liability of optic nerve (LON)) and blood flow in orbital vessels were assessed.

Results.—After surgery visual acuity increased in patients with the acute forms of OIS ($P < 0.05$). TES and LON also improved ($P < 0.01$). Mean indices of blood-flow velocities in the ophthalmic artery, the central retinal artery and the posterior ciliary arteries increased at 6 and 12 months after surgery ($P < 0.05$). There was ocular blood flow acceleration and decrease of vasoresistance in orbital arteries in both groups of patients.

Conclusions.—Carotid artery surgery effectively improved ocular blood flow in patients with acute and chronic forms of OIS in the late post operative period.

▶ In an attempt to determine the effect of carotid revascularization on ocular function and ocular blood flow in patients with ocular ischemic syndrome (OIS), Neroev et al retrospectively evaluated 180 patients who underwent carotid revascularization at a single institution over a 12-year period. Postoperatively, improvement in blood flow was noted in all patients with both acute and chronic forms of OIS after carotid revascularization. Clinically, however, only those patients with acute OIS uniformly experienced a significant increase in visual acuity postoperatively, accompanied by resolution of abnormal ophthalmoscopic findings and improvement in electrophysiologic characteristics of the visual system. In contrast, improvement of visual acuity occurred in only 16% of patients who had chronic forms of OIS. Whereas it has been shown that ocular symptoms, other than amaurosis fugax, are not associated with a high risk of hemispheric neurologic events,[1] carotid revascularization specifically for acute OIS may represent an indication that deserves more attention.

K. Hughes, MD

Reference

1. Dunlap AB, Kosmorsky GS, Kashyap VS. The fate of patients with retinal artery occlusion and Hollenhorst plaque. *J Vasc Surg.* 2007;46:1125-1129.

Comparing the Use of Diagnostic Imaging and Receipt of Carotid Endarterectomy in Elderly Black and White Stroke Patients

Martin KD, Naert L, Goldstein LB, et al (Yale School of Public Health, New Haven, CT; Iowa Foundation for Med Care, West Des Moines; Duke Univ and VA Med Ctr, Durham, NC)

J Stroke Cerebrovasc Dis 21:600-606, 2012

Background.—Previous studies show that black patients undergo carotid endarterectomy (CEA) less frequently than white patients. Diagnostic imaging is necessary to determine whether a patient is a candidate for the operation. We determined whether there were differences in the use of diagnostic carotid imaging and the frequency of CEA between elderly black and white ischemic stroke patients.

Methods.—Medicare fee-for-service beneficiaries with discharge diagnoses of ischemic stroke (*International Classification of Diseases, 9th revision* codes 433, 434, and 436) were randomly selected for inclusion in the National Stroke Project 1998-1999, 2000-2001. Receipt of at least one type of carotid imaging study was compared for black and white patients. Binomial logistic regression models were used to evaluate the associations between race and receipt of carotid imaging and CEA with adjustment for demographics, degree of carotid artery stenosis, and other clinical covariates.

Results.—Among 19,639 stroke patients (1974 black, 17,655 white), 69.6% received at least 1 diagnostic carotid imaging test (blacks 68.4%; whites 69.7%; $P = .233$). After risk adjustment, blacks were less likely to receive carotid imaging (adjusted odds ratio [OR] 0.87; 95% confidence interval [CI] 0.78-0.97). There was no relationship between race and the receipt of CEA after adjustment for degree of carotid stenosis and other covariates (adjusted OR 1.14; 95% CI 0.66-1.96).

Conclusions.—Black ischemic stroke patients were less likely to receive diagnostic carotid imaging than white patients, although the difference was small and only significant after risk adjustment. There was no difference in the proportion having CEA after adjustment for degree of carotid artery stenosis and other clinical factors.

▶ These authors have identified a difference in imaging studies performed but not the incidence of carotid endarterectomy in black vs white patients. Although it is reassuring that once the patients were diagnosed with severe carotid stenosis after stroke there was no difference in the rate of carotid intervention, this study does not provide information as to why black ischemic stroke patients were denied imaging studies. The randomized study of large numbers of patients from the Medicare database may guard against selection bias; however, incomplete assessment of all relevant factors that influence therapeutic decision making can inadvertently lead to incorrect conclusions. Although there were some demographic differences between white and black patients in this study, the difference in utilization of imaging studies for carotid stenosis was only statistically significant after risk adjustment. There are several problems with this study. First, of 19 629 stroke patients that were studied, only 1974 patients were black—more than an 8-fold difference in the study groups. It is possible that given the significant size difference between the black and white patient groups, different types of statistical analyses should be considered, such as propensity scoring. Second, in the methods section, the authors suggest that they assessed stroke severity in this patient population, but these data are never presented or discussed in the results or the discussion. Because it has been documented in many studies that black patients have more extensive intracranial vs extracranial vascular disease, the state of consciousness at the time of stroke is an essential factor to be considered in the decision analysis. In fact, the authors do mention in the discussion that they do not have data on whether the patients had contraindication to surgery and that they have no information regarding "clinical decision making." When it comes to assessment of interventions in patients who may be candidates for carotid intervention, it's essential to know all the variables that influence clinical decision making before suggesting a causal relationship between race and clinical decision making.

M. T. Watkins, MD

Ribosomal Protein L17, RpL17, is an Inhibitor of Vascular Smooth Muscle Growth and Carotid Intima Formation
Smolock EM, Korshunov VA, Glazko G, et al (Univ of Rochester School of Medicine & Dentistry, NY)
Circulation 126:2418-2427, 2012

Background.—Carotid intima-media thickening is associated with increased cardiovascular risk in humans. We discovered that intima formation and cell proliferation in response to carotid injury is greater in SJL/J (SJL) in comparison with C3HeB/FeJ (C3H/F) mice. The purpose of this study was to identify candidate genes contributing to intima formation.

Methods and Results.—We performed microarray and bioinformatic analyses of carotid arteries from C3H/F and SJL mice. Kyoto Encyclopedia of Genes and Genomes analysis showed that the ribosome pathway was significantly up-regulated in C3H/F in comparison with SJL mice. Expression of a ribosomal protein, RpL17, was >40-fold higher in C3H/F carotids in comparison with SJL. Aortic vascular smooth muscle cells from C3H/F grew slower in comparison to SJL. To determine the role of RpL17 in vascular smooth muscle cell growth regulation, we analyzed the relationship between RpL17 expression and cell cycle progression. Cultured vascular smooth muscle cells from mice, rats, and humans showed that RpL17 expression inversely correlated with growth as shown by decreased cells in S phase and increased cells in G_0/G_1. To prove that RpL17 acted as a growth inhibitor in vivo, we used pluronic gel delivery of RpL17 small interfering RNA to C3H/F carotid arteries. This resulted in an 8-fold increase in the number of proliferating cells. Furthermore, following partial carotid ligation in SJL mice, RpL17 expression in the intima and media decreased, but the number of proliferating cells increased.

Conclusions.—RpL17 acts as a vascular smooth muscle cell growth inhibitor (akin to a tumor suppressor) and represents a potential therapeutic target to limit carotid intima-media thickening.

▶ Using a no-flow carotid artery ligation model, this laboratory previously demonstrated that there are mouse strain—dependent differences in intima thickening that vary significantly among inbred mice. C3HeB/FeJ mice were resistant to intima formation, whereas SJL/J (SJL) mice exhibited a significant increase in intima thickening.

Using elegant microarray analysis and a combination of in vivo and in vitro techniques, these authors demonstrate a role for the ribosomal protein RpL17 in smooth muscle proliferation and possibly intimal thickening clinically associated with increased intimal-medial thickening (IMT), a clinical index of cardiovascular disease in humans. In the microarray analysis, RpL17 was the only gene that was significantly different in between-strain comparison and in sham and ligated comparisons. By using either scrambled small interfering RNA (siRNA) (siScr) or RpL17 siRNA (siRpL17) in vivo or in vitro, the authors provide convincing evidence that RpL17 inhibits vascular smooth muscle proliferation. They found that there is an inverse relationship between RpL17 expression and cell proliferation. In particular, in SJL, the number of RpL17-expressing cells was decreased and the number of proliferating cell nuclear antigen—expressing cells was increased after 1 week of injury. Thus, their in vivo data support a role for RpL17 in the regulation of intima and media cell proliferation.

The results also suggests that although RpL17 is part of the translational machinery, it is possible that its inhibitory effect on growth may exist outside the ribosome (extraribosomal) to alter cellular processes, such as cell cycle and gene transcription. These data provide evidence that RpL17 is a vascular smooth muscle cell (VSMC) growth inhibitor, akin to a tumor suppressor. This finding is significant because it is the first to show that a ribosomal protein functions to inhibit VSMC cell cycle progression and growth, making it a potential therapeutic target to limit carotid IMT. It remains to be determined whether RpL17 is downregulated in the carotid plaque of humans or whether this downregulation is related to hemodynamic or proinflammatory factors.

M. T. Watkins, MD

Cyclooxygenase-2—Derived Prostacyclin Regulates Arterial Thrombus Formation by Suppressing Tissue Factor in a Sirtuin-1—Dependent-Manner
Barbieri SS, Amadio P, Gianellini S, et al (IRCCS, Milan, Italy; Univ of Milan, Italy; et al)
Circulation 126:1373-1384, 2012

Background.—Selective inhibitors of cyclooxygenase (COX)-2 increase the risk of myocardial infarction and thrombotic events, but the responsible mechanisms are not fully understood.

Methods and Results.—We found that ferric chloride-induced arterial thrombus formation was significantly greater in COX-2 knockout compared with wild-type mice. Cross-transfusion experiments excluded the likelihood that COX-2 knockout platelets, despite enhanced aggregation responses to collagen and thrombin, are responsible for increased arterial thrombus formation in COX-2 knockout mice. Importantly, we observed that COX-2 deletion decreased prostacyclin synthase and production and peroxisome proliferator-activated receptor- and sirtuin-1 (SIRT1) expression, with consequent increased upregulation of tissue factor (TF), the primary initiator of blood coagulation. Treatment of wild-type mice with a prostacyclin receptor antagonist or a peroxisome proliferator-activated receptor-δ antagonist, which predisposes to arterial thrombosis, decreased SIRT1 expression and increased TF activity. Conversely, exogenous prostacyclin or peroxisome proliferator-activated receptor-δ agonist completely reversed the thrombotic phenotype in COX-2 knockout mice, restoring normal SIRT1 levels and reducing TF activity. Furthermore, inhibition of SIRT1 increased TF expression and activity and promoted generation of occlusive thrombi in wild-type mice, whereas SIRT1 activation was sufficient to decrease abnormal TF activity and prothrombotic status in COX-2 knockout mice.

Conclusions.—Modulation of SIRT1 and hence TF by prostacyclin/peroxisome proliferator-activated receptor-δ pathways not only represents a new mechanism in controlling arterial thrombus formation but also might be a useful target for therapeutic intervention in the atherothrombotic complications associated with COX-2 inhibitors.

▶ Selective inhibitors of cyclooxygenase-2 (COX-2) increase the risk of myocardial infarction and thrombotic events, but the responsible mechanisms are not fully understood. These authors hypothesized that COX-2 deletion in mice promotes arterial thrombosis and that this phenomenon is mediated by decreased plasma prostacyclin-2 levels, which in turn influence tissue factor (TF) expression. Expression of TF by the vessel wall or by circulating cells such as leukocytes or platelets may contribute to the generation of fibrin-rich thrombi. Circulating

TF-rich microparticles may also contribute to blood thrombogenicity. A role for TF, particularly for circulating TF, has been shown in a variety of pathologic conditions, including acute coronary syndromes, diffuse intravascular coagulopathy, endotoxinemia, and cancer.

Ferric chloride injury of the carotid artery was performed to induce thrombosis in wild-type and COX-2 deficient mice. They showed that deletion of COX-2 results in enhanced platelet aggregation in response to multiple stimuli. Cross-transfusion of wild-type platelets into thrombocytopenic COX-2 knockout mice did not reverse the increased propensity to occlusion. Moreover, when platelets derived from COX-2 knockout mice were transfused into wild-type mice, they still showed a normal thrombotic response to arterial injury.

The authors also show for the first time that endogenous plasma prostacyclin-2 strongly suppressed carotid artery thrombus formation induced by ferric chloride. Insights into the molecular mechanisms governing this phenomenon provide evidence that prostacyclin affects thrombus formation via a nonconventional pathway (ie, it inhibits TF expression via a sirtuin-1—mediated mechanism). This is an important study because COX-2 inhibitors continue to be used for management of arthritis in patients with vascular disease. It is an important follow-up to in vitro studies from our laboratory[1] that showed human microvascular endothelial cells only have COX-2, thereby suggesting that COX-2 inhibitions might promote a thrombogenic profile in vivo.

M. T. Watkins, MD

Reference

1. Watkins MT, Al-Badawi H, Russo AL, Soler H, Peterson B, Patton GM. Human microvascular endothelial cell prostaglandin E1 synthesis during in vitro ischemia-reperfusion. *J Cell Biochem.* 2004;92:472-480.

Wait times among patients with symptomatic carotid artery stenosis requiring carotid endarterectomy for stroke prevention
Jetty P, Husereau D, Kubelik D, et al (Ottawa Hosp and the Univ of Ottawa, Ontario, Canada; Univ of Ottawa, Ontario, Canada)
J Vasc Surg 56:661-667.e2, 2012

Background.—Current Canadian and international guidelines suggest patients with transient ischemic attack (TIA) or nondisabling stroke and ipsilateral internal carotid artery stenosis of 50% to 99% should be offered carotid endarterectomy (CEA) ≤2 weeks of the incident TIA or stroke. The objective of the study was to identify whether these goals are being met and the factors that most influence wait times.

Methods.—Patients who underwent CEA at the Ottawa Hospital for symptomatic carotid artery stenosis from 2008 to 2010 were identified. Time intervals based on the dates of initial symptoms, referral to and visit with a vascular surgeon, the decision to operate, and the date of surgery were recorded for each patient. The influence of various factors on wait times was explored, including age, sex, type of index event, referring physician, distance from the surgical center, degree of stenosis, and surgeon assigned.

Results.—Of the 117 patients who underwent CEA, 92 (78.6%) were symptomatic. The median time from onset of symptoms to surgery for all patients was 79 days (interquartile range [IQR], 34-161). The shortest wait times were observed in stroke patients (49 [IQR, 27-81] days) and inpatient referrals (66 [IQR, 25-103] days). Only 7 of the 92 symptomatic patients (8%) received care within the recommended 2 weeks. The median surgical wait time for all patients was 14 days (IQR, 8-25 days). In the multivariable analysis, significant predictors of longer wait times included retinal TIA ($P = .003$), outpatient referrals ($P = .004$), and distance from the center ($P = .008$). Patients who presented to the emergency department had the shortest delays in seeing a vascular surgeon and subsequently undergoing CEA ($P < .0001$). There was no difference between surgeons for wait times to be seen in the clinic; however, there were significant differences among surgeons once the decision was made to proceed with CEA.

Conclusions.—Our wait times for CEA currently do not fall within the recommended 2-week guideline nor does it appear feasible within the current system. Important factors contributing to delays include outpatient referrals, living farther from the hospital, and presenting with a retinal TIA (amaurosis fugax). Our findings also suggest better scheduling practices once a decision is made to operate can modestly improve overall and surgical wait times for CEA.

▶ In this article, the authors present an in-depth look into wait times associated with treating patients with symptomatic carotid artery disease at a tertiary referral center in Ottawa. The impetus of this study comes from a national and international recommendation that symptomatic carotid patients receive surgical treatment within 2 weeks from initial onset of symptoms.

The authors report that the median time from onset of symptoms to surgery for all patients was 79 days, and only 8% of patients were treated within the 2-week recommended timeframe. Patients with retinal transient ischemic attacks as their presenting symptom, patients referred to vascular surgeons by general practitioners or neurologists, and patients who lived farther from the referral center experienced the longest wait times. Predictors of shorter wait times were direct emergency department referrals to vascular surgeons.

The interval with the longest wait time was the interval the authors termed *T1*, defined as the time from initial symptoms to vascular referral. The median for this interval was 35 days. This study sheds light on the fact that the general public and perhaps even primary care physicians need to be better educated on the importance of timely referral to vascular surgeons when patients with carotid artery disease are symptomatic. This article encourages all physicians who treat patients with carotid artery disease to attempt to identify more efficient processes in an effort to treat symptomatic carotid artery disease sooner.

B. G. Peterson, MD

Comparison of renin and catecholamine release in patients undergoing eversion or conventional carotid endarterectomy
Demirel S, Macek L, Attigah N, et al (Ruprecht-Karls Univ, Heidelberg, Germany)
J Vasc Surg 56:324-333, 2012

Objective.—The two techniques for carotid endarterectomy (CEA)—conventional (C-CEA) and eversion (E-CEA)—have different effects on blood pressure. This study compared sympathetic activity after C-CEA and E-CEA, as measured by renin and catecholamine levels.

Methods.—E-CEA (n = 40) and C-CEA (n = 34) were performed in 74 patients with high-grade carotid stenosis. The choice of technique was made at the discretion of the operating surgeon. All patients received clonidine (150 µg) preoperatively. Regional anesthesia was used. The carotid sinus nerve was transected during E-CEA and preserved during C-CEA. Renin, metanephrine, and normetanephrine levels were measured preoperatively and at 24 and 48 hours postoperatively.

Results.—Compared with baseline, levels of renin, metanephrine, and normetanephrine decreased at 24 and 48 hours after C-CEA ($P < .0001$). After E-CEA, however, renin and normetanephrine levels were unchanged at 24 hours, and metanephrine levels were increased ($P < .0001$). At 48 hours, levels of renin ($P = .04$), metanephrine ($P < .0001$), and normetanephrine ($P = .02$) were increased. Compared with C-CEA, E-CEA was associated with significantly increased sympathetic activity at 24 and 48 hours ($P < .0001$). Although the use of vasodilators for postoperative hypertension did not differ in the postanesthesia care unit (E-CEA 35% vs C-CEA 18%, $P = .12$), vasodilator use on the ward was more frequent after E-CEA (60% vs 32%, $P = .02$).

Conclusions.—E-CEA appears to be associated with greater postoperative sympathetic activity and vasodilator requirements than C-CEA, findings likely related to sacrifice of the carotid sinus nerve during E-CEA but not C-CEA.

▶ Blood pressure and heart rate instability after carotid endarterectomy (CEA) have been extensively documented in the literature. Although the 2 techniques for CEA—conventional (C-CEA) and eversion (E-CEA)—have different effects on blood pressure, the ideal surgical technique for CEA has yet to be determined and the choice of the technique continues to be based on the personal experience and preference of the operating surgeon. E-CEA requires full mobilization of the carotid bifurcation and most often requires transection of the longitudinal nerve fibers of the carotid sinus nerve (CSN) with the loss of the baroreceptor reflex. However, disruption of the CSN fibers is less likely with conventional C-CEA because of the longitudinal arteriotomy commonly performed on the anterior surface of the vessels, with a less extensive dissection and mobilization of the carotid bifurcation. This prospective, nonrandomized study was performed in 74 patients undergoing either E-CEA, in which the carotid sinus nerve was transected, or C-CEA, in which it was preserved. Renin, metanephrine, and normetanephrine levels were measured preoperatively and at 24 and 48 hours postoperatively. They observed a differential neurohumoral effect on sympathetic nervous system activity, with an increase after E-CEA and a decrease after C-CEA. These findings add further credence to a decrease in baroreceptor sensitivity after E-CEA, a decrease most certainly the result of transection of the longitudinal CSN fibers during that procedure. Also, the observation of improved hemodynamic stability in the C-CEA group provides evidence that the metanephrine and norme-tanephrine findings may underlie the clinical manifestations observed in prior studies. As the authors state, longer-term comparative studies will be necessary to ascertain whether these effects persist and, if so, to determine any effect they might have on long-term cardiovascular morbidity. Other adverse events that should be examined are periprocedural stroke, death, restenosis, or local compli-cations. Indeed, many reviews comparing E-CEA and C-CEA have concluded that there is no evidence that one technique is superior to the other.

J. Cullen, PhD

Variability in Carotid Endarterectomy Practice Patterns Within a Metropolitan Area

Kansara A, Miller D, Damani R, et al (Wayne State Univ, Detroit, MI; Henry Ford Hosp, Detroit, MI; et al)
Stroke 43:3105-3107, 2012

Background and Purpose.—Previous clinical studies have suggested that patients with carotid stenosis with high surgical risk features may fare better with carotid artery stenting or aggressive medical therapy. The extent to which carotid endarterectomy is still being performed in this group of patients is unclear.

Methods.—A retrospective audit was performed among 4 hospitals over a 2-year period. The proportion of high surgical risk patients was compared and the in-hospital stroke, myocardial infarction, and death rates were compared among conventional and high surgical risk patients.

Results.—Three hundred thirty-five carotid endarterectomy operations were performed (63% asymptomatic) with 37.9% being high surgical risk subjects. The stroke, myocardial infarction, and death rate was 4.6% in conventional risk subjects and 10.2% in high surgical risk patients ($P < 0.05$). The only hospital with multidisciplinary carotid conferences had the lowest proportion of carotid endarterectomy operations in asymp-tomatic patients.

Conclusions.—A substantial proportion of carotid endarterectomy oper-ations are performed in patients with high surgical risk features. These patients experienced a 2-fold increase in major in-hospital complications, raising doubts about whether they benefit from carotid surgery. The use of preintervention multidisciplinary conferences may improve patient safety.

▶ This article is a must read for surgeons who perform carotid endarterectomy. In asymptomatic patients with a high-grade carotid stenosis, the debate continues on the value of surgical intervention. This study, which combined data from 4 institutions, had a very high rate of the composite endpoint (myocardial infarction, stroke, and death) in patients deemed to be at high surgical risk. The significance and safety of operating on asymptomatic patients once again is challenged. Perhaps we, as surgeons, need to be comfortable with the choice of best medical therapy and observation alone.

Hospitals that use multidisciplinary teaching conferences in which specific cases and individual patients are discussed among several specialties had a lower event rate and a lower percentage of asymptomatic patients who required surgical intervention. Neurologists should be included in the decision-making process. In addition, life expectancy is also discussed in this article as an important variable to consider when possible intervention may occur. To achieve benefit from carotid endarterectomy, a minimal life expectancy of 5 years is recommended by some current guidelines. I believe this well-written article adds to the overall uncertainty concerning intervention on asymptomatic stenoses.

R. L. Bush, MD, MPH

Very Urgent Carotid Endarterectomy Confers Increased Procedural Risk
Strömberg S, for the Swedish Vascular Registry (Swedvasc) Steering Committee (Sahlgrenska Univ Hosp, Gothenburg, Sweden; et al)
Stroke 43:1331-1335, 2012

Background and Purpose.—Current Swedish guidelines recommend that carotid endarterectomy should be performed within 14 days of a qualifying neurological event, but it is not clear if very urgent surgery after an event is associated with increased perioperative risk. The aim of this study was to determine how the time between the event and carotid endarterectomy affects the procedural risk of mortality and stroke.

Methods.—We prospectively analyzed data on all patients who underwent carotid endarterectomies for symptomatic carotid stenosis between May 12, 2008, and May 31, 2011, with records in the Swedish Vascular Registry (Swedvasc). Patients were divided according to time between the qualifying event and surgery (0–2 days, 3–7 days, 8–14 days, 15–180 days). Stroke rate and mortality at 30 days postsurgery were determined.

Results.—We analyzed data for 2596 patients and found that the combined mortality and stroke rate for patients treated 0 to 2 days after qualifying event was 11.5% (17 of 148) versus 3.6% (29 of 804), 4.0% (27 of 677), and 5.4% (52 of 967) for the groups treated at 3 to 7 days, 8 to 14 days, and 15 to 180 days, respectively. In a multivariate analysis, time was an independent risk factor for perioperative complications: patients treated at 0 to 2 days had a relative OR of 4.24 (CI, 2.07–8.70; $P < 0.001$) compared with the reference 3-to 7-day group.

Conclusions.—In this study of patients treated for symptomatic carotid disease, it was safe to perform surgery as early as Day 3 after a qualifying neurological event in contrast to patients treated within 0 to 2 days, which has a significantly increased perioperative risk.

▶ The timing of carotid endarterectomy following an ischemic neurologic event has been a moving target, ranging from immediate intervention to a delay of many weeks. Proponents of early intervention for carotid disease feel that way because of the high risk of a recurrent cerebrovascular event in the first few days after an initial ischemic event. This risk has to be balanced with the periprocedural risk associated with early intervention. Many of us have been taught that carotid endarterectomy (CEA) should be performed once a patient has been neurologically stabilized. This interesting population-based study of over 2700 patients with symptomatic carotid stenoses stratified patients according to timing of the CEA. The risk of stroke and death significantly decreased after day 2 following the initial neurologic event.

These data further support the current guidelines recommending early intervention from 3 to 14 days with the caveat that CEA performed from day 0 to day 2 was associated with a much higher risk. Furthermore, diabetes and female sex were also found to be independent risk factors, along with the timing of the operation. Thus, those of us who perform this particular operation have even more data to take away from this excellent article in terms of patient selection for early intervention. Guidelines for carotid revascularization are not set-in-stone protocols. Rather, they are recommended practices that allow some discretion or leeway in their interpretation, implementation, or use. Not all patients are created equal, as we know, so using our knowledge and experience supplemented by guidelines and published studies should translate into excellent patient outcomes.

R. L. Bush, MD, MPH

Perioperative Approach in the Surgical Management of Carotid Body Tumors
Zhang T-H, Jiang W-L, Li Y-L, et al (The Second Affiliated Hosp of Harbin Med Univ, People's Republic of China; et al)
Ann Vasc Surg 26:775-782, 2012

Background.—Now, surgical resection still remains the gold standard for the treatment of carotid body tumors (CBTs). Although advances in surgical techniques and the introduction of sensitive imaging modalities have significantly reduced mortality, the incidence of perioperative neurovascular complications, especially cranial nerve deficit and intraoperative hemorrhage, remains considerable. To solve these problems, preoperative embolization has been suggested; the reported benefits of preoperative embolization performed < 48 hours before surgery include a reduction in tumor size, decreased blood loss, and improved visualization, theoretically reducing neurologic morbidity by lessening the risk of stroke and damage to cranial nerves. The purpose of this study was to review our experience in the surgical management of CBTs with preoperative embolization and evaluate the outcomes and complications according to the Shamblin classification.

Methods.—Thirty-two patients who had been diagnosed with and surgically treated for CBTs were enrolled from January 2005 till July 2010. All perioperative scans were evaluated by computed tomography angiography. We reviewed patient demographics, radiographic findings, and surgical outcomes collected from medical records.

Results.—Thirty-two patients underwent surgical excision without mortality. Angiography with selective preoperative tumor embolization was performed on 21 patients. The median blood loss, operation time, and hospital stay for these patients were significantly reduced compared with those without embolization. There were no recurrences or delayed complications at the median follow-up of 20 months.

Conclusion.—Embolization as an adjunctive tool was beneficial for CBT surgery outcomes. Embolization should only be undertaken in those vessels that can be subselectively catheterized and determined not to allow free reflux of contrast medium into the internal carotid artery. Tumor embolization was performed on patients with Cook detachable coils, which are highly effective for supply artery closure if properly selected, and complications can be minimized by proper selection and positioning of the coil. Operation within 48 hours after embolization is recommended to minimize revascularization edema or a local inflammatory response.

▶ An uncommon entity seen in vascular practices, but one of the most interesting, is a carotid body tumor. Perioperative management, particularly whether or not to embolize the feeding artery, has been controversial. The advocates of preoperative embolization, including these authors, highlight decreased rates of intraoperative hemorrhage and cranial nerve injury. Others emphasize the unnecessary risks including difficulty in selecting small feeding vessels and reflux of embolic material into the internal carotid artery resulting in neurological damage. Other benefits seen in this small series included shorter operative times and hospital stays in the group that underwent embolization. However, to realize these benefits, one must have a truly skilled interventional radiologist or neuroradiologist who is familiar with microcatheter and super-selective techniques.

This article has many teaching points for vascular surgeons. The authors review the history of carotid body tumors and the Shamblin classification as well as surgical techniques and complications. They stress the importance of early detection and how this has been realized with the advent of rapid, high-resolution computed tomography. Thus, a team approach can be planned and coordinated with needed specialists for embolization, resection, head and neck dissection, and so on. Also, a teaching point made is that complete embolization is not necessary to decrease tumor size and vascularity. This technical tip should also result in a decrease in the overall risk of embolization procedure.

R. L. Bush, MD, MPH

Regional versus general anesthesia for carotid endarterectomy: The American College of Surgeons National Surgical Quality Improvement Program perspective

Schechter MA, Shortell CK, Scarborough JE (Duke Univ Med Ctr, Durham, NC)
Surgery 152:309-314, 2012

Background.—The ideal anesthetic technique for carotid endarterectomy remains a matter of debate. This study used the American College of Surgeons National Surgical Quality Improvement Program to evaluate the influence of anesthesia modality on outcomes after carotid endarterectomy.

Methods.—Postoperative outcomes were compared for American College of Surgeons National Surgical Quality Improvement Program patients undergoing carotid endarterectomy between 2005 and 2009 with either general or regional anesthesia. A separate analysis was performed on a subset of patients matched on propensity for undergoing carotid endarterectomy with regional anesthesia.

Results.—For the entire sample of 24,716 National Surgical Quality Improvement Program patients undergoing carotid endarterectomy and the propensity-matched cohort of 8,050 patients, there was no difference in the 30-day postoperative composite stroke/myocardial infarction/death rate based on anesthetic type. Within the matched cohort, the rate of other complications did not differ (2.8% regional vs 3.6% general anesthesia; $P = .07$), but patients receiving regional anesthesia had shorter operative (99 ± 36 minutes vs 119 ± 53 minutes; $P < .0001$) and anesthesia times (52 ± 29 minutes vs 64 ± 37 minutes; $P < .0001$) and were more likely to be discharged the next day (77.0% vs 64.4%; $P < .0001$).

Conclusion.—Anesthesia technique does not impact patient outcomes after carotid endarterectomy, but may influence overall cost of care.

▶ This study is an excellent example of using the American College of Surgeons National Surgical Quality Improvement Program (ACS-NSQIP) database to analyze a question or hypothesis with national prospectively collected data representing a wide variety of practices and surgeons. These authors examined outcomes following carotid endarterectomy (CEA) under either regional anesthesia (RA) or general anesthesia (GA). It has been stated in the literature that regional anesthesia is associated with lower cardiopulmonary complications. However, the effect of anesthetic type on postoperative outcomes has not been clear with varying outcomes. Using a large national dataset that has been validated and is tightly controlled, the ACS-NSQIP can offer insights into practices, outcomes, and may guide surgeons with their own decision-making.

In the centers participating in this database, the use of GA was more common (4:1) than RA. No differences were seen in postoperative morbidity and mortality rates. The major impact was seen in shorter operative times with patients who had RA. Because there is no time needed for anesthetic induction or waking the patient, the time needed for the surgical case is shortened. Furthermore, as I am a proponent of RA, time is saved in not placing an indwelling bladder catheter or other invasive monitoring lines. Additionally, the patient spends less time in the postoperative recovery room, may be easily admitted to a ward rather than an intensive care unit, and generally is more awake and tolerates a diet soon after the operation. The major caveat is that the surgeon and anesthesiologist must maintain open lines of communication about the patient's neurologic status, especially for selective shunt usage. This article is an excellent study and a must-read for surgeons who perform CEA. The major message is that one can select the type of anesthesia that will most benefit the patient and the surgeon without worry concerning the effect of anesthesia on perioperative outcomes.

R. L. Bush, MD, MPH

The need for emergency surgical treatment in carotid-related stroke in evolution and crescendo transient ischemic attack
Capoccia L, Sbarigia E, Speziale F, et al ("Sapienza" Univ of Rome, Italy)
J Vasc Surg 55:1611-1617, 2012

Objective.—The purpose of this study was to examine the safety of emergency carotid endarterectomy (CEA) in patients with carotid stenosis and unstable neurological symptoms.

Methods.—This prospective, single-center study involved patients with stroke in evolution (SIE) or fluctuating stroke or crescendo transient ischemic attack (cTIA) related to a carotid stenosis $\geq 50\%$ who underwent emergency surgery. Preoperative workup included National Institute of Health Stroke Scale (NIHSS) neurological assessment on admission, immediately before surgery and at discharge, carotid duplex scan, brain contrast-enhanced head computed tomography (CT) or magnetic resonance imaging (MRI). End points were perioperative (30-day) neurological mortality, NIHSS score variation, and hemorrhagic or ischemic stroke recurrence. Patients were evaluated according to clinical presentation (SIE or cTIA), timing of surgery, and presence of brain infarction on neuroimaging.

Results.—Between January 2005 and December 2009, 48 patients were submitted to emergency surgery. CEAs were performed from 1 to 24 hours from onset of symptoms (mean, 10.16 ± 7.75). Twenty-six patients presented an SIE with a worsening NIHSS score between admission and surgery, and 22 presented ≥ 3 cTIAs with a normal NIHSS score (= 0) immediately before surgery. An ischemic brain lesion was detected in four patients with SIE and eight patients with cTIA. All patients with cTIA presented a persistent NIHSS normal score before and after surgery. Twenty-five patients with SIE presented an NIHSS score improvement after surgery. Mean NIHSS score was 5.30 ± 2.81 before surgery and 0.54 ± 0.77 at discharge in the SIE group ($P < .0001$). One patient with SIE had a hemorrhagic transformation of an undetected brain ischemic lesion after surgery, with progressive neurological deterioration and death (2%).

Conclusions.—Due to the absence of randomized controlled trials of CEA for neurologically unstable patients, data currently available do not support a policy of emergency CEA in those patients. Our results suggest that a fast protocol, including CT scans and carotid duplex ultrasound scans in neurologically unstable patients, could help identify those that can be safely submitted to emergency CEA.

▶ The controversy and debate over when to operate on a symptomatic carotid lesion continues. We do know that waiting longer periods, up to 6 to 8 weeks, increases the chance of a recurrent cerebrovascular ischemic event. However, how early is too early? In patients with ongoing active symptoms, when should intervention occur? We know that the brain is at risk in these patients and the carotid plaque is unusually unstable with ongoing active ischemic events. This group from Italy has an aggressive approach to patients with unstable neurological symptoms and no evidence of brain infarct on imaging. Capoccia and colleagues choose to perform carotid endarterectomy within 24 hours of the onset of neurological symptoms, either crescendo transient ischemic attacks or strokes-in-evolution. Their results are commendable in the 47 patients included in the cohort, with most only suffering from hemorrhagic transformation.

Most interesting is the description of their strict postoperative care and hemodynamic monitoring. The patients were continued on intravenous heparin after carotid endarterectomy with very tight blood pressure management. I am very impressed with the strong collaboration with their neurology colleagues on a routine basis. Interdisciplinary approaches to patient care are becoming more commonplace and ensure all aspects of patient-centered care are identified.

R. L. Bush, MD, MPH

Carotid Endarterectomy Plus Medical Therapy or Medical Therapy Alone for Carotid Artery Stenosis in Symptomatic or Asymptomatic Patients: A Meta-Analysis
Guay J, Ochroch EA (Univ of Montréal, Quebec, Canada; Univ of Pennsylvania Health System, Philadelphia)
J Cardiothorac Vasc Anesth 26:835-844, 2012

Objective.—The purpose of this study was to compare carotid endarterectomy (CEA) plus medical therapy (MT) with MT alone for symptomatic and asymptomatic patients suffering from carotid artery stenosis in terms of long-term stroke/death rate.

Design.—A meta-analysis of parallel randomized, controlled trials (RCTs) (blind or open) published in English.

Setting.—A university-based electronic search.

Participants.—Patients suffering from carotid artery stenosis symptomatic or not.

Interventions.—Patients were subjected to CEA plus MT or MT alone.

Measurements and Main Results.—For asymptomatic patients, 6 RCTs comprising 5,733 patients (CEA = 2,853 and MT = 2,880) were included. CEA did not affect the stroke/death risk for asymptomatic patients (risk ratio [RR] = 0.93; 95% confidence interval [CI], 0.84 to 1.02; $I^2 = 0\%$;

$p = 0.14$). For symptomatic patients, 2 RCTs were included. They had 5,627 patients (CEA = 3,069 and MT = 2,558) of whom 2,295 patients (CEA = 1,213; MT = 1,082) had severe stenosis (North American Symptomatic Carotid Endarterectomy Trial [NASCET] technique ≥ 50% and European Carotid Surgery Trial technique ≥ 70%). CEA decreased the stroke/death risk only for patients with severe stenosis (RR = 0.69; 95% CI, 0.59-0.81; $p < 0.001$ [random effects model]; $I^2 = 0\%$ on the odds ratio and 17% on the RR [benefit or harm side]; number needed to treat = 11 [95% CI, 8-17]).

Conclusions.—CEA is helpful for recently symptomatic patients with carotid artery stenosis ≥ 50% (NASCET technique) but adds no benefit in terms of stroke/death for asymptomatic patients.

▶ The controversy being debated currently is whether intervention on an asymptomatic carotid artery stenosis is worth the risk to prevent a future neurological event. The past and very traditional recommendations have been that carotid artery endarterectomy (CEA) with the addition of medial therapy has been the gold standard for high-grade asymptomatic lesions. On the other hand, the evidence for early intervention in a person who has a symptomatic lesion is well established and does not spark any debate. This systematic review of randomized, controlled trials (RCT) published in English is a must-read for those involved and interested in this debate. Whether the article changes your mind, it is a well-written, concise amalgamation of all known data from the RCTs available. It is a good review of the RCTs, which the authors point out were all published prior to 2004, performed for both symptomatic and asymptomatic patients. It is also important to point out that medial management and pharmacotherapy has changed significantly in the interim since many of the RCTs were performed with new data, new drugs, and improved recommendations.

Critics of RCTs claim that this type of study design does not reflect real-world experience and what is actually happening in the community. Unfortunately, many of the real-world patients that one sees in a general vascular practice are older, frailer, and have many more comorbid conditions than that which would be allowed under most RCT inclusion criteria. Furthermore, women are not well represented in the trials, thus leaving one to wonder if the results can be extrapolated between genders. Despite these limitations, this meta-analysis is an excellent contribution to the literature, and it is very doubtful if RCTs randomizing CEA to best medical therapy will be repeated in the future.

R. L. Bush, MD, MPH

A 20-year Experience with Surgical Management of True and False Internal Carotid Artery Aneurysms

Pulli R, Dorigo W, Alessi Innocenti A, et al (Univ of Florence, Italy)
Eur J Vasc Endovasc Surg 45:1-6, 2013

Aim of the Study.—The aim of this study was to retrospectively analyse early and late results of surgical management of internal carotid artery (ICA) true and false aneurysms in a single-centre experience.

Materials and Methods.—From January 1988 to December 2011, 50 consecutive interventions for ICA aneurismal disease were performed; interventions were performed for true ICA aneurysm in 19 cases (group 1) and for ICA post-carotid endarterectomy (CEA) pseudo-aneurysm in the remaining 31 (group 2). Early results (<30 days) were evaluated in terms of mortality, stroke and cranial nerves' injury and compared between the two groups with χ^2 test.

Follow-up results (stroke free-survival, freedom from ICA thrombosis and reintervention) were analysed with Kaplan—Meier curves and compared with log-rank test.

Results.—All the patients in group 1 had open repair of their ICA aneurysm; in group 2 open repair was performed in 30 cases, while three patients with post-CEA aneurysm without signs of infection had a covered stent placed. There were no perioperative deaths. Two major strokes occurred in group 1 and one major stroke occurred in group 2 ($p = 0.1$). The rates of postoperative cranial nerve injuries were 10.5% in group 1 and 13% in group 2 ($p = 0.8$).

Median duration of follow-up was 60 months (range 1-276). Estimated 10-year stroke-free survival rates were 64% in group 1 and 37% in group 2 ($p = 0.4$, log rank 0.5); thrombosis-free survival at 10 years was 66% in group 1 and 34% in group 2 ($p = 0.2$, log rank 1.2), while the corresponding figures in terms of reintervention-free survival were 68% and 33%, respectively ($p = 0.2$, log rank 1.8).

Conclusions.—Surgical treatment of ICA aneurismal disease provided in our experience satisfactory early and long-term results, without significant differences between true and false aneurysms. In carefully selected patients with non-infected false aneurysm, the endovascular option seems to be feasible.

▶ This is an interesting article describing the treatment of 50 true and false carotid artery aneurysms over a 50-year timeframe at a single institution. Although practice patterns and approaches have changed in that lengthy period, many excellent teaching points can be extracted from this series. Although this series had 19 of 50 cases that were true aneurysms, I suspect most of us will mainly see post—carotid endarterectomy, or false, aneurysms. Because of distortion of structures in the neck from the aneurysm, mainly nerves, an endovascular approach has been stated to be the safer treatment modality. The authors' conclusion that "the endovascular option seems to be feasible" is rather weak given the excellent outcomes that they achieved. One should assume that endovascular repair in skilled hands should be feasible; the major question to answer in the article's conclusion is whether it is a superior treatment option.

A vascular surgeon needs to individualize care and be able to provide a full array of treatment options given a specific patient and disease. Having a large armamentarium of treatment modalities in one's skill set, including traditional open repair, will allow for directed patient care and, thus, first-rate outcomes. Another topic to guide care that can be gained from this study is the importance of serial follow-up studies in patients who have had carotid endarterectomies to assess not only for recurrent disease but also for the development of a false aneurysm. If found early after carotid endarterectomy, the surgeon needs to consider an occult infection as the etiology. Late development is most likely caused by degeneration of the artery at the suture line. Similarly, duplex scanning needs to be performed after open aneurysm repair to detect recurrent aneurismal disease.

R. L. Bush, MD, MPH

Modified Eversion Carotid Endarterectomy
Kumar S, Lombardi JV, Alexander JB, et al (Rowan Univ, Camden, NJ)
Ann Vasc Surg 27:178-185, 2013

Background.—Eversion carotid endarterectomy is a well-described technique for carotid endarterectomy (CEA). The advantage of this technique is a completely autogenous repair. We describe a modification of eversion endarterectomy (MEE) that expeditiously extracts the plaque through a linear incision over the common carotid artery and the proximal bulbous internal carotid artery (ICA) only, allowing primary closure. Selective shunting can also be performed without difficulty.

Methods.—A retrospective review of CEAs using MEE at two institutions by three vascular surgeons during a 5-year period was performed. Data were collected from the medical records, with institutional review board approval. Information regarding neurologic symptoms, degree of ICA stenosis, CEA technique, ICA clamp time, shunting, electroencephalographic monitoring, and postoperative complications was tabulated. Rate of significant restenosis (stenosis >50% by duplex criteria) was also calculated during the follow-up period.

Results.—Between 2005 and 2009, a total of 221 patients underwent MEE for carotid artery stenosis (CAS): 69 patients (31%) underwent MEE for symptomatic and 152 (68.8%) underwent MEE for asymptomatic CAS. Neuromonitoring in the form of electroencephalography was used in 85 (39%) patients, and an intraluminal shunt was used in 29 patients (13%) who had either severe contralateral disease or a previous ipsilateral cerebral infarction. Postoperative complications included transient ischemic attack (four, 2%), cerebral infarction (three, 1%), myocardial infarction (three, 1%), and hematoma (six, 3%). Four patients (2%) required a return to the operating room (OR). within 24 hours for hematoma (one, 1%) or postoperative neurologic deficit (three, %). The 30-day mortality was 1%. One patient (1%) required patch angioplasty because of the extent of disease and inability to obtain a good end point. Average cross-clamp time for MEE was 12.8 minutes. Two patients (1%) were reported to have hemodynamically significant restenosis within 2 years, with one patient requiring intervention.

Conclusions.—MEE is a safe and effective way of treating CAS, with acceptable morbidity, mortality, and low rate of recurrent stenosis despite the absence of a patch. Given the brief clamp time required, routine shunting and/or neuromonitoring for this technique may have questionable clinical value and expense.

▶ There are several techniques that one needs to be familiar with and comfortable performing when doing a carotid endarterectomy (CEA). Having an armamentarium of skills available allows one to individualize an operation to the patient, his/her anatomy and cerebral circulation, and the neurologic changes that can occur in the operating room. Whether one performs CEAs under regional or general anesthesia is immaterial to the technique that is used; the important aspect is the skill of the operating surgeon and the judgment involved in choosing a specific technique.

This article details a modification of a standard eversion technique without complete transection of the internal carotid artery. The authors have perfected this skill with very short clamp times with selective shunting. The clinical outcomes are similar to other studies of varying CEA techniques. These authors did use intraoperative electroencephalogram monitoring in a large percentage of patients, which greatly adds to nonreimbursable expenses and also involves preoperative setup time and additional personnel. One of the major controversies and challenges to achieving buy-in and widespread adoption of eversion CEA, regardless of whether it is modified, is the perceived risk of restenosis. Without the use of a patch, one may hypothesize that restenosis rates would be increased over patch angioplasty. However, this study, albeit with only 2-year data, had acceptable restenosis rates. Similarly, other published literature has shown no difference in comparing eversion with patch angioplasty. I recommend vascular surgeons read this article and study the technique. It is easy and expeditious to perform and may be a good option for select individual patients.

R. L. Bush, MD, MPH

Early versus delayed carotid endarterectomy in symptomatic patients

Annambhotla S, Park MS, Keldahl ML, et al (Northwestern Univ Feinberg School of Medicine, Chicago, IL)
J Vasc Surg 56:1296-1302, 2012

Background.—Delayed carotid endarterectomy (CEA) after a stroke or transient ischemic attack (TIA) is associated with risks of recurrent neurologic symptoms. In an effort to preserve cerebral function, urgent early CEA has been recommended in many circumstances. We analyzed outcomes of different time intervals in early CEA in comparison with delayed treatment.

Study Design.—Retrospective chart review from a single university hospital tertiary care center between April 1999 and November 2010 revealed 312 patients who underwent CEA following stroke or TIA. Of these 312 patients, 69 received their CEA within 30 days of symptom onset and 243 received their CEA after 30 days from symptom onset. The early CEA cohort was further stratified according to the timing of surgery: group A (27 patients), within 7 days; group B (17), between 8 and 14 days; group C (12), between 15 and 21 days; and group D (12), between 22 and 30 days. Demographic data as well as 30-day (mortality, stroke, TIA, and myocardial infarction) and long-term (all-cause mortality and stroke) adverse outcome rates were analyzed for each group. These were also analyzed for the entire early CEA cohort and compared against the delayed CEA group.

Results.—Demographics and comorbid conditions were similar between groups. For 30-day outcomes, there were no deaths, 1 stroke (1.4%), 0 TIAs, and 0 myocardial infarctions in the early CEA cohort; in the delayed CEA cohort, there were 4 (1.6%), 4 (1.6%), 2 (0.8%), and 2 (0.8%) patients with these outcomes, respectively ($P > .05$ for all comparisons). Over the long term, the early group had one ipsilateral stroke at 17 months and the delayed group had two ipsilateral strokes at 3 and 12 months. For long-term outcomes, there were 16 deaths in the early CEA cohort (21%) and 74 deaths in the delayed CEA cohort (30%, $P > .05$). Mean follow-up times were 4.5 years in the early CEA cohort and 5.8 years in the delayed CEA cohort.

Conclusions.—There were no differences in 30-day and long-term adverse outcome rates between the early and delayed CEA cohorts. In symptomatic carotid stenosis patients without evidence of intracerebral hemorrhage, carotid occlusion, or permanent neurologic deficits early carotid endarterectomy can be safely performed and is preferred over delaying operative treatment.

▶ This article is a fabulous example of one vascular group closely analyzing its outcomes when following different practice patterns in order to perform quality improvement. Every surgeon must periodically review his or her outcomes for the purposes of providing excellent care and assessing any need for change. The timing for performing a carotid endarterectomy (CEA) in a symptomatic patient has been argued with much controversy. The fear of a delayed approach is an increased rate of ischemic events, and the fear of an early intervention is intra-operative stroke and ischemic to hemorrhagic conversion. With several surgeons practicing either early or late surgical intervention for symptomatic carotid disease, this busy group from Northwestern University critically analyzed both practice patterns and reported their results.

We cannot control factors related to patient delays in presentation or provider to surgeon referral, but we can look at the overall individual patient and control our preference in operative timing. The results of this study, encompassing more than 300 patients with symptomatic disease, demonstrate no difference in adverse cardiovascular event rates between the early and late cohorts. Practice patterns in this group and many others have evolved toward an earlier, more aggressive approach to the symptomatic patient. Furthermore, the 2011 Society for Vascular Surgery guidelines advocate an early (within 2 weeks of the neurologic event) approach. I think it is safe to say that this study and others have put to rest the old recommendation of delaying CEA following an acute stroke from 4 to 6 weeks.

R. L. Bush, MD, MPH

Regional use of combined carotid endarterectomy/coronary artery bypass graft and the effect of patient risk

Jones DW, Stone DH, Conrad MF, et al (New York Presbyterian Hosp; Dartmouth-Hitchcock Med Ctr, Lebanon, NH; Massachusetts General Hosp, Boston; et al)
J Vasc Surg 56:668-676, 2012

Introduction.—Although carotid artery stenosis and coronary artery disease often coexist, many debate which patients are best served by combined concurrent revascularization (carotid endarterectomy [CEA]/coronary artery bypass graft [CABG]). We studied the use of CEA/CABG in New England and compared indications and outcomes, including stratification by risk, symptoms, and performing center.

Methods.—Using data from the Vascular Study Group of New England from 2003 to 2009, we studied all patients who underwent combined CEA/CABG across six centers in New England. Our main outcome measure was in-hospital stroke or death. We compared outcomes between all patients undergoing combined CEA/CABG to a baseline CEA risk group comprised of patients undergoing isolated CEA at non-CEA/CABG centers. Further, we compared in-hospital stroke and death rates between high and low neurologic risk patients, defining high neurologic risk patients as those who had at least one of the following clinical or anatomic features: (1) symptomatic carotid disease, (2) bilateral carotid stenosis >70%, (3) ipsilateral stenosis >70% and contralateral occlusion, or (4) ipsilateral or bilateral occlusion.

Results.—Overall, compared to patients undergoing isolated CEA at non-CEA/CABG centers (n = 1563), patients undergoing CEA/CABG (n = 109) were more likely to have diabetes (44% vs 29%; $P = .001$), creatinine > 1.8 mg/dL (11% vs 5%; $P = .007$), and congestive heart failure (23% vs 10%; $P < .001$). Patients undergoing CEA/CABG were also more likely to take preoperative beta-blockers (94% vs 75%; $P < .001$) and less likely to take preoperative clopidogrel (7% vs 25%; $P < .001$). Patients undergoing CEA/CABG had higher rates of contralateral carotid occlusion (13% vs 5%; $P = .001$) and were more likely to undergo an urgent/emergent procedure (30% vs 15%; $P < .001$). The risk of complications was higher in CEA/CABG compared to isolated CEA, including increased risk of stroke (5.5% vs 1.2%; $P < .001$), death (5.5% vs 0.3%; $P < .001$), and return to the operating room for any reason (7.6% vs 1.2%; $P < .001$). Of 109 patients undergoing CEA/CABG, 61 (56%) were low neurologic risk and 48 (44%) were high neurologic risk but showed no demonstrable difference in stroke

(4.9% vs 6.3%; $P = .76$), death, (4.9 vs 6.3%; $P = .76$), or return to the operating room (10.2% vs 4.3%; $P = .25$).

Conclusion.—Although practice patterns in the use of CEA/CABG vary across our region, the risk of complications with CEA/CABG remains significantly higher than in isolated CEA. Future work to improve patient selection in CEA/CABG is needed to improve perioperative results with combined coronary and carotid revascularization.

▶ This article should be read both because of its scientific value and as an emphasis on the ongoing controversy about combined concurrent carotid endarterectomy (CEA) and coronary artery bypass graft (CABG) procedures. This topic has been much debated in the past, with most studies demonstrating worse outcomes when the 2 procedures are performed in the same setting as compared with separately. The Vascular Study Group of New England has provided many valuable additions to the literature, and this manuscript highlights another accomplishment from this dataset. The results from this cohort show that combined CEA/CABG procedures are not common and that the patients having concurrent operations have a higher burden of concomitant comorbidities. No doubt this sicker, frailer subset of patients is at much higher risk for adverse perioperative events, including stroke and death. This may be a risk that is not due to the procedures themselves but to the additive comorbid factors. Unfortunately for these patients who need combined CEA/CABG, a higher operative risk profile is present along with increased rates of complications, including possible stroke and death. As seen by the fact that less than 2% of the CEAs from this dataset involve a concomitant CABG, patient selection is with much trepidation.

Again, I congratulate the Vascular Study Group of New England and its participating institutions for critically analyzing their outcomes, actively publishing the results, and providing guidance to practitioners. An interesting fact to contemplate is that three-fourths of the patients having combined CEA/CABG had asymptomatic carotid disease. As far as a take-home message concerning patient selection, a surgeon needs to truly consider the implications of subjecting a patient with asymptomatic carotid disease to a combined procedure unless one can demonstrate equivalent outcomes regardless of symptomatic status.

R. L. Bush, MD, MPH

Eversion Carotid Endarterectomy—Our Experience After 20 Years of Carotid Surgery and 9897 Carotid Endarterectomy Procedures
Radak D, Tanasković S, Matić P, et al (Univ of Belgrade, Republic of Serbia)
Ann Vasc Surg 26:924-928, 2012

Background.—The aim of this article is to review our experience in surgical treatment of carotid atherosclerosis using eversion carotid endarterectomy (eCEA) in 9,897 patients performed in the last 20 years, with particular attention to diagnostic approach, surgical technique, medical therapy, and final outcome.

Methods.—From January 1991 to December 2010, 9,897 primary eCEAs were performed for high-grade carotid stenosis. Patients treated for restenosis after previous carotid surgery were excluded from the analysis. Follow-up included routine clinical evaluation and noninvasive surveillance, with duplex scanning, 1 and 6 months after surgery, and annually afterward.

Results.—The majority of the patients were symptomatic (stroke, 42.8%; transient ischemic attack, 55.1% [focal cerebral and retinal ischemia]), whereas only 2.1% of the patients were asymptomatic. For the final diagnosis, duplex scanning was performed in 83.4% of patients and angiography in only 16.3% ($P < 0.001$). Average carotid artery clamping time was 11.9 ± 3.2 minutes, and the majority of the patients were operated under general anesthesia (99.4%). Intraoperative shunting and local anesthesia were rarely performed; 0.6% of the patients were operated under local anesthesia, and in 0.5% of the patients, intraluminal shunt was used. Neurological and total morbidity showed a steady decline over time, with rate of neurological morbidity of 1.1% and total morbidity of 3.9% at the end of 2010. Neurological mortality and total mortality also showed a steady decline over time, with rate of neurological mortality of 0.3% and total mortality of 0.8% at the end of 2010. There was a low rate of both, nonsignificant restenosis (<50%), which was verified in 2.1% of the patients, and significant restenosis (>50%), which was observed in 4.3% of the patients.

Conclusion.—Our data show that eCEA is a reliable surgical technique for the treatment of atherosclerotic carotid disease, with low morbidity and mortality. The specificity of our experience is the significant number of patients with preoperative stroke, but despite this fact, results are comparable with previously published series. It also highlights the importance of comprehensive surgical training in reducing complications.

▶ This is a very large experience of eversion carotid endarterectomy (eCEA) spanning 20 years at the University of Belgrade in the Republic of Serbia. Not often are we entitled to a glimpse into the practice patterns of this country, which compare drastically with those of the United States. Including almost 10 000 patients, this cohort is quite unique in that it contains 97.9% symptomatic patients and 2.1% asymptomatic patients. Also distinctive is that 83.4% of the patients had a Duplex scan as their sole preoperative imaging study. Furthermore, the operative data are also worth mentioning with an average carotid clamp time of 11.9 minutes and only 0.5% of the cohort having an intraluminal shunt. This is a much shorter clamp time needed than when a patch is routinely used. The rate of neurological complications was low at 1.1% overall, and the restenosis rate that is often a concern after eCEA was 4.3%.

This study is impressive in many ways, including the cohort size, the very high percentage of symptomatic patients treated, the low shunt rate, and the short- and long-term outcomes rates. The authors justify the low shunt rate based on the very short carotid clamp time, and this ideology is further justified by the superior outcomes they achieve. This may seem like an arbitrary decision-making process, but there are complications associated with routine shunting. One question that I do have is the need to stop all antiplatelet therapy 1 week before the eCEA.

Maintaining patients on at least aspirin has not been shown to be associated with increased bleeding or postoperative hematoma rates. Aspirin protects the carotid, the brain and, ultimately, the heart. With the exception of this practice pattern, this series should be commended for its outcomes and perfection of a specific technique.

R. L. Bush, MD, MPH

The impact of race and ethnicity on the outcome of carotid interventions in the United States
Schneider EB, Black JH III, Hambridge HL, et al (The Johns Hopkins Hosp, Baltimore, MA)
J Surg Res 177:172-177, 2012

Objective.—Previous studies have demonstrated an adverse impact of African American race and Hispanic ethnicity on the outcomes of carotid endarterectomy (CEA), although little is known about the influence of race and ethnicity on the outcome of carotid angioplasty and stenting (CAS). The present study was undertaken to examine the influence of race and ethnicity on the outcomes of CEA and CAS in contemporary practice.

Methods.—The nationwide inpatient sample (2005—2008) was queried using International Classification of Diseases-9 codes for CEA and CAS in patients with carotid artery stenosis. The primary outcomes were postoperative death or stroke. Multivariate analysis was performed adjusting for age, gender, race, comorbidities, high-risk status, procedure type, symptomatic status, year, insurance type, and hospital characteristics.

Results.—Overall, there were 347,450 CEAs and 47,385 CASs performed in the United States over the study period. After CEA, Hispanics had the greatest risk of mortality ($P < 0.001$), whereas black patients had the greatest risk of stroke ($P = 0.02$) compared with white patients on univariate analysis. On multivariable analysis, Hispanic ethnicity remained an independent risk factor for mortality after CEA (relative risk 2.40; $P < 0.001$), whereas the increased risk of stroke in black patients was no longer significant. After CAS, there were no racial or ethnic differences in mortality. On univariate analysis, the risk of stroke was greatest in black patients after CAS ($P = 0.03$). However, this was not significant on multivariable analysis.

Conclusion.—Hispanic ethnicity is an independent risk factor for mortality after CEA. While black patients had an increased risk of stroke after CEA and CAS, this was explained by factors other than race. Further studies are warranted to determine if Hispanic ethnicity remains an independent risk factor for mortality after discharge.

▶ This is an interesting must read for vascular surgeons who treat diverse populations. Using the National Inpatient Sample, a large national database, these authors from Johns Hopkins demonstrated both racial and ethnic differences in outcomes following carotid revascularization, either carotid endarterectomy, or stenting. In particular, Hispanic ethnicity was associated with a higher mortality after endarterectomy and African-American race was associated with an increased stroke risk after both endarterectomy and stenting, though this risk was not significant after multivariate analyses. Even though the National Inpatient Sample is inpatient data only, there are many important points to be gained from this study.

Delving further into the data, Hispanic ethnicity was an independent risk factor regardless of the presence or absence of comorbid conditions also associated with worse outcomes. This suggests an environmental or genetic component that may also influence surgical risk. Not known are the details about these particular Hispanic patients and how they fared after discharge. Because patients undergoing carotid endarterectomy are most likely to be discharged the day after the procedure, it is unclear whether this increase in mortality would be sustained or disappear. Additionally, one needs to consider other variable such as socioeconomic status, number of generations established in this country, geographic variables, time to presentation, prior health care influences or lack of health care, insurance status, and so on, in more detail. Though area of the country and private insurance were not found to be significant independent variables on univariate analysis, a more thorough dissection of the data is needed. Furthermore, these variables are also going to come into play and be important as this country moves forward with health care reform. Perhaps some of the ethnic and racial disparities will diminish, though this will take years or decades to realize.

R. L. Bush, MD, MPH

Outcomes of carotid endarterectomy under general and regional anesthesia from the American College of Surgeons' National Surgical Quality Improvement Program
Leichtle SW, Mouawad NJ, Welch K, et al (Saint Joseph Mercy Health System, Ann Arbor, MI; Univ of Michigan, Ann Arbor)
J Vasc Surg 56:81-88.e3, 2012

Objective.—Despite multiple studies over more than 3 decades, there still is no consensus about the influence of anesthesia type on postoperative outcomes following carotid endarterectomy (CEA). The objective of this study was to investigate whether anesthesia type, either general anesthesia (GA) or regional anesthesia (RA), independently contributes to the risk of postoperative cardiovascular complications or death using the American College of Surgeons' National Surgical Quality Improvement Program (ACS NSQIP) database.

Methods.—Retrospective analysis of elective cases of CEA from 2005 through 2009 was performed. A propensity score model using 45 covariates, including demographic factors, comorbidities, stroke history, measures of general health, and laboratory values, was used to adjust for bias and to determine the independent influence of anesthesia type on postoperative stroke, myocardial infarction (MI), and death.

Results.—Of 26,070 cases listed in the ACS NSQIP database, GA and RA were used in 22,054 (84.6%) and 4016 (15.4%) cases, respectively. Postoperative stroke, MI, and death occurred in 360 (1.63%), 133 (0.6%), and 154

(0.70%) patients of the GA group, respectively, and in 58 (1.44%), 11 (0.27%), and 27 (0.67%) patients of the RA group, respectively. Stratification by propensity score quintile and adjustment for covariates demonstrated GA to be a significant risk factor for postoperative MI with an adjusted odds ratio (OR) and confidence interval (CI) of 2.18 (95% CI, 1.17-4.04), $P = .01$ in the entire study population. The OR for MI was 5.41 (95% CI, 1.32-22.16; $P = .019$) in the subgroup of patients with preoperative neurologic symptoms, and 1.44 (95% CI, 0.71-2.90; $P = .31$) in the subgroup of patients without preoperative neurologic symptoms.

Conclusions.—This analysis of a large, prospectively collected and validated multicenter database indicates that GA for CEA is an independent risk factor for postoperative MI, particularly in patients with preoperative neurologic symptoms.

▶ The choice of what type of anesthesia, general (GA) or local/regional (RA), has been written about in the literature, with many studies showing no difference and some showing improved outcomes with RA. This study used a large validated national database, the American College of Surgeons' National Quality Improvement Program, of more than 22 000 cases with GA and more than 4000 with RA. The main conclusion was that GA was an independent risk factor for perioperative myocardial infarction. Patients who had symptomatic carotid disease were particularly at increased risk for myocardial infarction. This study emphasizes the need for surgeons as well as anesthesiologists to be comfortable with performing carotid endarterectomy (CEA) under either type of anesthesia. Perhaps, more individualization of anesthesia to the particular patient needs to be emphasized. The take-home message of this important study needs to be that symptomatic patients should be considered for a regional or local anesthetic option. Many anesthesiologists are not adept at performing cervical blocks, but this is not necessary in every case. One can perform a CEA under simple direct local anesthesia with monitored anesthesia during the operation.

The surgeon can easily learn this technique and how to maintain patient comfort and decrease anxiety during the operation. Personally, I position the patient without heavy blankets or warmers, as the patient may become nervous and warm during the case. I use no cervical roll or Foley catheter, which also adds to discomfort. My anesthesia team has learned to use mainly narcotics and few benzodiazepines during the case and to keep the blood pressure on the higher side to promote contralateral cerebral circulation. Shunts are rarely necessary. I encourage all trainees and practicing surgeons to be familiar with CEA under RA and to individualize their care to improve outcomes and decrease adverse cardiovascular events.

R. L. Bush, MD, MPH

Analysis of Florida and New York state hospital discharges suggests that carotid stenting in symptomatic women is associated with significant increase in mortality and perioperative morbidity compared with carotid endarterectomy

Vouyouka AG, Egorova NN, Sosunov EA, et al (Mount Sinai Med School, NY; Columbia Univ, NY)
J Vasc Surg 56:334-342.e2, 2012

Background.—Although large randomized studies have established the efficacy and safety of carotid endarterectomy (CEA) and, recently, carotid artery stenting (CAS), the under-representation of women in these trials leaves the comparison of risks to benefits of performing these procedures on women an open question. To address this issue, we reviewed the hospital outcomes and delineated patient characteristics predicting outcome in women undergoing carotid interventions using New York and Florida statewide hospital discharge databases.

Methods.—We analyzed in-hospital mortality, postoperative stroke, cardiac postoperative complications, and combined postoperative stoke and mortality in 20,613 CEA or CAS hospitalizations for the years 2007 to 2009. Univariate and multiple logistic regression analyses of variables were performed.

Results.—CEA was performed in 16,576 asymptomatic and 1744 symptomatic women and CAS in 1943 asymptomatic and 350 symptomatic women. Compared with CAS, CEA rates, in asymptomatic vs symptomatic, were significantly lower for in-hospital mortality (0.3% vs 0.8% and 0.4% vs 3.4%), stroke (1.5% vs 2.6% and 3.5% vs 9.4%), and combined stroke/mortality (1.7% vs 3.1% and 3.8% vs 10.9%). In cohorts matched by propensity scores, the same trend favoring CEA remained significant in symptomatic women. There was no difference in cardiac complication rates among asymptomatic women, but among symptomatic woman cardiac complications were more frequent after CAS (10.6% vs 6.5%; $P = .0077$). Among symptomatic women, the presence of renal disease, coronary artery disease, or age ≥ 80 years increased the risk of CAS over CEA threefold for the composite end point of stroke or death. For asymptomatic women only in those with coronary artery disease or diabetes, there was a statistical difference in the composite mortality/stroke rates favoring CEA (1.9% vs 3.3% and 1.7% vs 3.4%, respectively). After adjusting for relevant clinical and demographic risk factors and hospital annual volume, for CAS vs CEA, the risk of the composite end point of stroke or mortality was 1.7-fold higher in symptomatic and 3.4-fold higher in asymptomatic patients. Medicaid insurance, symptomatic patient, history of cancer, and presence of heart failure on admission were among other strong predictors of composite stroke/mortality outcome.

Conclusions.—Databases reflecting real-world practice performance and management of carotid disease in women suggest that CEA compared with CAS has overall better perioperative outcomes in women. Importantly, CAS is associated with significantly higher morbidity in certain clinical settings and this should be taken into account when choosing a revascularization procedure.

▶ This article is a great example of how retrospective studies using large registries can be useful in identifying trends and eliciting important clinical information, especially when data from prospective studies are lacking. Registries, though often thought of as second-rate data, represent real-world experience that is not subject to the stringent inclusion/exclusion criteria of many prospective clinical trials. There are limitations, such as data validation and consistency, but the large cohort sizes often overcome some of these limitations.

The current prospective randomized trials that analyze outcomes after carotid artery revascularization, either carotid endarterectomy or carotid artery stenting, for atherosclerotic occlusive disease were not designed to detect gender-specific differences. However, given that the prevalence of > 50% carotid stenosis is 6% in elderly women (age greater than 68 years) compared with 8% in similarly aged men, diagnosing disease and studying the outcomes of various procedures in women is paramount. Women tend to have different patterns of atherosclerotic disease and may have different responses to therapy than men. Because data from all male studies may not be able to be extrapolated to women, it is crucial for investigators to separate out this population for study.

I commend the authors for analyzing more than 20 000 women who underwent stenting or endarterectomy for symptomatic and asymptomatic carotid disease in either New York or Florida. They found in this large cohort that women fared better in terms of stroke and mortality rates after endarterectomy in all circumstances, particularly so in those with symptomatic disease. This article should be read by all who perform carotid revascularization.

R. L. Bush, MD, MPH

The European Society for Vascular Surgery Guidelines for Carotid Intervention: An Updated Independent Assessment and Literature Review
Kakisis JD, Avgerinos ED, Antonopoulos CN, et al (Attikon Univ Hosp, Haidari, Athens, Greece)
Eur J Vasc Endovasc Surg 44:238-243, 2012

Background and Purpose.—Many medical societies now recommend carotid stenting as an alternative to endarterectomy which raises the question of whether the ESVS guidelines are still valid. This review addresses the validity of the ESVS guidelines that refer to carotid stenting based on the evidence available today.

Methods.—We conducted a review and meta-analysis based on the original ESVS guidelines paper and articles published over the past 2 years.

Results.—For symptomatic patients, surgery remains the best option, since stenting is associated with a 61% relative risk increase of periprocedural stroke or death compared to endarterectomy. However, centres of excellence in carotid stenting may achieve comparable results. In asymptomatic patients, there is still no good evidence for any intervention because the stroke risk from an asymptomatic stenosis is very low, especially with the best modern medical treatment. CREST and CAVATAS have verified that mid-term stroke prevention after successful stenting is similar to endarterectomy. EVA-3S, SPACE, ICSS and CREST have provided additional evidence regarding the role of age in choosing therapeutic modality. The role of the cerebral protection devices is challenged by the imaging findings of small randomised trials but supported by large systematic reviews.

Conclusions.—The ESVS guidelines that refer to carotid stenting not only remain valid but also have been further strengthened by the latest available clinical data. An update of these guidelines including all of the recent evidence is needed to provide an objective and up-to-date interpretation of the data.

▶ This article provides the latest, evidence-based update on the guidelines for carotid intervention and is a must-read for physicians treating patients who have carotid artery disease. The European Society for Vascular Surgery (ESVS) last submitted their guidelines for carotid intervention in 2008, based on the literature available at that time. Since this publication, 14 societies have published recommendations in contrast to ESVS guidelines, and several additional publications have become available in the literature prompting the need for an updated analysis of the data. This article provides that much-needed analysis.

This article takes into consideration the latest available data concerning carotid interventions, and rather than refuting the original ESVS recommendations, it adds evidence to support the Society's recommendations. Including International Carotid Stenting Study[1] and CREST[2] data, this group provides an updated meta-analysis that further strengthens the role of carotid endarterectomy (CEA) over carotid artery stenting (CAS) in symptomatic patients (improved odds ratio of 1.61 from 1.39, and statistical significance of $P = .007$ from .02). Moreover, although not reaching statistical significance, the latest meta-analysis favors CEA over CAS in the treatment of asymptomatic patients, with the correct observation that offering CAS to asymptomatic patients is advisable in centers with high volume and proven low periprocedural complication rates.

The authors also acknowledge the need for a triple-armed study comparing the role of best medical management, CEA, and CAS in the treatment of asymptomatic carotid artery disease but correctly state that current evidence is not available to provide level A recommendations in this patient population. Overall, this article is a succinct synopsis of the latest available evidence-based data concerning carotid artery interventions in patients with carotid artery disease.

B. G. Peterson, MD

References

1. International Carotid Stenting Study investigators, Ederle J, Dobson J, Featherstone RL, et al. Carotid artery stenting compared with endarterectomy in patients with symptomatic carotid stenosis (International Carotid Stenting Study): an interim analysis of a randomised controlled trial. *Lancet.* 2010;375:985-997.
2. Brott TG, Hobson RW II, Howard G, et al; CREST Investigators. Stenting versus endarterectomy for treatment of carotid-artery stenosis. *N Engl J Med.* 2010;363:11-23.

The Impact of Gender on In-hospital Outcomes after Carotid Endarterectomy or Stenting

Bisdas T, Egorova N, Moskowitz AJ, et al (Mount Sinai Med School, NY; et al)
Eur J Vasc Endovasc Surg 44:244-250, 2012

Aim.—We sought to better define the impact of sex on 'in-hospital outcomes' after carotid endarterectomy (CEA) or stenting (CAS).

Methods.—Hospital discharge databases for all carotid interventions obtained from the New York State (NYS) Department of Health, Statewide Planning and Research Cooperative System between 2000 and 2009 (29,917 women, 39,771 men) were analysed. Mortality, stroke and composite event (stroke/death) were compared between procedures after matching of patients by propensity score. Acute myocardial infarction (AMI) was our secondary 'end' point.

Results.—More than 90% of patients in both sexes were asymptomatic (27,439 women and 36,295 men). Compared to men, asymptomatic women experienced more strokes after CEA (women: 1.38%, men: 1.16%, $P = 0.03$) and higher AMI rates after both procedures (CEA; women: 0.75%, men: 0.51%, $P = 0.0009$, CAS; women: 0.96%, men: 0.28%, $P = 0.01$). Between procedures, symptomatic women undergoing CAS showed higher rates of mortality (CAS: 4.19%, CEA: 0.47%, $P = 0.01$) and combined (stroke/mortality) events (CAS: 12.09%, CEA: 6.05%, $P = 0.02$). In all other cohorts, no statistically significant difference was found between the procedures.

Conclusions.—Compared to CEA, CAS led to inferior in-hospital outcomes only in symptomatic women in the last decade in NYS. Men and asymptomatic women showed comparable outcomes after both procedures, whereas asymptomatic females were more prone to AMI after both interventions. These sex-associated differences should be taken into account for the treatment of carotid artery disease.

▶ Randomized, controlled trials (RCTs) comparing carotid endarterectomy (CEA) and carotid artery stenting (CAS) often do not have sufficient numbers to assess outcome differences between gender groups. This report attempts to overcome this power limitation by utilizing a New York State administrative database with about 70 000 patients who underwent either CEA or CAS to ascertain in-hospital/procedural outcomes according to preoperative symptom status and gender.

Similar to post-hoc analyses of RCTs comparing CEA and CAS, this group found symptomatic women to be at almost 2-fold higher risk of periprocedural stroke when undergoing CAS compared with CEA. This large dataset reconfirms that symptomatic women undergoing CAS are at significantly higher perioperative stroke risk and should preferentially undergo CEA when appropriately indicated. However, given that these administrative databases have limited clinical data, it is difficult to pin down a mechanism responsible for the cause of the higher stoke rate.

B. G. Peterson, MD

A Simplified Murine Intimal Hyperplasia Model Founded on a Focal Carotid Stenosis

Tao M, Mauro CR, Yu P, et al (Brigham and Women's Hosp, Boston, MA; et al)
Am J Pathol 182:277-287, 2013

Murine models offer a powerful tool for unraveling the mechanisms of intimal hyperplasia and vascular remodeling, although their technical complexity increases experimental variability and limits widespread application. We describe a simple and clinically relevant mouse model of arterial intimal hyperplasia and remodeling. Focal left carotid artery (LCA) stenosis was created by placing 9-0 nylon suture around the artery using an external 35-gauge mandrel needle (middle or distal location), which was then removed. The effect of adjunctive diet-induced obesity was defined. Flowmetry, wall strain analyses, biomicroscopy, and histology were completed. LCA blood flow sharply decreased by ~85%, followed by a responsive right carotid artery increase of ~71%. Circumferential strain decreased by ~2.1% proximal to the stenosis in both dietary groups. At 28 days, morphologic adaptations included proximal LCA intimal hyperplasia, which was exacerbated by diet-induced obesity. The proximal and distal LCA underwent outward and negative inward remodeling, respectively, in the mid-focal stenosis (remodeling indexes, 1.10 and 0.53). A simple, defined common carotid focal stenosis yields reproducible murine intimal hyperplasia and substantial differentials in arterial wall adaptations. This model offers a tool for investigating mechanisms of hemodynamically driven intimal hyperplasia and arterial wall remodeling.

▶ Murine models of human disease remain an important source of mechanistic information regarding potential mechanisms of disease and therapeutic interventions. For cardiovascular researchers interested in intimal hyperplasia, the existing murine models are of controversial importance. Intimal hyperplasia cannot be reliably created in the most common murine strain, that is, the C57BL6 mouse. To reliably obtain morphologic evidence of intimal hyperplasia, investigators need to use either of the $ApoE^{-/-}$ strains, which, because of the presence of genetic deletions, have questionable relevance. Second, flow-dependent models of intimal hyperplasia resulting from mechanical denudation of the intimal are technically challenging and often result in an asymmetric distribution of disease. Finally, the most reliable murine model of intimal hyperplasia is actually a no-flow model in which the common carotid artery is completely ligated; that is, it is a no-flow model that is again of questionable clinical relevance. Thus, the report by Tao et al represents a major departure from the available literature. It is a flow model that can be generated in the most common murine model without genetic or systemic hemodynamic intervention (hypertension). The pattern of disease generated by this model is symmetric and very consistent. Unlike the murine models of intimal injury, which require special wires and multiple intravascular manipulations, this model does not require any intravascular manipulations. It is a partial ligation model in which a fine suture is used to narrow the common carotid artery of the mouse. In very short order, this model will become the standard for molecular and histologic analysis of intimal hyperplasia in mice.

M. T. Watkins, MD

Carotid artery stenting outcomes are equivalent to carotid endarterectomy outcomes for patients with post-carotid endarterectomy stenosis

AbuRahma AF, Abu-Halimah S, Hass SM, et al (West Virginia Univ, Charleston; et al)
J Vasc Surg 52:1180-1187, 2010

Background.—Carotid artery stenting (CAS) has been advocated as an alternative to redo surgery for patients with post-carotid endarterectomy (CEA) stenosis. This study compares early and late clinical outcomes for both groups.

Methods.—This study analyzes 192 patients: 72 had reoperation (Group A) and 120 had CAS for post-CEA stenosis (Group B). Patients were followed prospectively and had duplex ultrasounds at 1 month, and every 6 to 12 months thereafter. The perioperative complications (perioperative stroke, myocardial infarction/death, cranial nerve injury) and 4-year end points were analyzed. A Kaplan-Meier lifetable analysis was used to estimate rates of freedom from stroke, stroke-free survival, $\geq 50\%$ restenosis, and $\geq 80\%$ restenosis.

Results.—Demographic/clinical characteristics were comparable for both groups, except for diabetes mellitus and coronary artery disease, which were significantly higher in Group B. The indications for reoperations were transient ischemic attacks/stroke in 72% for Group A versus 57% for Group B ($P = .0328$). The mean follow-up was 33 months (range, 1-86 months) for Group A and 24 months (range, 1-78 months) for Group B ($P = .0026$). The proportion of early (<24 months) carotid restenosis prior to intervention was 51% in Group A versus 27% in Group B ($P = .0013$). The perioperative stroke rates were 3% and 1%, respectively ($P = .5573$). There were no myocardial infarctions or deaths in either group. The overall incidence of cranial nerve injury was 14% for Group A versus 0% for Group B ($P < .0001$). However, there was no statistical difference between the groups relating to permanent cranial nerve injury (1% versus 0%). The combined early and late stroke rates for Groups A and B were 3% and 2%, respectively ($P = .6347$). The stroke-free rates at 1, 2, 3, and 4 years for Groups A and B were 97%, 97%, 97%, and 97% and 98%, 98%, 98%, and 98%, respectively ($P = .6490$). The stroke-free survival rates were not significantly different. The rates of freedom from $\geq 50\%$ restenosis at 1, 2, 3, and 4 years were 98%, 95%, 95%, and 95% for Group A versus 95%, 89%, 80%, and 72% for Group B ($P = .0175$). The freedom from $\geq 80\%$ restenosis at 1, 2, 3, and 4 years for Groups A and B were 98%, 97%, 97%, and 97% versus 99%, 96%, 92%, and 87%, respectively ($P = .2281$). Four patients (one symptomatic) in Group B had reintervention for $\geq 80\%$ restenosis. The rate of freedom from reintervention for Groups A and B were

100%, 100%, 100%, and 100% versus 94%, 89%, 83%, and 79%, respectively ($P = .0634$).

Conclusions.—CAS is as safe as redo CEA. Redo CEA has a higher incidence of transient cranial nerve injury; however, CAS has a higher incidence of $\geq 50\%$ in-stent restenosis.

▶ Patients who have significant, recurrent stenoses after carotid endarterectomy (CEA) historically have been treated with redo-CEA, and some have argued that carotid artery stenting (CAS) is an equally effective treatment option in this challenging group. Until now, this argument was largely based on small case series. This is the largest study to compare redo-CEA with CAS in patients with significant, recurrent stenoses after CEA, and it finally adds credence to the practice of addressing significant, recurrent disease, whether secondary to neointimal hyperplasia or progressive atherosclerosis, with CAS.

With postprocedure stroke, death, and myocardial infarction rates not statistically different between groups, redo-CEA was not surprisingly shown to have a significantly higher risk of cranial nerve injury compared with CAS; however, all but one of these injuries was transient in nature. On the other hand, CAS was shown to be less durable than redo-CEA in follow-up. The CAS group saw a significantly higher incidence of greater than 50% restenosis, and there was a trend toward more reinterventions in the CAS group. Nevertheless, this is the largest comparative study to show equivalence between redo-CEA and CAS in terms of freedom from greater than 80% restenosis at 4 years, and the details here certainly deserve to be mentioned when discussing treatment options with patients found to have significant, recurrent lesions after CEA.

B. G. Peterson, MD

Characteristics of Ischemic Brain Lesions After Stenting or Endarterectomy for Symptomatic Carotid Artery Stenosis: Results From the International Carotid Stenting Study—Magnetic Resonance Imaging Substudy
Gensicke H, on behalf of the ICSS-MRI Substudy Investigators (Univ Hosp Basel, UK; et al)
Stroke 44:80-86, 2013

Background and Purpose.—In a substudy of the International Carotid Stenting Study (ICSS), more patients had new ischemic brain lesions on diffusion-weighted magnetic resonance imaging (MRI) after stenting (CAS) than after endarterectomy (CEA). In the present analysis, we compared characteristics of diffusion-weighted MRI lesions.

Methods.—Number, individual and total volumes, and location of new diffusion-weighted MRI lesions were compared in patients with symptomatic carotid stenosis randomized to CAS (n = 124) or CEA (n = 107) in the ICSS-MRI substudy.

Results.—CAS patients had higher lesion numbers than CEA patients (1 lesion, 15% vs 8%; 2-5 lesions, 19% vs 5%; >5 lesions, 16% vs 4%). The overall risk ratio for the expected lesion count with CAS versus CEA was 8.8 (95% confidence interval, 4.4–17.5; $P < 0.0001$) and significantly increased among patients with lower blood pressure at randomization, diabetes mellitus, stroke as the qualifying event, left-side stenosis, and if patients were treated at centers routinely using filter-type protection devices during CAS. Individual lesions were smaller in the CAS group than in the CEA group ($P < 0.0001$). Total lesion volume per patient did not differ significantly. Lesions in the CAS group were more likely to occur in cortical areas and subjacent white matter supplied by leptomeningeal arteries than lesions in the CEA group (odds ratio, 4.2; 95% confidence interval, 1.7–10.2; $P = 0.002$).

Conclusions.—Compared with patients undergoing CEA, patients treated with CAS had higher numbers of periprocedural ischemic brain lesions, and lesions were smaller and more likely to occur in cortical areas and subjacent white matter. These findings may reflect differences in underlying mechanisms of cerebral ischemia.

Clinical Trial Registration.—URL: http://www.isrctn.org. Unique identifier: ISRCTN25337470.

▶ This study, which is a subanalysis from the International Carotid Stenting Study, demonstrates that carotid angioplasty and stenting (CAS) results in a higher number of periprocedural magnetic resonance imaging (MRI) lesions than carotid endarterectomy. Many studies have now been published that document a higher number of embolic episodes as defined by new diffusion-weighted lesions on MRI. The current study takes the information a bit further and also reports the volume of lesions and location in the brain. Interestingly, the CAS lesions were smaller and more likely to occur in the cortical or subjacent white matter areas. This resulted in no difference being seen in total lesion volume because of the small size of the lesions with CAS. Additionally, symptomatic patients undergoing carotid revascularization had more diffusion-weighted imaging (DWI) lesions identified, thus signifying a potential role of plaque instability.

The risk factors the authors found associated with an increase in DWI lesions were diabetes, low blood pressure, stroke, and left-sided lesions. One issue not raised in this study, or the analyses, was any difference in overall neurologic status or a detailed cognitive examination. Having a neurologist participate would have determined the significance of the increased number of lesions and any potential decline in functionality of the patient. Are these clinically silent lesions? Is there an association between neurologic function and increased numbers of DWI lesions? These important questions have yet to be answered, although I believe we all agree that luminal manipulation of the carotid artery during CAS results in increased risk of emboli.

R. L. Bush, MD, MPH

Carotid Artery Surgery: High-Risk Patients or High-Risk Centers?

Bouziane Z, Nourissat G, Duprey A, et al (St Etienne Univ Hosp, France)
Ann Vasc Surg 26:790-796, 2012

Background.—Carotid angioplasty and stenting has been proposed as an alternative to carotid endarterectomy (CEA) in patients deemed as at high risk for this surgical procedure. To date, definitely accepted criteria to identify "high-risk" patients for CEA do not exist. Our objective was to assess the relevance of numerous supposed high-risk factors in our experience, as well as their possible effect on our early postoperative results.

Methods.—A retrospective review of 1,033 consecutive CEAs performed during a 5.6-year period at a single institution was conducted (Vascular Surgery Department, St. Etienne University Hospital, France). Early results in terms of mortality and neurologic events were recorded. Univariate and multivariate analyses for early risk of stroke, myocardial infarction, and death were performed, considering the influence of age, sex, comorbidities, clinical symptoms, and anatomic features.

Results.—The cumulative 30-day stroke and death rate was 1.2%. A total of 10 strokes occurred and resulted in three deaths. The postoperative stroke risk was significantly higher in the subgroup of patients treated for symptomatic carotid artery disease: 2,6% ($P = 0,004$). Univariate analysis and logistic regression did not show statistical significance for 30-day results in any of the considered variables.

Conclusion.—Patients with significant medical comorbidities, contralateral carotid occlusion, and high carotid lesions can undergo surgery without increased complications. Those parameters should not be used as exclusion criteria for CEA.

▶ This well-written retrospective study from Bouziane and colleagues in France states what most vascular surgeons know to be true: anatomic characteristics and medical comorbidities should not deter a physician from recommending carotid endarterectomy (CEA). Prior to the introduction of carotid angioplasty and stenting as an alternative to traditional surgical intervention for carotid stenosis, one would not consider such issues. The patient was either a candidate for interventional treatment or not. Surgical maneuvers for dealing with anatomical challenges exist and are well tolerated by the patients. Medical management was maximized prior to the operation. Local anesthesia can be used in patients who are at high risk for general anesthesia. If a patient was deemed at too high of a surgical risk compared with observational management alone, none was undertaken. If a surgeon has experience and technical expertise, as well as a first-class anesthetic and surgical team, then the patient is likely to benefit from CEA.

This should be the treatment algorithm for carotid artery surgery as well. One needs to first determine whether the patient warrants intervention on the basis of a carotid lesion. Questions arise as to the efficacy of intervening on asymptomatic lesions given the superior atherosclerotic medical management that currently exists and did not in the old, frequently quoted trials concerning asymptomatic disease. The take-home message from these authors is that the individual surgeon needs to tailor his or her treatment to the individual patient and the clinical setting. Only the vascular surgeon has the experience and training to perform either CEA or carotid artery surgery and be able to talk honestly and candidly with the patient about both procedures.

R. L. Bush, MD, MPH

The Impact of Gender on In-hospital Outcomes after Carotid Endarterectomy or Stenting
Bisdas T, Egorova N, Moskowitz AJ, et al (Mount Sinai Med School, NY; Mount Sinai School of Medicine, NY; et al)
Eur J Vasc Endovasc Surg 44:244-250, 2012

Aim.—We sought to better define the impact of sex on 'in-hospital outcomes' after carotid endarterectomy (CEA) or stenting (CAS).

Methods.—Hospital discharge databases for all carotid interventions obtained from the New York State (NYS) Department of Health, State-wide Planning and Research Cooperative System between 2000 and 2009 (29,917 women, 39,771 men) were analysed. Mortality, stroke and composite event (stroke/death) were compared between procedures after matching of patients by propensity score. Acute myocardial infarction (AMI) was our secondary 'end' point.

Results.—More than 90% of patients in both sexes were asymptomatic (27,439 women and 36,295 men). Compared to men, asymptomatic women experienced more strokes after CEA (women: 1.38%, men: 1.16%, $P = 0.03$) and higher AMI rates after both procedures (CEA; women: 0.75%, men: 0.51%, $P = 0.0009$, CAS; women: 0.96%, men: 0.28%, $P = 0.01$). Between procedures, symptomatic women undergoing CAS showed higher rates of mortality (CAS: 4.19%, CEA: 0.47%, $P = 0.01$) and combined (stroke/mortality) events (CAS: 12.09%, CEA: 6.05%, $P = 0.02$). In all other cohorts, no statistically significant difference was found between the procedures.

Conclusions.—Compared to CEA, CAS led to inferior in-hospital outcomes only in symptomatic women in the last decade in NYS. Men and asymptomatic women showed comparable outcomes after both procedures, whereas asymptomatic females were more prone to AMI after both interventions. These sex-associated differences should be taken into account for the treatment of carotid artery disease.

▶ This is an interesting article that may raise more questions than it answers using the New York Department of Health Statewide dataset (SPARCS), which collects discharge data from all hospitals in the state. It is comprehensive in its variable list and also separates comorbidities present on admission from those that arose during a hospital stay. Both types of carotid revascularization, stenting (CAS) and endarterectomy (CEA), are analyzed over a multiyear period. Interestingly, over 9 years, there were > 27 000 women compared with > 36 000 men who had carotid interventions. This is an unusually high proportion of women compared with other published studies, especially the prospective randomized trials for either intervention. The first question arises: why are there so many women undergoing CAS and CEA in the state of New York? Or are men being operated on at lesser rates?

The second question occurs during the actual data analysis and specifics concerning members of each cohort. Less than 9% of the cohorts of men and women were intervened on for symptomatic carotid disease. In other words, in New York State, the vast majority of patients having a carotid operation or stent are asymptomatic. This is well above the usual proportions of 70% asymptomatic and 30% symptomatic lesions. Why are so many patients with asymptomatic disease being intervened on given the known natural history of carotid disease? It is very hard to justify the combined stroke and death rates of about 2.5% in men or women when associated with only an asymptomatic lesion. Given the vast improvement in medical management for atherosclerotic disease over the past decade, it would be interesting for these authors to further analyze the data by year to see if the proportion of asymptomatic/symptomatic patients changed over time. It is disturbing to think that with the current body of knowledge, data, publications, and medical guidelines, surgeons and interventionalists are still recommending intervention over observation. The medical community needs more data to support this premise.

R. L. Bush, MD, MPH

Contralateral occlusion is not a clinically important reason for choosing carotid artery stenting for patients with significant carotid artery stenosis
Brewster LP, Beaulieu R, Kasirajan K, et al (Emory Univ Hosp, Atlanta, GA; Johns Hopkins Hosp, Baltimore, MD; East Bay Cardiovascular and Thoracic Associates, Concord, CA)
J Vasc Surg 56:1291-1295, 2012

Objective.—Contralateral carotid artery occlusion by itself carries an increased risk of stroke. Carotid endarterectomy (CEA) in the presence of contralateral carotid artery occlusion has high reported rates of perioperative morbidity and mortality. Our objective was to determine if there is a clinical benefit to patients who receive carotid artery stenting (CAS) compared to CEA in the presence of contralateral carotid artery occlusion.

Methods.—We conducted a retrospective medical chart review over a 4.5-year institutional experience of persons with contralateral carotid artery occlusion and ipsilateral carotid artery stenosis who underwent CAS or CEA. The main outcome measures were 30-day cardiac, stroke, and mortality rate, and midterm mortality.

Results.—Of a total of 713 patients treated for carotid artery stenosis during this time period, 57 had contralateral occlusion ($\sim$8%). Thirty-nine of these patients were treated with CAS, and 18 with CEA. The most common indications for CAS were prior neck surgery (18), contralateral internal carotid occlusion (nine), and prior neck radiation (seven). The average age was 70 ± 8.5 for CEA and 66.7 ± 9.3 for CAS ($P = .20$).

Both groups were predominantly men (CEA 12 of 18; CAS 28 of 39; $P = .76$), with similar prevalence of symptomatic lesions (CEA 8 of 18, CAS 20 of 39; $P = .77$). Two patients died within 30 days in the CAS group (5%). No deaths occurred within 30 days in the CEA group ($P = .50$); the mortality rate for CAS and CEA combined was 3.5%. No perioperative strokes or myocardial infarction occurred in either group. Two transient ischemic attacks occurred after CAS. At mean follow-up of 29.4 ± 16 months (CEA) and 28 ± 14.4 months (CAS; range, 1.5-48.5 months), seven deaths occurred in the CAS group and one in the CEA group (17.9% vs 5.5%; $P = .40$). There were two reinterventions in the CAS group for in-stent restenosis and there were no reoperations in the CEA group.

Conclusions.—Although CEA and CAS can both be performed with good perioperative results and acceptable midterm mortality, the observed outcomes do not support use of contralateral carotid artery occlusion as a selection criterion for CAS over CEA in the absence of other indications.

▶ The controversy over the significance of contralateral carotid occlusion in the setting of ipsilateral significant carotid artery disease continues. Does this truly represent a high-risk anatomical situation? Many have described a contralateral carotid artery occlusion as 1 of the high-risk criteria that then warrant consideration of carotid stent (CAS) placement to avoid cerebral ischemia, shunt placement, and any need for deep or general anesthesia. This study is another necessary addition to the current body of knowledge looking at whether carotid stenting bestows a clinical benefit over carotid endarterectomy (CEA) in patients with contralateral carotid occlusion.

This experienced group from Emory demonstrates in their large institutional cohort of patients undergoing carotid interventions (both CEA and CAS), 57 (8%) of whom had contralateral carotid artery occlusion, there were similar outcomes in both groups. No clinical advantage in either the perioperative or follow-up period was observed by choosing 1 procedure over the other. Their conclusion is basically that the presence of contralateral occlusion should not be considered an anatomical selection criterion to designate a patient as "high risk for CEA."

Many interventionalists recommend an interdisciplinary team approach to patients with symptomatic carotid artery disease; this includes neurologists to evaluate the patients' neurologic status in a specific and focused manner both pre- and postintervention. Small cognitive or other neurologic deficits may be identified with more detailed examinations. This type of data may give more insight into the effects of CEA or CAS in patients with clinical or anatomic variables such as contralateral occlusion. In any event, this study adds credence to not including contralateral occlusion as a high-risk criterion necessitating carotid stenting but rather looking at the patient as a whole in terms of the numbers of comorbidities that exist.

R. L. Bush, MD, MPH

Carotid endarterectomy is more cost-effective than carotid artery stenting

Sternbergh WC III, Crenshaw GD, Bazan HA, et al (Ochsner Clinic Foundation, New Orleans, LA)
J Vasc Surg 55:1623-1628, 2012

Objective.—Cost-effectiveness has become an important end point in comparing therapies that may be considered to have clinical equipoise. While controversial, some feel that recent multicenter randomized controlled trials have codified clinical equipoise between carotid endarterectomy (CEA) and carotid artery stenting (CAS).

Methods.—A retrospective analysis of hospital cost and 30-day clinical outcomes was performed on patients undergoing CEA and CAS between January 1, 2008 and September 30, 2010 at a single tertiary referral institution. Cost, not charges, of the index hospitalization was divided into supply, labor, facility, and miscellaneous categories. All costs were normalized to 2010 values.

Results.—A total of 306 patients underwent either CEA (n = 174) or CAS (n = 132). Mean hospital cost for CAS was \$9426 ± \$5776 while CEA cost was \$6734 ± \$3935 (*P* < .0001). This cost differential was driven by the significantly higher direct supply costs for CAS (\$5634) vs CEA (\$1967) (*P* ≤ .0001). The higher costs for CAS were seen consistently in symptomatic, asymptomatic, elective, and urgent subgroups. Patients undergoing CAS who were enrolled in a trial or registry (53.8%) incurred significantly less cost (\$7779 ± \$3525) compared to those who were not (\$11,279 ± \$7114; *P* = .0004). Patients undergoing CEA trended toward a higher prevalence of being symptomatic (44.8%) compared to CAS (34.0%; *P* = .058). Age was not significantly different between patients undergoing CEA and CAS (70.2 vs 72.0, respectively; *P* = .36). Coronary artery disease was more common in patients undergoing CAS (60.3% vs 39%; *P* = .0001). The prevalence of chronic obstructive pulmonary disease, renal failure, hypertension, and diabetes was not significantly different between cohorts. Thirty-day combined stroke/death/myocardial infarction rate was 2.3% (4 of 174) in the CEA group and 3.8% (5 of 132) in the CAS group, *P* = .5. Overall length of stay (LOS) was 2.1 days in both groups (*P* = .9). LOS was higher for urgent interventions (7.3-7.5 days) and symptomatic status (2.9-3.5 days) when compared to patients treated electively (1.3-1.4 days).

Conclusions.—Treatment of carotid disease with CAS was 40% more costly than CEA and did not provide better clinical outcomes or a reduction in LOS. These trends were consistent in symptomatic, asymptomatic, urgent, and elective subgroups At present, CAS cannot be considered a cost-effective treatment for carotid disease.

▶ This is an excellent study looking at the cost effectiveness of 2 different procedures, carotid endarterectomy (CEA) and carotid stenting (CAS), that have seemingly equal outcomes for carotid artery disease. As the data gathers on clinical outcomes for differing procedures to treat the same disease, one has to look at the cost to the institution and the patient. As we consider health care reform and the rising costs of health care in the United States, more attention will have to be given to reducing the cost of health care delivery while preserving excellent clinical outcomes. The personal cost to the patient will also have to be included such as pain, time spent in the hospital, missed time from work, and recuperation or rehabilitation time necessary. Some procedures such as endovascular aneurysm repair (EVAR) have an increased clinical or device cost over open surgery, but the personal cost is much less to the patient. Such consideration must be made in the final health care cost calculation, but unfortunately they are not. Many countries have decreased or eliminated EVAR because of the high device-related expenses. However, with CEA and CAS, the personal costs are fairly equal and many recent trials such as the SAPPHIRE (Stenting and Angioplasty with Protection in Patients at High Risk for Endarterectomy) and CREST (Carotid Revascularization Endarterectomy vs Stenting Trial) studies have demonstrated clinical equipoise. Thus, a cost analysis of the procedure itself is fundamental.

Sternbergh and co-authors showed that in their institution CAS was 40% more expensive than CEA, and there was no difference regardless of symptomatology or urgency of the operation. Given these results, one needs to consider if health care reform should include coverage of the lowest cost, but equal, procedure, with any extra costs for personal preferences going to the patient. This is a politically charged question that will be difficult to answer in our society, which values choice above all.

R. L. Bush, MD, MPH

R.L. Bush, MD, MPH

12 Vascular Trauma

An outcome analysis of endovascular versus open repair of blunt traumatic aortic injuries

Azizzadeh A, Charlton-Ouw KM, Chen Z, et al (Univ of Texas Health Science Ctr and Memorial Hermann Heart and Vascular Inst, Houston)

J Vasc Surg 57:108-115, 2013

Background.—Aortic injury is the second most common cause of death after blunt trauma. Thoracic endovascular aortic repair (TEVAR) has been rapidly adopted as an alternative to the traditional open repair (OR) for treatment of traumatic aortic injury (TAI). This paradigm shift has improved the outcomes in these patients. This study evaluated the outcomes of TEVAR compared with OR for patients with TAI.

Methods.—We analyzed prospectively collected data from the institutional trauma registry between April 2002 and June 2010. These data were supplemented with a retrospective review of hospital financial accounts. The primary outcome was the presence or absence of any complication, including in-hospital death. Secondary outcomes included fixed, variable, and total hospital costs and intensive care unit (ICU), preoperative, postoperative and total hospital length of stay (LOS).

Results.—Amongst 106 consecutive patients (74 men; mean age, 36.4 years), 56 underwent OR and 50 underwent TEVAR for treatment of TAI. The proportion of patients who underwent TEVAR compared with OR increased from 0% to 100% during the study period. The TEVAR patients were significantly older than the OR patients (41.1 vs 32.2 years, $P = .012$). For patients who underwent TEVAR, the estimated odds ratio (95% confidence interval) of complications, including in-hospital mortality was 0.33 (0.11-0.97; $P = .045$) compared with the OR group. The average number of complications, including in-hospital death, was higher in the OR group than in the TEVAR group (adjusted means, 1.29 vs 0.94). The OR group had a higher proportion of patients with complications, including in-hospital death, compared with the TEVAR group (69.6% vs 48%). Although, the mean adjusted variable costs were higher for TEVAR than for OR ($P = .017$), the mean adjusted fixed and total costs were not significantly different. Owing to a policy of delayed selective management, the adjusted preoperative LOS was significantly higher for TEVAR (9.8 vs 3.0 days, $P = .022$). The difference in the ICU or total hospital LOS was not significant. Although the proportion of uninsured patients was similar in both groups, the cohort (n = 106) had a significantly higher proportion of uninsured patients (29% vs 5%) compared with the general vascular

231

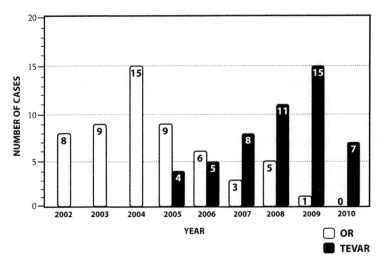

FIGURE 3.—Treatment of traumatic aortic injury: the proportion of patients undergoing thoracic endovascular aortic repair (*TEVAR*) increased from 0% to 100% from April 2, 2002 to June 2, 2010. *OR*, Open repair. (Reprinted from the Journal of Vascular Surgery. Azizzadeh A, Charlton-Ouw KM, Chen Z, et al. An outcome analysis of endovascular versus open repair of blunt traumatic aortic injuries. *J Vasc Surg.* 2013;57:108-115, Copyright 2013, with permission from the Society for Vascular Surgery.)

TABLE 3.—Descriptive Results: Proportion of Individual Complications and In-Hospital Death by Study Group

Variable[a]	OR (n = 56) No. (%)	TEVAR (n = 50) No. (%)
Complication + death	39 (69.64)	24 (48.00)
Complication + death, mean	1.29	0.94
Death	5 (8.9)	2 (4.0)
Cardiac	5 (8.93)	3 (6.00)
Respiratory	32 (57.14)	18 (36.00)
Gastrointestinal	4 (7.14)	2 (4.00)
Stroke	2 (3.57)	1 (2.00)
Paraplegia	0	0
Other neurologic	4 (7.14)	1 (2.00)
All neurologic	6 (10.71)	2 (4)
Hematologic	7 (12.7)	5 (10.00)
Peripheral vascular	2 (3.57)	0
Infectious	6 (10.71)	6 (12.00)
Renal	10 (17.86)	4 (8.00)
Other	6 (10.71)	5 (10.00)

OR, Open repair; *TEVAR*, thoracic endovascular aortic repair.
[a]Data are shown as number (%) except where indicated.

surgical population at our institution (0.29 vs 0.051, 95% confidence interval for difference in proportions, 0.22-0.40; *P* < .0001).

Conclusions.—Compared with TEVAR, patients who underwent OR had three times higher odds to face a complication or in-hospital death. The mean total cost of TEVAR was not significantly different than OR. The findings support the use of TEVAR over OR for patients with TAI (Fig 3, Table 3).

▶ From a leading group in the management of blunt aortic injury comes this report comparing open with endovascular repair. These authors, with a deep experience in open surgical approaches to thoraco-abdominal aortic pathology, saw a shift in their own practice patterns over the course of a decade (Fig 3) from 100% open repair in 2002 to 100% thoracic endovascular aortic repair today.

The results should be of no surprise to anyone who has a pulse and is even remotely involved in the treatment of these severely injured patients. TEVAR is better than open repair.[1] Period. Open repair had a 3-fold higher complication profile including death (Table 3).

One interesting data point here is that at cost analysis, there was no difference in mean total cost. These authors are to be congratulated on adopting this endovascular strategy in the 21st century.

B. W. Starnes, MD

Reference

1. Tang GL, Tehrani HY, Usman A, et al. Reduced mortality, paraplegia, and stroke with stent graft repair of blunt aortic transections: a modern meta-analysis. *J Vasc Surg.* 2008;47:671-675.

Epidemiology and Outcome of Vascular Trauma at a British Major Trauma Centre
Perkins ZB, De'Ath HD, Aylwin C, et al (The Royal London Hosp, UK)
Eur J Vasc Endovasc Surg 44:203-209, 2012

Objectives.—In the United Kingdom, the epidemiology, management strategies and outcomes from vascular trauma are unknown. The aim of this study was to describe the vascular trauma experience of a British Trauma Centre.

Methods.—A retrospective observational study of all patients admitted to hospital with traumatic vascular injury between 2005 and 2010.

Results.—Vascular injuries were present in 256 patients (4.4%) of the 5823 total trauma admissions. Penetrating trauma caused 135 (53%) vascular injuries whilst the remainder resulted from blunt trauma. Compared to penetrating vascular trauma, patients with blunt trauma were more severely injured (median ISS 29 [18−38] vs. ISS 11 [9−17], $p < 0.0001$), had greater mortality (26% vs. 10%; OR 3.0, 95% CI 1.5−5.9; $p < 0.01$) and higher limb amputation rates (12% vs. 0%; $p < 0.0001$). Blunt vascular trauma patients were also twice as likely to require a massive blood transfusion (48% vs. 25%; $p = 0.0002$) and had a five-fold longer hospital length of stay (median 35 days (15−58) vs. 7 (4−13), $p < 0.0001$) and critical care stay (median 5 days (0−11) vs. 0 (0−2), $p < 0.0001$) compared to patients with penetrating trauma. Multivariate regression analysis showed that age, ISS,

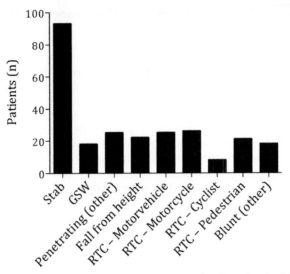

FIGURE 2.—Mechanisms of vascular injury amongst our study cohort. (Reprinted from European Journal of Vascular and Endovascular Surgery. Perkins ZB, De'Ath HD, Aylwin C, et al. Epidemiology and outcome of vascular trauma at a British major trauma Centre. *Eur J Vasc Endovasc Surg.* 2012;44:203-209, Copyright 2012, with permission from European Society for Vascular Surgery.)

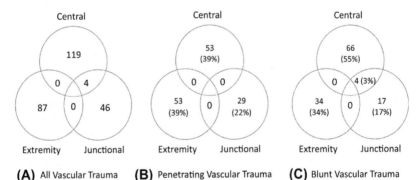

FIGURE 3.—Venn diagrams demonstrating numbers of vascular injury per anatomical zone. A) 256 patients with vascular trauma, B) 135 patients with penetrating vascular trauma and C) 121 patients with blunt vascular trauma. (Reprinted from European Journal of Vascular and Endovascular Surgery. Perkins ZB, De'Ath HD, Aylwin C, et al. Epidemiology and outcome of vascular trauma at a British major trauma Centre. *Eur J Vasc Endovasc Surg.* 2012;44:203-209, Copyright 2012, with permission from European Society for Vascular Surgery.)

shock and zone of injury were independent predictors of death following vascular trauma.

Conclusion.—Traumatic vascular injury accounts for 4% of admissions to a British Trauma Centre. These patients are severely injured with high mortality and morbidity, and place a significant demand on hospital resources. Integration of vascular services with regional trauma systems will be an essential part of current efforts to improve trauma care in the UK (Figs 2 and 3).

▶ Historically, the United Kingdom has not had an organized system for trauma care. As a result, little is known about the epidemiology, management, and outcomes for vascular trauma. This 6-year review from the first British major trauma center is the largest description of civilian vascular trauma in Britain. The results show that vascular trauma is not uncommon, is associated with high mortality and morbidity, and places a significant burden on hospital resources.

Of 5823 trauma admissions over a 5-year period, vascular injuries were present in 256 patients (4.4%). This compares with a rate of 1.5% in the United States. The authors divided vascular injuries into three categories: (a) junctional (axillo-subclavian or femoral), (b) central, and (c) extremity (Fig 3). Interestingly, over half of the injuries were of penetrating mechanism, with the overwhelming majority being stab wounds (as compared with gunshot wounds in South Africa) (Fig 2).

The overall mortality rates for vascular-injured patients was 18%, which compares favorably with major urban trauma centers worldwide. Even with expert care, these injuries are associated with a high morbidity and mortality and place substantial burden on hospital resources. These results will improve our understanding of vascular trauma and aid resource planning for future trauma and vascular systems.

B. W. Starnes, MD

A Ten Year Review of Civilian Iliac Vessel Injuries from a Single Trauma Centre

Oliver JC, Bekker W, Edu S, et al (Univ of Cape Town, South Africa)
Eur J Vasc Endovasc Surg 44:199-202, 2012

Objective.—To report the surgical management and outcome of iliac vessel (IV) injuries in a civilian trauma centre with a high incidence of penetrating trauma.

Design, Patients and Methods.—A retrospective record review of patients with IV injuries treated between January 2000 and December 2009.

Results.—Sixty nine patients, 59 with gunshot wounds, sustained 108 iliac vessel injuries. Mean revised trauma and injury severity scores was 7.06 and 28.4, respectively. Twenty nine patients required damage control laparotomy. Common or external iliac arteries were repaired by primary repair (10), temporary shunt with delayed graft (6), interposition graft (5) or ligation if limb non-viable (3). Forty-seven patients had injuries to the common or external iliac vein, 42 were ligated. Mortality was 25% and 6 survivors required amputation.

Conclusions.—In a stable patient a primary arterial repair is preferred but a temporary shunt can be a life and limb saving option in the unstable

TABLE 2.—Outcome Related to Type of Vessel Injured

Vessel Injured	N	Fasciotomy	Amputation	Survive with Amputation	Deaths
Artery only					
Common/external	12	3	3	2	1
Internal	5	0	0	0	1
Vein & artery					
Common/external artery & vein	17	6	7	4	7
Internal artery & common/external v	6	0	0	0	0
Common/external a & internal vein	1	1	0	0	0
Internal artery & vein	1	0	0	0	1
Vein only					
Common/external	25	1	1	0	7
Internal	3	0	0	0	0
Total	69	11	11	6	17

patient. Ligating the common or external iliac veins is associated with a low incidence of prolonged leg swelling (Table 2).

▶ Groote Schuur is one of Cape Town's premier tertiary academic hospitals and was officially opened in 1938. The hospital is internationally renowned for trauma (penetrating trauma, in particular).

Reported herein is a 10-year experience in the management of penetrating iliac vessel trauma in a young population, mostly secondary to gunshot wounds. One hundred eight iliac vessel injuries were examined. There are several lessons to be learned from this experience:

1. The overall mortality rate is noteworthy at 25%.

2. Combined iliac artery and vein injuries are highly lethal, and prophylactic fasciotomy should be routinely done in these cases. Amputation rates are highest in this category (Table 2).

3. Temporary intraluminal shunts can be life and limb saving in the profoundly coagulopathic patient with multiple injuries.

4. Because of a high incidence of associated bowel injury, primary repair or interposition vein graft should be preferred over prosthetic repair.

B. W. Starnes, MD

Anatomic distribution and mortality of arterial injury in the wars in Afghanistan and Iraq with comparison to a civilian benchmark
Markov NP, DuBose JJ, Scott D, et al (United States Army Inst for Surgical Res, San Antonio, TX; Air Force Ctr for the Sustainment of Trauma Readiness and Skills C-STARS, Baltimore, MD)
J Vasc Surg 56:728-736, 2012

Objective.—The purpose of this study was to examine the anatomic distribution and associated mortality of combat-related vascular injuries comparing them to a contemporary civilian standard.

Design.—The Joint Trauma Theater Registry (JTTR) was queried to identify patients with major compressible arterial injury (CAI) and noncompressible arterial injury (NCAI) sites, and their outcomes, among casualties in Iraq and Afghanistan from 2003 to 2006. The National Trauma Data Bank (NTDB) was then queried over the same time frame to identify civilian trauma patients with similar arterial injuries. Propensity score-based matching was used to create matched patient cohorts from both populations for analysis.

Results.—Registry queries identified 380 patients from the JTTR and 7020 patients from the NTDB who met inclusion criteria. Propensity score matching for age, elevated Injury Severity Score (ISS; >15), and hypotension on arrival (systolic blood pressure [SBP] <90) resulted in 167 matched patients from each registry. The predominating mechanism of injury among matched JTTR patients was explosive events (73.1%), whereas penetrating injury was more common in the NTDB group (61.7%). In the matched cohorts, the incidence of NCAI did not differ (22.2% JTTR vs 26.6% NTDB; *P* =.372), but the NTDB patients had a higher incidence of CAI (73.7% vs 59.3%; *P* =.005). The JTTR cohort was also found to have a higher incidence of associated venous injury (57.5% vs 23.4%; *P* <.001). Overall, the matched JTTR cohort had a lower mortality than NTDB counterparts (4.2% vs 12.6%; *P* =.006), a finding that was also noted among patients with NCAI (10.8% vs 36.4%; *P* =.008). There was no difference in mortality between matched JTTR and NTDB patients with CAI overall (2.0% vs 4.1%; *P* =.465), or among those presenting with Glasgow Coma Scale (GCS) <8 (28.6% vs 40.0%; *P* = 1.00) or shock (SBP <90; 10.5% vs 7.7%; *P* = 1.00). The JTTR mortality rate among patients with CAI was, however, lower among patients with ISS >15 compared with civilian matched counterparts (10.7% vs 42.4%; *P* =.006).

Conclusions.—Mortality of injured service personnel who reach a medical treatment facility after major arterial injury compares favorably to a matched civilian standard. Acceptable mortality rates within the military cohort are related to key aspects of an organized Joint Trauma System, including prehospital tactical combat casualty care, rapid medical evacuation to forward surgical capability, and implementation of clinical practice guidelines. Aspects of this comprehensive combat casualty care strategy may translate and be of value to management of arterial injury in the civilian sector.

▶ In the wake of the Boston bombings, it seems especially appropriate to review this article regarding the "Anatomic distribution and mortality of arterial injury in the wars in Afghanistan and Iraq with comparison to a civilian benchmark." In this article, Markov et al review the data now amassed in the Joint Theater Trauma Registry (JTTR) to the American College of Surgeon's National Trauma Data Bank (NTDB). The authors point out that although vascular injuries affect the minority of trauma victims, they are responsible for most amputations and death from exsanguination. Initial reports on vascular trauma from the current military conflict involved several smaller databases generated by individual surgeons. Review of initial databases, including ones on the mechanisms of death, led Cordts et al at the US Army Surgeon General's office to issue self-applied tourniquets to all soldiers, profoundly decreasing the number of soldiers exsanguinating from compressible extremity injuries. The creation of the JTTR in 2008 has now allowed the Department of Defense to more formally analyze patterns of injury in an effort to increase the survival of our military. In this article, the authors perform a propensity scoring and matching technique using age, injury severity score, and initial hemodynamics to control for the differences between civilian and military trauma populations. Despite the limitations of not including injuries from the first 2 years of the war when no tourniquets were available, the authors perform an excellent comparison of the 2 trauma populations. They showed that the mortality of injured service personnel who reach a medical treatment facility after major arterial injury is 8% and compares favorably with a matched civilian standard. The authors are to be congratulated for accomplishing the monumental task of a JTTR. It is this reviewer's hope that through such thoughtful analysis continued improvements in combat casualty care will continue. At the moment, this database is focusing on several projects that will accomplish this, including new approaches to the control of noncompressible torso hemorrhage and the treatment of junctional vascular injuries.

D. L. Gillespie, MD, RVT, FACS

13 Venous Thrombosis and Pulmonary Embolism

Quantity of Residual Thrombus after Successful Catheter-directed Thrombolysis for Iliofemoral Deep Venous Thrombosis Correlates with Recurrence

Aziz F, Comerota AJ (Jobst Vascular Inst, Toledo, OH)

Eur J Vasc Endovasc Surg 44:210-213, 2012

Objectives.—Iliofemoral deep venous thrombosis (IFDVT) is an independent risk factor for recurrent DVT. It has been observed that recurrent DVT correlates with residual thrombus. This study evaluates whether risk of recurrence is related to the amount of residual thrombus following catheter-directed thrombolysis (CDT) for IFDVT.

Methods.—Patients who underwent CDT for IFDVT had their degree of lysis quantified by a reader blind to the patients' long-term clinical outcome. Patients were classified into two groups, ≥50% and <50% residual thrombus. Recurrence was defined as a symptomatic presentation with image verification of new or additional thrombus.

Results.—A total of 75 patients underwent CDT for IFDVT. Median follow-up was 35.9 months. Sixty-eight patients (91%) had no evidence of recurrence and seven (9%) developed recurrence. Of the patients who had ≥50% (mean 80%) residual thrombus, 50% (4/8) experienced recurrence, but in those with <50% (mean 35%) residual thrombus, only 5% (3/67) had recurrent DVT ($P = 0.0014$).

Conclusion.—The burden of residual thrombus at completion of CDT correlates with the risk of DVT recurrence. Patients having CDT for IFDVT had a lower risk of recurrence than expected. Successful clearing of acute clot in IFDVT patients significantly reduces the recurrence risk compared to patients with a large residual thrombus burden.

▶ There has been expansion of catheter-directed clot removal options for iliofemoral deep venous thrombosis over recent years. However, catheter-directed thrombolysis continues to be effective as a sole therapy, but it is limited by the potential for recurrence over time. The key finding in this study is the correlation of residual thrombus burden with recurrence. Although this study is limited to inclusion of catheter-directed thrombolysis only, the need to remove as much clot as possible is clear. Whether strategies that include concomitant pharmacomechanical or ultrasound-enhanced options can help with more rapid and thorough clot removal remains unclear from this study's scope and is pending further ongoing investigation in larger randomized trials.

M. A. Passman, MD

Symptomatic venous thromboembolism after femoral vein harvest

Dhanisetty RV, Liem TK, Landry GJ, et al (Oregon Health and Science Univ, Portland)
J Vasc Surg 56:696-702, 2012

Objective.—The femoral vein is increasingly utilized as a conduit in major arterial and venous reconstruction. However, perioperative complications, especially venous thromboembolism (VTE) associated with femoral vein harvest (FVH), are not well described. The purpose of this study was to determine the incidence and risk factors for the development of symptomatic VTE in patients who undergo FVH.

Methods.—We conducted a retrospective cohort study of all patients who underwent FVH over a 5-year period at a single institution. Patient clinical characteristics, indications for surgery, postoperative venous duplex scans, and computerized tomography scans of the chest were gathered and reviewed from an electronic medical record query. Statistical analysis was performed to determine which factors correlate with development of perioperative complications after FVH.

Results.—There were 57 patients (53% male; mean age, 62 years) who underwent 58 FVHs. Of the procedures, 53% were performed for arterial reconstruction and 47% for vascular reconstruction after cancer resection (85% portomesenteric reconstruction). Perioperative VTEs were diagnosed in 17 of 58 (29%) FVH procedures. Sixteen ipsilateral deep vein thromboses (DVTs) occurred distal to the FVH site and five (9%) occurred proximal to the FVH site. The incidence of VTE was significantly greater in patients with malignancy (52% vs 10%; $P = .001$), and 88% of all VTEs in this series were diagnosed in patients with cancer. All DVTs proximal to the FVH site and all DVTs in the contralateral extremity occurred in patients with malignancy. Pulmonary embolism occurred in two patients. No patients developed compartment syndrome or limb loss. Eight patients (14%) required FVH site wound debridement.

Conclusions.—VTE after FVH occurs more frequently in patients with malignancy. Aggressive and prolonged thromboprophylaxis and routine venous ultrasound surveillance are warranted after FVH in patients with malignancy.

▶ The femoral vein has been used with increasing frequency for both arterial and venous reconstruction when a larger autogenous conduit is needed. Although most of the literature reports reasonable outcomes and low venous morbidity in aortoiliac and femoral-femoral arterial reconstruction, there is less information regarding its wider use in venous reconstructions. While this study looks at the overall experience using femoral vein conduit, when used for the venous reconstruction population, there may be added potential risk for venous morbidity, especially when femoral vein is used in the setting of malignancy, a known risk factor for venous thromboembolism. Although routine thromboprophylaxis was used in this study population, standard protocols may be insufficient in this group, thereby suggesting a role for more extended prophylaxis and routine ultrasound surveillance as advocated by the authors but not necessarily supported by the study design. Regardless, this study does highlight a higher risk group that requires special considerations for venous thromboembolism prevention.

M. A. Passman, MD

Dedicated tracking of patients with retrievable inferior vena cava filters improves retrieval rates
Lucas DJ, Dunne JR, Rodriguez CJ, et al (Walter Reed Natl Military Med Ctr, Bethesda, MD)
Am Surg 78:870-874, 2012

Retrievable IVC filters (R-IVCF) are associated with multiple complications, including filter migration and deep venous thrombosis. Unfortunately, most series of R-IVCF show low retrieval rates, often due to loss to follow-up. This study demonstrates that actively tracking R-IVCF improves retrieval. Trauma patients at one institution with R-IVCF placed between January 2007 and January 2011 were tracked in a registry with a goal of retrieval. These were compared to a control group who had R-IVCF placed previously (December 2005 to December 2006). Outcome measures include filter retrieval, retrieval attempts, loss to follow-up, and time to filter retrieval. We compared 93 tracked patients with R-IVCF with 20 controls. The baseline characteristics of the groups were similar. Tracked patients had significantly higher rates of filter retrieval (60% *vs* 30%, $P = 0.02$) and filter retrieval attempts (70% *vs* 30%, $P = 0.002$) and were significantly less likely to be lost to follow-up (5% vs 65%, $P < 0.0001$). Time to retrieval attempt was 84 days in the registry versus 210 days in the control group, which trended towards significance ($P = 0.23$). Tracking patients with R-IVCF leads to improved retrieval rates, more retrieval attempts, and decreased loss to follow up. Institutions should consider tracking R-IVCF to maximize retrieval rates.

▶ With the US Food and Drug Administration warning regarding the need to remove retrievable vena cava filters,[1] there has been a growing need to incorporate mechanisms to follow patients with vena cava filters to increase opportunities to remove the filters when indicated. Passive efforts have been well documented to fail, with many patients lost to follow-up. This study is one of several recent publications that have shown the benefit of active tracking to improve filter retrieval rates. It is the responsibility of those placing retrievable filters to have a system in place to close the loop on retrieving the filter when clinically indicated, and active tracking and reminder systems are imperative to this effort. Although this particular study is based on a military-based study population, it presents a system that can easily be translated to meet the needs of civilian health care systems. As interest to improve filter retrievable rates increases, more centralized registry and notification efforts coordinated through patient safety organizations are on the near horizon.

M. A. Passman, MD

Reference

1. Inferior Vena Cava (IVC) Filters: Initial Communication: Risk of Adverse Events with Long Term Use. August 2010. Available at http://www.fda.gov/Safety/MedWatch/SafetyInformation/SafetyAlertsforHumanMedicalProducts/ucm221707.htm. Accessed June 4, 2013.

Pulmonary Embolism Without Deep Venous Thrombosis
Schwartz T, Hingorani A, Ascher E, et al (Maimonides Med Ctr, Brooklyn, NY)
Ann Vasc Surg 26:973-976, 2012

Background.—To identify patients with pulmonary embolism (PE) without deep venous thrombosis (DVT), and to compare them with those with an identifiable source on upper (UED) and lower-extremity venous duplex scans (LED).

Methods.—We performed a retrospective review of 2700 computed tomography angiograms of the chest between January 2008 and September 2010 and identified 230 patients with PE. We then evaluated the results of UED and LED and divided the patients into four groups based on the results of their duplex studies. We compared patients with PE and DVT with those with PE and no DVT in terms of age, gender, size and location of PE, critical illness, malignancy, and in-hospital mortality.

Results.—We identified 152 women and 78 men (mean age, 68 years) with PE. One hundred thirty-one patients had a documented source of PE (group 1). Fifty-three patients had negative LED results, but did not undergo UED (group 2). Thirty-one patients did not undergo either LED or UED (group 3). Seven men and eight women had no documented source of PE on UED and LED (group 4). Ten of 15 patients in group 4 had a documented malignancy listed as one of their diagnoses. Because patients in groups 2 and 3 did not undergo complete duplex studies, we excluded them from our analysis. We then reviewed the discharge summaries of patients in groups 1 and 4. There was no statistically significant difference in age and gender distribution, size and location of PE, critical illness, smoking status, cardiovascular disease, trauma, and in-hospital mortality between patients in group 1 and 4. Patients in group 4 had a statistically significant increased prevalence of malignancy (67% vs. 40%, $P = 0.046$). Patients in group 4 also had a higher percentage of active cancer than those in group 1 (47% vs. 24%, $P = 0.084$), although not statistically significant. We defined active cancer as either a metastatic disease or a malignancy diagnosed shortly before or after the diagnosis of PE. Patients who were undergoing treatment for cancer at the time of diagnosis of PE were also considered to have active cancer.

Conclusion.—We demonstrated a statistically significant increased prevalence of malignancy in patients with PE without DVT. However, pathophysiology and clinical significance are the aspects that remain to be understood after accrual of more patients and further research. Possibilities such as de novo thrombosis of pulmonary arteries, complete dislodgement of thrombi from peripheral veins, or false-negative venous duplex need to be explored.

▶ Pulmonary embolism (PE) without an identifiable source of deep venous thrombosis (DVT) as a clinical entity is poorly defined. Although de novo pulmonary artery thrombosis, complete embolization from the source vein, or false-negative extremity imaging are all possibilities, the need for anticoagulation remains regardless of whether the source is identified. With the noted increased prevalence in patients with malignancy, the potential for hypercoagulability may also play a role, thereby emphasizing the need for anticoagulation. The only clinical dilemma involves patients who cannot be anticoagulated and in whom there may be a consideration for a vena cava filter. Without a defined source, the decision of where to locate the filter, inferior, superior vena cava, or both, becomes even more problematic. Although the scope of this study did not address vena cava filters, in general, unless circumstances indicate ongoing PE without an identifiable source, avoiding filters would be preferred. Clearly, further evidence on this poorly defined entity is needed to help provide clinical guidance when anticoagulation cannot be used.

M. A. Passman, MD

Comparison of vein valve function following pharmacomechanical thrombolysis versus simple catheter-directed thrombolysis for iliofemoral deep vein thrombosis
Vogel D, Walsh ME, Chen JT, et al (Jobst Vascular Inst, Toledo, OH; Bowling Green State Univ, OH)
J Vasc Surg 56:1351-1354, 2012

Background.—Successful catheter-directed thrombolysis (CDT) for iliofemoral deep vein thrombosis (IFDVT) reduces post-thrombotic morbidity and is a suggested treatment option by the American College of Chest Physicians for patients with IFDVT. Pharmacomechanical thrombolysis (PMT) is also suggested to shorten treatment time and reduce the dose of plasminogen activator. However, concern remains that mechanical devices might damage vein valves. The purpose of this study is to examine whether PMT adversely affects venous valve function compared to CDT alone in IFDVT patients treated with catheter-based techniques.

Methods.—Sixty-nine limbs in 54 patients (39 unilateral, 15 bilateral) who underwent catheter-based treatment for IFDVT form the basis of this study. Lytic success and degree of residual obstruction were analyzed by reviewing postprocedural phlebograms. All patients underwent bilateral postprocedure duplex to evaluate patency and valve function. Phlebograms and venous duplex examinations were interpreted in a blinded fashion. Limbs were analyzed based on the method of treatment: CDT alone (n = 20), PMT using rheolytic thrombolysis (n = 14), and isolated pharmacomechanical thrombolysis (n = 35). The validated outcome measures were compared between the treatment groups.

Results.—Sixty-nine limbs underwent CDT with or without PMT. The average patient age was 47 years (range, 16-78). Venous duplex was performed 44.4 months (mean) post-treatment. Of the limbs treated with CDT with drip technique, 65% demonstrated reflux vs 53% treated with PMT ($P = .42$). There was no difference in long-term valve function between patients treated with rheolytic and isolated pharmacomechanical thrombolysis. In the bilateral group, 87% (13/15) demonstrated reflux in at least one limb. In the unilateral group, 64% (25/39) had reflux in their treated limb and 36% (14/39) in their contralateral limb. There was no correlation effect of residual venous obstruction on valve function, although few patients had >50% residual obstruction.

Conclusions.—In patients undergoing catheter-based intervention for IFDVT, PMT does not adversely affect valve function compared with CDT alone. A higher than expected number of patients had reflux in their uninvolved limb.

▶ Preservation of venous valve function and prevention of postthrombotic venous reflux is one of the goals of catheter-based clot removal. Based on concern for potential secondary valve damage from intraluminal pharmacomechanical thrombolysis (PMT) techniques that use larger profile catheters, this study compares follow-up venous valve testing with ultrasound scan in patients with iliofemoral deep vein thrombosis undergoing catheter-directed thrombolysis (CDT) vs PMT. Although there was no significant difference noted between both groups, there was a high rate of venous reflux noted across the study populations (65% in CDT group, and 53% in PMT group; $P = .42$), while small sample size and retrospective study design limit the strength of these findings. However, this study shows that although preservation of valve function is not necessarily influenced by catheter size and intraluminal manipulation, the concept of expanding techniques that allow more rapid and complete clot removal should be the focus of catheter clot removal efforts independent of concern for secondary valve damage from catheter instrumentation.

M. A. Passman, MD

Management of the Thrombosed Filter-Bearing Inferior Vena Cava

Sildiroglu O, Ozer H, Turba UC (Univ of Virginia Health System, Charlottesville)
Semin Intervent Radiol 29:57-63, 2012

Inferior vena cava (IVC) filter thrombosis is a complex problem. Thrombus within an IVC filter may range from an asymptomatic small thrombus to critical IVC occlusion that affects both lower extremities. The published experience of IVC thrombosis management in relation to filters is either anecdotal or limited to a small group of patients; however, endovascular treatment methods appear to be safe and effective in patients with IVC thrombosis. This review focuses on filter-related IVC thrombosis and its endovascular management.

▶ The almost exponential increase in the use of inferior vena cava (IVC) filters over the past decade has led to an increase in several new pathologic entities that require therapy. One such problem, as detailed in this article, is IVC filter thrombosis. IVC and iliac vein thrombosis is a feared complication of IVC filters. Among all models of filters deployed, the OptEase is associated with the highest postplacement deep vein thrombosis (DVT) rate, 4.4% in the British Society of Interventional Radiology's report. Further, the similarly designed TrapEase filter was associated with a significantly higher rate of IVC thrombosis in a randomized trial comparing it with the Greenfield filter. The OptEase and TrapEase are unique among IVC filters because of their double-basket design as opposed to the single-cylinder design found in most IVC filters. Computational and imaging studies of this unique design suggest that alterations in flow dynamics and shear stress with thrombus trapped against the vein wall may be at least partially responsible for this increase in IVC thrombosis. This article reports that even with the paucity of published data, endovascular treatment methods appear to be safe and effective in patients with filter-related IVC thrombosis, with results comparable to those reported for catheter-directed iliofemoral DVT therapy.

D. L. Gillespie, MD, RVT, FACS

Dedicated tracking of patients with retrievable inferior vena cava filters improves retrieval rates

Lucas DJ, Dunne JR, Rodriguez CJ, et al (Walter Reed Natl Military Med Ctr, Bethesda, MD)
Am Surg 78:870-874, 2012

Retrievable IVC filters (R-IVCF) are associated with multiple complications, including filter migration and deep venous thrombosis. Unfortunately, most series of R-IVCF show low retrieval rates, often due to loss to follow-up. This study demonstrates that actively tracking R-IVCF improves retrieval. Trauma patients at one institution with R-IVCF placed between January 2007 and January 2011 were tracked in a registry with a goal of retrieval. These were compared to a control group who had R-IVCF placed previously (December 2005 to December 2006). Outcome measures include filter retrieval, retrieval attempts, loss to follow-up, and time to filter retrieval. We compared 93 tracked patients with R-IVCF with 20 controls. The baseline characteristics of the groups were similar. Tracked patients had significantly higher rates of filter retrieval (60% vs 30%, $P = 0.02$) and filter retrieval attempts (70% vs 30%, $P = 0.002$) and were significantly less likely to be lost to follow-up (5% vs 65%, $P < 0.0001$). Time to retrieval attempt was 84 days in the registry versus 210 days in the control group, which trended towards significance ($P = 0.23$). Tracking patients with R-IVCF leads to improved retrieval rates, more retrieval attempts, and decreased loss to follow up. Institutions should consider tracking R-IVCF to maximize retrieval rates.

▶ Because the touted benefit of temporary inferior vena cava filters (IVCFs) is in their short-term use, their overall retrieval rate is of importance. In Karmy-Jones's American Association for the Surgery of Trauma multicenter study of 446 patients receiving retrievable IVCFs, there was a 20% overall retrieval rate, with 34% left for ongoing indications and 31% lost to follow-up.[1] However, even in the United States, where wounded servicemen and servicewomen are followed closely in a centralized military health care system, the retrieval rates have been equally low. In a study by Johnson et al of US soldiers injured in Iraq and Afghanistan, the overall retrieval rate was 18%, with 63% left for ongoing indications and only 11% lost to follow-up.[2]

In this study at the same institution, retrievable IVCFs placed between January 2007 and January 2011 were tracked in a registry with a goal of retrieval. These were compared with a control group who had a retrievable IVCF placed previously (December 2005 to December 2006). They compared 93 tracked patients with retrievable IVCFs with 20 controls. The baseline characteristics of the groups were similar. Tracked patients had significantly higher rates of filter retrieval (60% vs 30%; $P = .02$) and filter retrieval attempts (70% vs 30%; $P = .002$) and were significantly less likely to be lost to follow-up (5% vs 65%; $P < .0001$). It certainly seems that tracking patients with retrievable IVCFs leads to improved retrieval rates, more retrieval attempts, and decreased loss to follow-up. Institutions should consider tracking retrievable IVCFs to maximize retrieval rates.

D. L. Gillespie, MD, RVT, FACS

References

1. Karmy-Jones R, Jurkovich GJ, Velmahos GC, et al. Practice patterns and outcomes of retrievable vena cava filters in trauma patients: an AAST multicenter study. *J Trauma.* 2007;62(1):17-24; discussion 24-25.
2. Johnson ON 3rd, Gillespie DL, Aidinian G, White PW, Adams E, Fox CJ. The use of retrievable inferior vena cava filters in severely injured military trauma patients. *J Vasc Surg.* 2009;49(2):410-416; discussion 416.

British Society of Interventional Radiology (BSIR) Inferior Vena Cava (IVC) Filter Registry
Uberoi R, Tapping CR, Chalmers N, et al (Oxford Univ Hosp, Headington, UK)
Cardiovasc Intervent Radiol 2013 [Epub ahead of print]

Purpose.—The British Society of Interventional Radiology (BSIR) Inferior Vena Cava (IVC) Filter Registry was produced to provide an audit of current United Kingdom (UK) practice regarding placement and retrieval of IVC filters to address concerns regarding their safety.

Methods.—The IVC filter registry is a web-based registry, launched by the BSIR on behalf of its membership in October 2007. This report is based on prospectively collected data from October 2007 to March 2011. This report contains analysis of data on 1,434 IVC filter placements and 400 attempted retrievals performed at 68 UK centers. Data collected included patient demographics, insertion and retrieval data, and patient follow-up.

Results.—IVC filter use in the majority of patients in the UK follows accepted CIRSE guidelines. Filter placement is usually a low-risk procedure, with a low major complication rate (<0.5%). Cook Gunther Tulip (560 filters: 39%) and Celect (359 filters: 25%) filters constituted the majority of IVC filters inserted, with Bard G2, Recovery filters, Cordis Trapease, and OptEase constituting most of the remainder (445 filters: 31%). More than 96% of IVC filters deployed as intended. Operator inexperience (<25 procedure) was significantly associated with complications ($p < 0.001$). Of the IVC filters initially intended for temporary placement, retrieval was attempted in 78%. Of these retrieval was technically successful in 83%. Successful retrieval was significantly reduced for implants left in situ for >9 weeks versus those with a shorter dwell time. New lower limb deep vein thrombosis (DVT) and/or IVC thrombosis was reported in 88 patients following filter placement, there was no significant difference of incidence between filter types.

Conclusions.—This registry report provides interventional radiologists and clinicians with an improved understanding of the technical aspects of IVC filter placement to help improve practice, and the potential consequences of IVC filter placement so that we are better able to advise patients. There is a significant learning curve associated with IVC filter insertion, and when a filter is placed with the intention of removal, procedures should be in place to avoid the patient being lost to follow-up.

▶ A fundamental question underlying the use of newer retrievable inferior vena cava filters (IVCFs) is whether they are safe and effective. Retrospective review data on the long-term safety and efficacy of permanent filters is relatively robust, while long-term studies of newer retrievable filters are comparatively lacking. In 2010, the US Food and Drug Administration issued an alert to remove retrievable IVCFs as soon as possible. The British Society of Interventional Radiology recently published the First UK Inferior Vena Cava Filter Registry Report 2011, which is aimed to gain insight into the use of retrievable IVCFs. In it, preprocedural, procedural, and outcomes are reported for 5 retrievable filters. From it, some general recommendations have been formed. First, when right femoral access is unavailable for access, a jugular approach should be used when possible. Second, when a filter is placed with the intention of removal, procedures should be in effect to prevent the patient from being lost to follow-up. And third, filter retrieval is most successful within weeks and should be scheduled within this timeframe.

D. L. Gillespie, MD, RVT, FACS

Caval Penetration by Retrievable Inferior Vena Cava Filters: A Retrospective Comparison of Option and Günther Tulip Filters

Olorunsola OG, Kohi MP, Fidelman N, et al (Univ of California, San Francisco)
J Vasc Interv Radiol 24:566-571, 2013

Purpose.—To compare the frequency of vena caval penetration by the struts of the Option and Günther Tulip cone filters on postplacement computed tomography (CT) imaging.

Materials and Methods.—All patients who had an Option or Günther Tulip inferior vena cava (IVC) filter placed between January 2010 and May 2012 were identified retrospectively from medical records. Of the 208 IVC filters placed, the positions of 58 devices (21 Option filters, 37 Günther Tulip filters [GTFs]) were documented on follow-up CT examinations obtained for reasons unrelated to filter placement. In cases when multiple CT studies were obtained after placement, each study was reviewed, for a total of 80 examinations. Images were assessed for evidence of caval wall penetration by filter components, noting the number of penetrating struts and any effect on pericaval tissues.

Results.—Penetration of at least one strut was observed in 17% of all filters imaged by CT between 1 and 447 days following placement. Although there was no significant difference in the overall prevalence of penetration when comparing the Option filter and GTF (Option, 10%; GTF, 22%), only GTFs showed time-dependent penetration, with penetration becoming more likely after prolonged indwelling times. No patient had damage to pericaval tissues or documented symptoms attributed to penetration.

Conclusions.—Although the Günther Tulip and Option filters exhibit caval penetration at CT imaging, only the GTF exhibits progressive penetration over time.

▶ In this study, the authors found there was penetration of at least one strut in 17% of all filters imaged by CT between 1 and 447 days following placement. Although there was no significant difference in the overall prevalence of penetration when comparing the Option filter and Günther Tulip filter (GTF; Option, 10%; GTF, 22%), only GTFs showed time-dependent penetration, with penetration becoming more likely after prolonged indwelling times. No patient had damage to pericaval tissues or documented symptoms attributed to penetration. Although the GTF and Option filter exhibit caval penetration at CT imaging, only the GTF exhibits progressive penetration overtime.

Specifically related to the issue of retrievability is the issue of migration and fracture. Filter migration and fracture can lead to life-threatening embolization or vessel perforation. It can be argued that in order to maintain retrievability, stability is sacrificed. Most retrievable inferior vena cava filters (IVCFs) have a migration rate of approximately 1%; however, the G2 filter is associated with a much higher migration rate of 4.5%. Additionally, of 188 reports of IVCF fracture in the Manufacturer and User Facility Device Experience Database from 2000 to 2010, 127 were with the G2. This was higher than for any other IVCF. This high rate of filter fracture has been found in other studies as well.

D. L. Gillespie, MD, RVT, FACS

Comparison of vein valve function following pharmacomechanical thrombolysis versus simple catheter-directed thrombolysis for iliofemoral deep vein thrombosis
Vogel D, Walsh ME, Chen JT, et al (Jobst Vascular Inst, Toledo, OH; Bowling Green State Univ, OH)
J Vasc Surg 56:1351-1354, 2012

Background.—Successful catheter-directed thrombolysis (CDT) for ilio-femoral deep vein thrombosis (IFDVT) reduces post-thrombotic morbidity and is a suggested treatment option by the American College of Chest Physicians for patients with IFDVT. Pharmacomechanical thrombolysis (PMT) is also suggested to shorten treatment time and reduce the dose of plasminogen activator. However, concern remains that mechanical devices might damage vein valves. The purpose of this study is to examine whether PMT adversely affects venous valve function compared to CDT alone in IFDVT patients treated with catheter-based techniques.

Methods.—Sixty-nine limbs in 54 patients (39 unilateral, 15 bilateral) who underwent catheter-based treatment for IFDVT form the basis of this study. Lytic success and degree of residual obstruction were analyzed by reviewing postprocedural phlebograms. All patients underwent bilateral postprocedure duplex to evaluate patency and valve function. Phlebograms and venous duplex examinations were interpreted in a blinded fashion. Limbs were analyzed based on the method of treatment: CDT alone (n = 20), PMT using rheolytic thrombolysis (n = 14), and isolated pharmacomechanical thrombolysis (n = 35). The validated outcome measures were compared between the treatment groups.

Results.—Sixty-nine limbs underwent CDT with or without PMT. The average patient age was 47 years (range, 16-78). Venous duplex was performed 44.4 months (mean) post-treatment. Of the limbs treated with CDT with drip technique, 65% demonstrated reflux vs 53% treated with PMT ($P = .42$). There was no difference in long-term valve function between patients treated with rheolytic and isolated pharmacomechanical thrombolysis. In the bilateral group, 87% (13/15) demonstrated reflux in at least one limb. In the unilateral group, 64% (25/39) had reflux in their treated limb and 36% (14/39) in their contralateral limb. There was no correlation effect of residual venous obstruction on valve function, although few patients had >50% residual obstruction.

Conclusions.—In patients undergoing catheter-based intervention for IFDVT, PMT does not adversely affect valve function compared with CDT alone. A higher than expected number of patients had reflux in their uninvolved limb.

▶ The use of pharmacomechanical thrombolysis (PMT) has been shown to increase the safety of catheter-directed thrombolysis (CDT) of deep venous thrombosis by decreasing time to treat and dosage of thrombolytic drugs. Early encouraging results from studies seem to indicate that patients' quality of life is improved by reopening their acutely thrombosed iliofemoral veins. As we await more robust data from the ATTRACT trial, several questions remain. In this article, the authors attempt to compare the effect of catheter-directed thrombolysis with that of pharmacomechanical thrombolysis on valvular function. The authors used a continuous patient cohort and blinded the review of postlysis phlebograms and valve closure times. Their results show no difference in valve function using PMT compared with CDT. In addition, there was no difference in PMT technique and valve function. The study results should be interpreted with the under-standing that this is a small study of only 54 patients. Whether any of these patients had pre-existing valvular incompetence is not known. In addition, valve closure times were performed with the patients in reverse Trendelenburg position and not standing. Lastly, venous stenosis after thrombolysis was deter-mined using single planar phlebography, which is notoriously inaccurate for detecting venous stenoses compared with multiplanar phlebography or intravas-cular ultrasound. Despite the limitations, these results would seem to indicate that vein valve competence may not be salvageable using thrombolysis. We anxiously await the results of larger prospective studies to give us a better understanding of the role of thrombolysis in preserving vein valve function and ultimately prevent-ing the postthrombotic syndrome.

D. L. Gillespie, MD, RVT, FACS

14 Chronic Venous and Lymphatic Disease

High Compression Pressure over the Calf is More Effective than Graduated Compression in Enhancing Venous Pump Function
Mosti G, Partsch H (Clinica MD Barbantini, Lucca, Italy; Med Univ of Vienna, Austria)
Eur J Vasc Endovasc Surg 44:332-336, 2012

Background.—Graduated compression is routinely employed as standard therapy for chronic venous insufficiency.

Aim.—The study aims to compare the haemodynamic efficiency of a multi-component graduated compression bandage (GCB) versus a negative graduated compression bandage (NGCB) applied with higher pressure over the calf.

Methods.—In 20 patients, all affected by greater saphenous vein (GSV) incompetence and candidates for surgery (Clinical, etiologic, anatomic and pathophysiologic data, CEAP C2-C5), the ejection fraction of the venous calf pump was measured using a plethysmographic method during a standardised walking test without compression, with GCB and NGCB, all composed of the same short-stretch material. Sub-bandage pressures were measured simultaneously over the distal leg and over the calf.

Results.—NGCBs with median pressures higher at the calf (62 mmHg) than at the distal leg (50 mmHg) achieved a significantly higher increase of ejection fraction (median + 157%) compared with GCB, (+115%) with a distal pressure of 54 mmHg and a calf pressure of 28 mmHg ($P < 0.001$).

Conclusions.—Patients with severe venous incompetence have a greater haemodynamic benefit from NGCB, especially during standing and walking, than from GCB.

▶ Use of compression in patients with venous insufficiency is clearly established. However, contrary to traditional dogma favoring graduated compression with reduced pressure profile from ankle to calf, there is growing evidence that negative compression stockings with higher pressure at the calf are more effective than standard compression stockings. This study extends this work to evaluate the hemodynamic efficiency of negative compression bandages showing a greater benefit when compared with multicomponent graduated compression bandages in patients with severe venous incompetence. Although challenging prior perceptions is important, more evidence is needed to evaluate whether this hemo-dynamic benefit extends to clinical outcome measures.

M. A. Passman, MD

Randomized clinical trial of ultrasound-guided foam sclerotherapy *versus* surgery for the incompetent great saphenous vein
Shadid N, Ceulen R, Nelemans P, et al (Maastricht Univ Med Centre, The Netherlands; Albert Schweitzer Hosp, Dordrecht, The Netherlands; Maastricht Univ, The Netherlands; et al)
Br J Surg 99:1062-1070, 2012

Background.—New minimally invasive treatment modalities, such as ultrasound-guided foam sclerotherapy (UGFS), are becoming more popular. In a multicentre randomized controlled non-inferiority trial, the effectiveness and costs of UGFS and surgery for treatment of the incompetent great saphenous vein (GSV) were compared.

Methods.—Patients with primary great saphenous varicose veins were assigned randomly to either UGFS or surgical stripping with high ligation. Recurrence, defined as reflux combined with venous symptoms, was determined on colour duplex scans at baseline, 3 months, 1 year and 2 years after initial treatment. Secondary outcomes were presence of recurrent reflux (irrespective of symptoms), reduction of symptoms, health-related quality of life (EQ-5D™), adverse events and direct hospital costs.

Results.—Two hundred and thirty patients were treated by UGFS and 200 underwent GSV stripping. The 2-year probability of recurrence was similar in the UGFS and surgery groups: $11 \cdot 3$ per cent (24 of 213) and $9 \cdot 0$ per cent (16 of 177) respectively ($P = 0 \cdot 407$). At 2 years, reflux irrespective of venous symptoms was significantly more frequent in the UGFS group ($35 \cdot 0$ per cent) than in the surgery group ($21 \cdot 0$ per cent) ($P = 0 \cdot 003$). Mean(s.d.) hospital costs per patient over 2 years were €774(344) per patient for UGFS and €1824(141) for stripping.

Conclusion.—At 2-year follow-up, UGFS was not inferior to surgery when reflux associated with venous symptoms was the clinical outcome of interest. UGFS has the potential to be a cost-effective approach to a common health problem. Registration numbers: NCT01103258 (http://www.clinicaltrials.gov) and NTR654 (http://www.trialregister.nl).

▶ Although this randomized study shows that ultrasound-guided foam sclerotherapy (UGFS) is not inferior to surgery (high ligation and stripping) in terms of measured clinical outcomes at 2 years, there are significant limitations, including an unblinded study population, enrollment falling short of intended sample size to achieve statistical power, some patients declining treatment especially in the surgery group, and disparate need for additional varicose vein phlebectomies in the surgery group. More importantly, with current expanding minimally invasive venous treatment options, including endothermal ablation techniques in most centers, comparison of UGFS to surgery is less relevant in current venous practice.

M. A. Passman, MD

Influence of high-heeled shoes on venous function in young women
Tedeschi Filho W, Dezzotti NRA, Joviliano EE, et al (Univ of São Paulo, Brazil)
J Vasc Surg 56:1039-1044, 2012

Background.—Walking with high-heeled shoes is a common cause of venous complaints such as pain, fatigue, and heavy-feeling legs. The aim of the study was to clarify the influence of high-heeled shoes on the venous return and test the hypothesis that women wearing different styles of high-heeled shoes present an impaired venous return when compared with their values when they are barefoot.

Methods.—Thirty asymptomatic women (mean age, 26.4 years) wearing appropriately sized shoes were evaluated by air plethysmography (APG), a test that measures changes in air volume on a cuff placed on the calf, while they performed orthostatic flexion and extension foot movements and altered standing up and lying down. The test was repeated in four situations: barefoot (0 cm), medium heels (3.5 cm), stiletto high heels (7 cm), and platform high heels (7 cm). The APG values of venous filling index (VFI), ejection fraction (EF), and residual volume fraction (RVF) were divided into four groups according to heel height and compared by repeated-measures analysis of variance.

Results.—RVF was increased in the groups wearing high heels (stiletto and platform) compared with the barefoot group ($P < .05$). RVF was increased in the medium-heel group (3.5 cm) compared with the barefoot group ($P < .05$), and despite the lack of statistical significance, the medium-heel group showed lower values of RVF compared with the two high-heel groups. The EF parameter followed the opposite tendency, showing higher values for the barefoot group compared with the other three groups ($P < .05$). Values for VFI were similar in the three situations evaluated.

Conclusions.—High heels reduce muscle pump function, as demonstrated by reduced EF and increased RVF values. The continuous use of high heels tends to provoke venous hypertension in the lower limbs and may represent a causal factor of venous disease symptoms.

▶ The negative impact of high-heeled shoes on venous function shown in this study is an interesting association in that it highlights the importance of the interaction of foot and calf muscle pump, which is hindered by elevating heel levels. From an evolutionary standpoint, humans were not designed to walk on high heels, so this negative physiologic finding is not a surprise. However, although this study concludes that continuous use of high heels tends to provoke venous hypertension, any causal relationship to development of symptomatic venous disease is an overreach. Although venous disease is more common in women, this association is likely multifactorial and not solely caused by the ergonomics of footwear. Interestingly, the impact of high-heeled shoes was not tested in men. What may also be of interest to both men and women is extending the same physiologic venous evaluation to the current controversy between traditional running shoes, which are designed for heel-to-toe movement, vs barefoot (forefoot) running gait and whether there is a difference in venous function between different running shoe designs.

M. A. Passman, MD

Great saphenous vein diameter does not correlate with worsening quality of life scores in patients with great saphenous vein incompetence
Gibson K, Meissner M, Wright D (Lake Washington Vascular Surgeons, Bellevue; Univ of Washington, Seattle; BTG PLLC, London)
J Vasc Surg 56:1634-1641, 2012

Objective.—Previous studies have correlated increasing great saphenous vein (GSV) diameter with increasing CEAP clinical classification. Some insurance carriers are currently using specific GSV diameters to determine coverage for treatment of axial venous insufficiency. The aim of this study was to investigate the correlation of patient quality of life (QOL) measures with GSV diameters in varicose vein patients with GSV reflux.

Methods.—Data were collected from the records of 91 patients prospectively enrolled in two varicose vein trials. The patients had symptomatic varicose veins with saphenofemoral junction and proximal GSV reflux. Maximum GSV diameter was measured on duplex ultrasound imaging, with the patient standing, within 5 cm of the saphenofemoral junction. Chronic Venous Insufficiency Questionnaire 2 (CIVIQ-2; Servier, Neuilly-sur-Seine, France), Venous Insufficiency Epidemiological and Economic Study (VEINES) Symptom (Sym) and QOL assessments, and the Venous Clinical Severity Score (VCSS) assessment were completed before treatment of GSV insufficiency. Demographic information, patient weight, height, and body mass index were collected. Correlations between pairs of data were done using Pearson product-moment and Spearman correlation coefficients.

Results.—The 91 study patients (19 men, 72 women) were a mean age of 45 years (range, 18-65 years). The mean GSV diameter was 6.7 mm (range, 2.2-14.1 mm). The mean VCSS score was 7.8 (range, 3-12). There was a weak correlation between increasing GSV diameter and VCSS ($r = 0.23$; $P = .03$) and no correlation between GSV diameter and the CIVIQ-2 score ($r = 0.01$), VEINES-QOL ($r = -0.07$), and VEINES-Sym ($r = -0.1$).

Conclusions.—GSV diameter is a poor surrogate marker for assessing the effect of varicose veins on a patient's QOL; thus, using GSV diameter as a sole criterion for determining medical necessity for the treatment of GSV reflux is inappropriate. Further correlations between QOL measures and duplex-derived objective findings are warranted.

▶ Although there has been some correlation of great saphenous vein (GSV) diameter with symptomatic varicose veins and physician-derived outcome measures, such as the CEAP (Clinical, Etiologic, Anatomic, Pathophysiologic) and VCSS (Venous Clinical Severity Scoring) and objective measurement of reflux with ultrasound, this relationship is not absolute. As shown in this study, when using quality-of-life venous assessment tools, GSV diameter is a poor surrogate marker for assessing the clinical impact of varicose veins on patient-derived outcome measures. Because GSV diameter is a variable marker for severity of venous disease, recent efforts by insurance carriers to restrict approval of venous operation coverage based on GSV diameter as a sole parameter in determining medical necessity is flawed and should be challenged.

M. A. Passman, MD

Saphenous pulsation on duplex may be a marker of severe chronic superficial venous insufficiency
Lattimer CR, Azzam M, Kalodiki E, et al (Ealing Hosp and Imperial College London, UK)
J Vasc Surg 56:1338-1343, 2012

Background.—Pulsatile flow in deep, perforating veins and varicose veins (VVs) has been described previously to support a hypothesis of arteriovenous (AV) fistulae in the pathogenesis of VVs. Its presence has also been suggested as a cause of failure of VV treatments. However, AV communications have never been adequately visualized and direct pressure tracings within leg veins have been inconclusive. The present study was observational aiming to investigate the prevalence and rate of spontaneous pulsation within the great saphenous vein (GSV) in volunteers and patients using color duplex and compare this to reflux and markers of disease severity.

Methods.—Twenty-seven consecutive patients (32 legs, median Venous Clinical Severity Score (VCSS) = 5 [0-11]) attending the VV clinic and 23 consecutive ambulatory normal volunteers (46 legs) had their GSV assessed at midthigh using color duplex. Subjects were examined standing with the hips resting against an adjustable couch, bearing weight on the contralateral leg, with the test leg touching the ground. The presence of flow and reflux were initially determined using manual calf compression. Saphenous pulsation (SP) was defined as a cyclical change in velocity. The GSV diameter and SP rate were then recorded after 2 minutes of dependency. The number of pulsations was counted from video recordings.

Results.—The resting SP, if present, was discrete, monophasic, of variable amplitude, antegrade, and irregular, irrespective of respiration. Pulsation was detected in 2/44 (4.5%) legs with C_{0-1} (C part of CEAP), 9/17 (52.9%) legs with C_{2-3}, and 16/17 (94.1%) legs with C_{4-6} ($P < .05$, z test of column proportions). Reflux occurred in 8/32 (25%) legs without SP ($C_0 = 2$, $C_1 = 1$, $C_2 = 3$, $C_3 = 2$). The median GSV diameter was significantly elevated in the presence of SP (no pulse: 3.5 [range, 1.5-8.1] mm; pulse: 7 [range, 4-9.4] mm; $P < .0005$). The median refluxing GSV diameter in GSV pulsators compared with nonpulsators was 7 (range, 4-9.4) mm; vs

5.1 (range, 2.7-8.1) mm, respectively ($P = .003$). The median SP rate in refluxing GSVs was 52 (range, 22-95) beats per minute.

Conclusions.—The high prevalence of pulsatile antegrade saphenous flow is a novel observation in patients with severe superficial chronic venous insufficiency. It is detectable in 75% of patients with GSV reflux and significantly increases with clinical severity and saphenous diameter. It may be a marker of advanced venous disease and, as it is easy to record, it could supplement duplex evaluations of reflux. Further work is needed to establish the clinical relevance of the SP in terms of disease progression, recurrence after treatment, and as a hemodynamic marker of severity.

▶ Pulsatile flow in varicose veins has been previously described, but its source and physiologic significance remains unclear. The observation in this study of a high prevalence of pulsatile antegrade flow in the great saphenous vein, using the techniques described, and its correlation with severe superficial chronic venous insufficiency highlights a potentially useful adjunct ultrasound parameter that could be used in conjunction with standard duplex evaluation of reflux. However, the clinical relevance of this finding as it relates to natural history of venous disease, venous severity outcome measures, correlation with venous symptoms, and predictors of treatment failure or recurrence have yet to be defined.

M. A. Passman, MD

Generic Health-related Quality of Life is Significantly Worse in Varicose Vein Patients with Lower Limb Symptoms Independent of Ceap Clinical Grade

Darvall KAL, Bate GR, Adam DJ, et al (Birmingham Univ, UK)
Eur J Vasc Endovasc Surg 44:341-344, 2012

Objectives.—To determine the relationship between lower limb symptoms and generic health-related quality of life (HRQL) in patients with varicose veins (VV).

Methods.—284 patients on the waiting list for VV treatment completed the Short Form-12 (SF12) and a questionnaire asking about the presence of lower limb symptoms commonly attributed to venous disease (pain or ache, itching, tingling, cramp, restless legs, a feeling of swelling, and heaviness).

Results.—Median age was 57 years (interquartile range 45–67); 100 (35%) were male, and 182 (64%) had CEAP clinical grade 2 or 3 disease. Jonckheere–Terpstra test for trend revealed that both physical ($P < .0005$) and mental ($P = .001$) HRQL worsened as the reported number of symptoms increased. Patients reporting tingling ($P = .016$, Mann–Whitney U test), cramp ($P = .001$), restless legs ($P < .0005$), swelling ($P < .0005$), and heaviness ($P < .0005$) had a significantly worse physical HRQL than those who did not. Mental HRQL was also significantly worse in patients with tingling ($P = .010$), cramp ($P = .008$), restless legs ($P = .040$), swelling ($P = .001$), and heaviness ($P = .035$). These significant relationships remained, and pain was also correlated with worse physical HRQL ($P = .011$), when linear regression was performed to control for CEAP clinical grade, age and sex.

Conclusions.—Physical and mental HRQL is significantly worse in VV patients with lower limb symptoms irrespective of the clinical stage of disease. This observation confirms that VV are not primarily a cosmetic problem and that NHS rationing of treatment to those with CEAP C4-6 disease excludes many patients who would benefit from intervention in terms of HRQL. Generic HRQL instruments also allow comparison with interventions for other chronic conditions.

▶ For patients with varicose veins, correlation of lower limb symptoms with clinical or ultrasound evidence of chronic venous insufficiency can be variable and may lead to limited coverage for varicose vein interventions. Although health-related quality of life (HRQL) questionnaires have been used to show benefit of venous operation, correlation with limb symptoms has been inconsistent. The findings of this study of significantly worse HRQL parameters in patients with varicose veins and lower limb symptoms, irrespective of clinical stage of venous disease, suggest a potential expanded role of HRQL measures to help determine those who may benefit most from venous intervention, but further investigation, including outcome assessment, would be required to make this connection.

M. A. Passman, MD

A randomized double-blind trial of upward progressive versus degressive compressive stockings in patients with moderate to severe chronic venous insufficiency

Couzan S, Leizorovicz A, Laporte S, et al (Clinique Mutualiste, Saint-Étiennea, France; Université de Lyon, France; Université Jean Monnet Saint-Étienne, France; et al)
J Vasc Surg 56:1344-1350, 2012

Background.—The present randomized double-blind multicenter study was designed to assess the efficacy of a progressive compressive stocking (new concept with maximal pressure at calf), compared to a degressive compressive stocking graded 30 mm Hg, evaluating the improvement of lower leg symptoms of chronic venous insufficiency (CVI) in ambulatory patients with moderate to severe chronic venous disease.

Methods.—Both gender outpatients presenting symptomatic moderate to severe CVI were eligible for a treatment by compressive stockings. Patients were randomly assigned to receive either degressive compressive stockings (30 mm Hg at ankle, 21 mm Hg at upper calf) or progressive compressive stockings (10 mm Hg at ankle, 23 mm Hg at upper calf). The primary outcome, evaluated after 3 months, was a composite success outcome, including improvement of pain or heavy legs without onset of either ulcer, deep or superficial vein thrombosis of the lower limbs, or pulmonary embolism. The ease of application of the compressive stockings reported by patients was one of secondary outcome.

Results.—Overall, 401 patients (199 in the progressive compressive stocking group and 202 in the degressive compressive stocking group) were randomized by 44 angiologists in France. Among them, 66% were classified in the C3 CEAP category. The rate of success was significantly higher in the progressive compressive stocking group compared to the degressive compressive stocking group (70.0% vs 59.6%; relative risk, 1.18; 95% confidence interval, 1.02-1.37; $P = .03$). This was mainly due to more frequent symptom improvement in the progressive compressive stocking group. The compressive stockings were considered easy to apply by 81.3% of patients in the progressive compressive stocking group vs 49.7% of patients in the degressive compressive stocking group ($P < .0001$). The rate of related serious adverse events was low and similar in both groups.

Conclusions.—This trial has demonstrated that progressive compressive stockings are more effective than usual degressive compressive stockings in the improvement of pain and lower leg symptoms in patients with CVI. Moreover, progressive compressive stockings were easier to apply, raising no safety concern at 3 months.

▶ This randomized, double-blind trial applies a novel functional concept to compression stockings, a therapeutic intervention for chronic venous insufficiency in which device innovation has been uncommon and primarily focused on cosmetic factors. The trial was powered for statistical assessment for superiority and utilized a thoughtful and detailed approach to blinding both patients and participating angiologists. The observed success advantage associated with use of upward progressive stockings was primarily attributed to symptomatic improvement and suggests that a change in stocking design may lead to improved outcomes without significant additional risk (or, hopefully, costs). By including ease of stocking application as an endpoint, the investigators were able to evaluate a factor potentially influencing treatment effectiveness (which is commonly difficult to assess from randomized trial results). It is surprising to note that although the upward compressive stockings were easier to apply, compliance was similar between groups. Delving further into noncompliance with future studies will hopefully identify influential factors that can be used to individualize treatment selection. It is interesting to note that although both deep vein thrombosis (DVT) and pulmonary embolism were included in the aggregate endpoint, screening was not performed for either of these outcomes as part of the study protocol. Given the history of venous thromboembolism in nearly one-fourth and baseline C3-grade venous insufficiency among two-thirds of patients, it is hard to know what criteria might have prompted a diagnostic workup for DVT in this cohort with such a high prevalence of extremity symptoms at baseline. Because the study was powered based on symptomatic response,[1] the adverse event outcomes, therefore, may require further verification through additional studies utilizing larger cohorts or routine screening.

M. A. Corriere, MD, MS

Reference

1. Couzan S, Assante C, Laporte S, Mismetti P, Pouget JF. Booster study: comparative evaluation of a new concept of elastic stockings in mild venous insufficiency. *Presse Med.* 2009;38:355-361.

Increased activation of the hypoxia-inducible factor pathway in varicose veins
Lim CS, Kiriakidis S, Paleolog EM, et al (Imperial College London, UK)
J Vasc Surg 55:1427-1439.e1, 2012

Background.—Venous hypoxia has been postulated to contribute to varicose vein (VV) formation. Direct measurements of vein wall oxygen tension have previously demonstrated that the average minimum oxygen tensions were significantly lower in VVs compared with non-varicose veins (NVVs). Hypoxia-inducible factors (HIFs) are nuclear transcriptional factors that regulate the expression of several genes of oxygen homeostasis. This study aimed to investigate if hypoxia was associated with VVs by assessing the expression of HIF-1α, HIF-2α, HIF target genes, and upstream HIF regulatory enzymes in VVs and NVVs, and their regulation by hypoxia.

Methods.—VVs and NVVs were surgically retrieved and immediately snap-frozen or used for organ culture preparation. The relative expression of HIF-1α, HIF-2α, HIF target genes, and HIF regulatory enzymes in VVs and NVVs was analyzed with quantitative polymerase chain reaction (Q-PCR) and Western blot. VV and NVV organ ex vivo cultures were exposed to 16 hours of normoxia, hypoxia (oxygen tension 1%), or the hypoxia mimetic dimethyloxallyl glycine (DMOG) 1 mM in normoxia. The vein organ cultures were then analyzed for HIF-1α, HIF-2α, and their target gene expression with Q-PCR and Western blot.

Results.—HIF-1α and HIF-2α mRNA were significantly upregulated in VVs compared with NVVs (89.8 ± 18.6 vs 10.4 ± 7.2 and 384.9 ± 209.4 vs 8.1 ± 4.2, respectively). HIF target gene mRNA expression was also significantly elevated in VVs compared with NVVs, namely glucose transporter-1 (GLUT-1; 8.7 ± 2.1 vs 1.0 ± 0.3), carbonic anhydrase-9 (CA9; 8.5 ± 2.1 vs 2.8 ± 1.2), vascular endothelial growth factor (VEGF; 7.5 ± 2.1 vs 0.9 ± 0.2), and BCL2/adenovirus E1B 19-kDa protein-interacting protein 3 (BNIP-3; 4.5 ± 0.7 vs 1.4 ± 0.3). The upregulation of HIF-1α, HIF-2α, and HIF target genes in VVs was also reflected at protein level. Of the HIF regulatory enzymes, the expression of prolyl-hydroxylase domain (PHD)-2 and PHD-3 was found to be elevated in VVs compared with NVVs. Exposure of VV and NVV organ cultures to hypoxia or DMOG was associated with increases in HIF-1α and HIF-2α protein and HIF target gene expression compared with normoxia only.

Conclusions.—The study concluded, we believe for the first time, an increased activation of the HIF pathway, with upregulation of the expression of HIF-1α and HIF-2α transcription factors, and HIF target genes, in VVs compared with NVVs. Exposure of VVs and NVVs to hypoxic conditions was associated with increased expression of HIF-1α and HIF-2α protein and HIF target genes. The data suggest that the HIF pathway may be associated with several pathophysiologic changes in the VV wall, and that hypoxia may be a feature contributing to VV pathogenesis.

▶ Varicose veins represent one of the most common vascular conditions in the adult population. They can lead to chronic venous insufficiency of the lower extremity and are an enormous health burden to millions of patients in the United States. Despite their prevalence and tremendous impact on the quality of life of patients, the mechanism of their formation is still unclear. Hypoxia is known to be a key factor in the regulation of various physiologic responses, and venous hypoxia secondary to blood stasis in patients with chronic venous disease has been postulated to contribute to varicose vein wall changes. This regulation is partially mediated by transcription factors of the hypoxia inducible factor (HIF) family, which are transcription complexes that respond to changes in oxygen, providing cells with a master regulator that coordinates changes in gene transcription. The mechanism of the regulation of the HIF pathway by oxygen has been well reported in the literature in various cells and tissues. Given that vein wall changes are now thought to be the primary events of varicose vein formation, understanding the upstream regulation of these changes may help identify new therapeutic targets for varicose veins. The authors of this study showed an increased activation of the HIF pathway, with upregulation of the expression of HIF-1α and HIF-2α transcription factors, together with increased expression of HIF target genes, including the expression of the HIF regulating enzymes (PHD and FIH) in varicose veins when compared with nonvaricose veins. Given that varicose veins affect more than 25 million individuals in the US and the causes of their formation still remain unclear, the potential of pharmacologic therapy using HIF as a target could be useful in the management of varicose veins.

J. Cullen, PhD

Endothelium-dependent nitric oxide and hyperpolarization-mediated venous relaxation pathways in rat inferior vena cava
Raffetto JD, Yu P, Reslan OM, et al (Brigham and Women's Hosp, Boston, MA)
J Vasc Surg 55:1716-1725, 2012

Introduction.—The vascular endothelium plays a major role in the control of arterial tone; however, its role in venous tissues is less clear. The purpose of this study was to determine the role of endothelium in the control of venous function and the relaxation pathways involved.

Methods.—Circular segments of inferior vena cava (IVC) from male Sprague–Dawley rats were suspended between two wires and isometric contraction to phenylephrine (Phe; 10^{-5} M) and 96 mM KCl was measured. Acetylcholine (Ach; 10^{-10} to 10^{-5} M) was added and the percentage of venous relaxation was measured. To determine the role of nitric oxide (NO) and prostacyclin (PGI_2), vein relaxation was measured in the presence of the nitric oxide synthase inhibitor N_ω-nitro-L-arginine methyl ester (L-NAME; 3×10^{-4} M) and the cyclooxygenase inhibitor indomethacin (10^{-5} M). To measure the role of hyperpolarization, vein relaxation was measured in the presence of K^+ channel activator cromakalim (10^{-11} to 10^{-6} M), and the nonselective K^+ channel blocker tetraethylammonium (TEA; 10^{-3} M). To test for the contribution of a specific K^+ channel, the effects of K^+ channel blockers: glibenclamide (adenosine triphosphate [ATP]-sensitive K_{ATP}, 10^{-5} M), 4-aminopyridine (4-AP; voltage-dependent K_v, 10^{-3} M), apamin (small conductance Ca^{2+}-dependent SK_{Ca}, 10^{-7} M), and iberiotoxin (large conductance Ca^{2+}-dependent BK_{Ca}, 10^{-8} M) on Ach-induced relaxation were tested.

Results.—Ach caused concentration-dependent relaxation of Phe contraction (maximum 49.9 ± 4.9%). Removal of endothelium abolished Ach-induced relaxation. IVC treatment with L-NAME partially reduced Ach relaxation (32.8 ± 4.9%). In IVC treated with L-NAME plus indomethacin, significant Ach-induced relaxation (33.6 ± 3.2%) could still be observed, suggesting a role of endothelium-derived hyperpolarizing factor (EDHF). In IVC treated with L-NAME, indomethacin and TEA, Ach relaxation was abolished, supporting a role of EDHF. In veins stimulated with high KCl, Ach caused relaxation (maximum 59.5 ± 3.5%) that was abolished in the presence of L-NAME and indomethacin suggesting that any Ach-induced EDHF is blocked in the presence of high KCl depolarizing solution, which does not favor outward movement of K^+ ion and membrane hyperpolarization. Cromakalim, an activator of KATP, caused significant IVC relaxation when applied alone or on top of maximal Ach-induced relaxation, suggesting that the Ach response may not involve K_{ATP}. Ach-induced relaxation was not inhibited by glibenclamide, 4-AP, or apamin, suggesting little role of K_{ATP}, K_v or SK_{Ca}, respectively. In contrast, iberiotoxin significantly inhibited Ach-induced relaxation, suggesting a role of BK_{Ca}.

Conclusions.—Thus, endothelium-dependent venous relaxation plays a major role in the control of venous function. In addition to NO, an EDHF pathway involving BK_{Ca} may play a role in endothelium-dependent venous relaxation.

▶ The vascular endothelium serves as an autocrine and paracrine organ that regulates vascular wall function by controlling vasomotor tone and preventing atherosclerosis and thrombosis. Although the pathways of vascular relaxation in the arterial system have been well characterized, the role of nitric oxide (NO), cyclic guanosine monophosphate, prostacyclin-cyclic adenosine monophosphate, and endothelium-derived hyperpolarizing factor in venous relaxation is less defined. Although the majority of K^+ channels have been characterized in the arterial system, little is known regarding the K^+ channels involved in venous hyperpolarization and relaxation.

These authors provide a detailed analysis of the endothelium-dependent venous relaxation pathway using circular segments of rat inferior vena cava. They demonstrate that acetylcholine causes significant endothelium-dependent relaxation to a magnitude that is similar to that in arterial segments. In addition to being mediated by NO, this Ach-induced relaxation also seems to involve the large conductance Ca^{2+}-dependent K^+ channel. As the authors point out, we need to be careful in extrapolating these data from rat veins to human veins.

Further studies should characterize relaxation pathways in the control of greater saphenous veins but also the changes in the venous relaxation mechanisms in varicose veins. Even with the determination of the cellular pathways responsible for venous dilation, the elucidation of the triggers responsible for activation of these pathways remains imperative. The identification of the mechanisms of venous relaxation could be important in the management of venous disease, which can range from vein restenosis and graft failure to venous dilation and varicose veins. Given that varicose veins affect over 25 million individuals in the United States and are not only associated with incompetent valves but also vasodilation, the potential of pharmacologic therapy using specific blockers of the NO pathway and K^+ channels could be useful in the management of varicose veins.

J. Cullen, PhD

Long-term results of a randomized controlled trial on ultrasound-guided foam sclerotherapy combined with saphenofemoral ligation vs standard surgery for varicose veins
Kalodiki E, Lattimer CR, Azzam M, et al (Ealing Hosp, London, UK)
J Vasc Surg 55:451-457, 2012

Background.—The long-term results of a prospective, randomized controlled trial in patients with primary varicose veins are reported.

Methods.—Saphenofemoral ligation (SFL) was done in 73 patients (82 legs). In addition, 43 (23 women; age, 47) underwent stripping and multiple phlebectomies under general anesthesia (group S), and 39 (32 women; age, 49) had concurrent sclerotherapy under local anesthesia (group F). Assessments included CEAP C status, Venous Clinical Severity Score (VCSS), Venous Segmental Disease Score (VSDS), Aberdeen Varicose Vein Questionnaire (AVVQ), and 36-Item Short-Form (SF-36) scores.

Results.—CEAP C was similar between groups (C_{2-6}). In group S, 40% of legs required 25 additional foam sessions (mean volume, 11 mL). In group F, 47.5% of legs required 33 sessions (mean volume, 9 mL) The groups had equivalent preoperative VCSS scores and similar changes at 3 ($P=.504$) and 5 years ($P=.484$), as were the absolute VCSS scores at 3 ($P=.313$) and 5 years ($P=.104$; Mann-Whitney U). The VSDS score improved (median [interquartile range]) preoperatively vs 3 years (group S, 16.32 [14.7] vs 8.94 [11.51], $P=.003$; group F, 12.28 [10.37] vs 4.97 [6.19]; $P<.0005$, Wilcoxon). Above knee obliteration occurred in 17 of 26 (65.4%) for group S and in 16 of 33 (48.5%) for group F at 3 years, and in 14 (53.8%) and 19 (57.6%) at 5 years. AVVQ scores were similar before and at 3 years ($P =.703$) but significantly favored group S at 5 years ($P =.015$; Mann-Whitney U). The AVVQ also improved within both groups. The SF-36 mental summary score over 3 years deteriorated in group S ($P =.04$). However, the physical summary scores did not change between groups (S, $P =.361$; F, $P =.889$) or the mental score in group F ($P =.285$). Changes in the physical ($P =.724$) and mental ($P =.354$, Mann-Whitney U) scores did not differ between the groups due to treatment.

Conclusion.—At 3 and 5 years of follow-up, the treatment was equally effective in the surgical and foam groups, as demonstrated with VCSS, VSDS, and the SF-36 physical component score. At 5 years, the AVVQ was significantly better in the surgical group. The additional foam sessions were also similar. Because traditional surgery for varicose veins does not provide a definitive treatment, foam sclerotherapy could be offered as in a dental care treatment model: "treat as and when the problem appears."

▶ There are many modalities in the treatment of varicose veins; however, appropriate randomized trials to evaluate the effectiveness, safety, clinical outcome, and patient-observed improvement of different treatments are scarce. In addition, long-term data are usually hampered by costs, patient accrual, institutional limitations, and patient-related factors. The authors in this study are to be congratulated for performing a well-designed, randomized, clinical trial, with clinician-derived and patient-derived outcomes and 3-year and 5-year follow-up.

The study randomized 43 limbs to saphenofemoral ligation and stripping with stab phlebectomies vs 39 limbs to saphenofemoral ligation with foam sclerotherapy (3% sodium tetradecyl sulfate prepared by the Tessari method 1.2 mL of sodium tetradecyl sulfate mixed with 4.8 mL of air) of the varicosed great saphenous vein under ultrasound guidance. The parameters measured were the C (clinical) component of the CEAP classification, the Venous Clinical Severity Score (VCSS), and the Venous Segmental Disease Score. In addition, patients completed 2 questionnaires, including the disease-specific Aberdeen Varicose Veins Questionnaire (AVVQ) and the generic 36-Item Short-Form (SF-36). Both groups were equally matched for clinical class CEAP score and disease severity. Following treatment, the VCSS improved significantly for both treatment groups and had similar changes at 3 and 5 years. The AVVQ score was similar between both groups before and at 3 years, but it significantly favored the surgical group at 5 years ($P =.015$; Mann-Whitney U test). The SF-36 mental component score over 3 years decreased (deteriorated) in the surgical group ($P =.04$). However, there was no change in the physical component scores between the surgical group ($P =.361$) and the foam group ($P =.889$) or in the mental component score in the foam group ($P =.285$). In both groups (surgical 40% and foam 48%) during follow-up, repeat sessions of foam sclerotherapy were required to treat recurrent varicose veins, with no serious adverse outcomes.

The authors concluded from this study that at 3 and 5 years' of follow-up, the treatment was equally effective between the surgical and foam groups.

Although at 5 years, the AVVQ was significantly better in the surgery group, the margins were small and may not have had any clinical significance.

Other studies have randomized patients to compare laser ablation, radiofrequency ablation, foam sclerotherapy, and surgical stripping for great saphenous reflux and found similar efficacy. However, they also found higher technical failure after foam sclerotherapy and faster recovery after radiofrequency ablation and foam sclerotherapy compared with the results from laser ablation and surgery.[1] It may be that ligating the saphenofemoral junction and then infusing foam under ultrasound guidance may offer some advantages, as determined in this study. A randomized controlled trial comparing recurrences, VCSS, and quality of life in patients treated with either endovenous laser ablation vs ligation and stripping demonstrated no difference in these outcomes at 2-year midterm follow-up, and other published results up to 5 years demonstrated similar findings.[2] Given the many modalities to treat the saphenous system and its varicose veins, future well-designed trials are required as new developments in technology advance the treatment of primary venous disease, so that clinicians are guided by the best evidence-based data.

J. D. Raffetto, MD

References

1. Rasmussen LH, Lawaetz M, Bjoern L, Vennits B, Blemings A, Eklof B. Randomized clinical trial comparing endovenous laser ablation, radiofrequency ablation, foam sclerotherapy and surgical stripping for great saphenous varicose veins. *Br J Surg*. 2011;98:1079-1087.
2. Rasmussen LH, Bjoern L, Lawaetz M, Lawaetz B, Blemings A, Eklöf B. Randomised clinical trial comparing endovenous laser ablation with stripping of the great saphenous vein: clinical outcome and recurrence after 2 years. *Eur J Vasc Endovasc Surg*. 2010;39:630-635.

Failure of microvenous valves in small superficial veins is a key to the skin changes of venous insufficiency
Vincent JR, Jones GT, Hill GB, et al (Univ of Otago, Dunedin, New Zealand)
J Vasc Surg 54:62S-69S.e3, 2011

Objective.—To determine the role of microvenous valves in the superficial venous system in the prevention of reflux and skin changes in the progression of venous insufficiency.

Methods.—The venous anatomy of 15 amputated lower limbs, eight free from clinical venous disease and seven with varicose veins and ulcers, was examined using retrograde venography corrosion casting. Prior to amputation, all limbs were scanned by duplex ultrasound to confirm the presence or absence of reflux in the great (GSV) and small saphenous veins or their tributaries. The resulting resin casts were photographed and mapped to show the position, orientation, and competency of valves in the superficial venous network. Casts were also examined by scanning electron microscopy.

Results.—Retrograde venous filling was demonstrated in the "normal" limbs despite a competent GSV. Microvalves were identified down to the sixth generation of tributaries from the GSV. Only in regions where incompetence existed in microvalves out to the third (ie, the "boundary") generation was the resin able to penetrate deeper into microvenous networks of the dermis. This was despite the presence of subsequent competent valves, which were able to be bypassed in the network. In limbs with varicose veins and venous ulcers, reflux into the small venous networks and capillary loops was more extensive with more dense networks and greater tortuosity.

Conclusions.—This study demonstrates that valvular incompetence can occur independently in small superficial veins in the absence of reflux within the GSV and the major tributaries. We have shown that once there is incompetence of the third generation "boundary" microvalves, reflux can extend into the microvenous networks in the skin. These effects are markedly worse in the presence of GSV incompetence. We propose that degenerative changes with valve incompetence are required in both the larger proximal vessels and the small superficial veins, in particular at the "boundary" valve level, for the severe skin changes in venous insufficiency to occur (Figs 1D, 4, 6, 7C, D and 8).

▶ Chronic venous disease (CVD) leads to a spectrum of clinical manifestations, from varicose veins to venous edema to skin changes, including hyperpigmentation, lipodermatosclerosis, and the most severe problem of venous ulceration. The pathophysiology is complex and includes leukocytes activation, endothelial activation, migration of macrophages into the extracellular tissues, release of cytokines and growth factors, activation of transcription pathways, alterations in apoptosis, activation of metalloproteinases, collagen alterations, and tissue degradation. Central to these events are the pressure changes that affect the

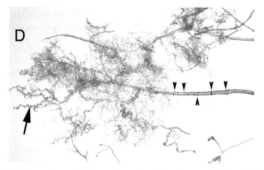

FIGURE 1.—D. Varying patterns of retrograde resin casting in normal limbs (CEAP 0 or 1). All limbs had competent great saphenous veins (GSVs) as determined by ultrasound. D, Multiple territories of small vein network filling and dilated tortuous (*arrow*) veins (63-year-old female). Of note, the GSV was intact with numerous competent valves and tributaries (*arrowheads*). (Reprinted from the Journal of Vascular Surgery. Vincent JR, Jones GT, Hill GB, et al. Failure of microvenous valves in small superficial veins is a key to the skin changes of venous insufficiency. *J Vasc Surg.* 2011;54:62S-69S.e3, Copyright 2011, with permission from the Society for Vascular Surgery.)

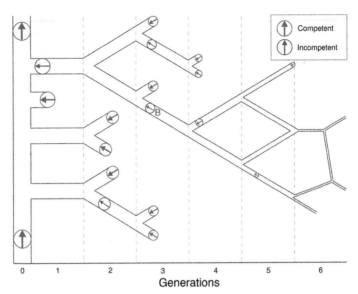

	Generation								
	0	**1**	**2**	**3**	**4**	**5**	**6**	**undetermined***	**Total**
Competent	12	39	62	71	48	9	2	4	247
Incompetent	0	13	16	19	1	0	0	2	51
Total	12	52	78	90	49	9	2	6	298
Proportion Incompetent (%)	0	25	21	21	2	0	0	33	17

FIGURE 4.—Schematic representation of valve distribution and effect of competency on resin filling with table of actual total valve counts by generation and competency. As shown in the table, competent valves were found through all six generations, while the vast majority of incompetent valves were observed in generations one to three (94%). The concept of a "boundary" valve is represented in the schematic by an incompetent valve in generation 3 (B). Reflux through this valve results in widespread filling of the subsequent generations of tributaries, despite the presence of a more distal competent valve. The two other incompetent valves shown in generations two and three are not boundary, as subsequent competent valves prevent further resin reflux. *Generation could not be determined, usually due to cast breakage. (Reprinted from the Journal of Vascular Surgery. Vincent JR, Jones GT, Hill GB, et al. Failure of microvenous valves in small superficial veins is a key to the skin changes of venous insufficiency. *J Vasc Surg.* 2011;54:62S-69S.e3, Copyright 2011, with permission from the Society for Vascular Surgery.)

microcirculation in the venous system. Our understanding and unification of all these events is not well understood.

In this elegant study, the authors addressed the question of the microcirculation in the skin, specifically assessing microvenous valves and their role in CVD. The authors examined venous anatomy of 15 amputated lower limbs, 8 free from clinical venous disease and 7 with varicose veins and ulcers and performed retrograde venography with corrosion casting. Retrograde resin infusion, from the venous aspect in the great saphenous vein, is cannulated with a 20-gauge needle at the level of the medial malleolus and is akin to

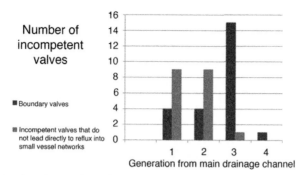

FIGURE 6.—"Boundary" and "non-boundary" incompetent valves in areas of reflux by generation. (Reprinted from the Journal of Vascular Surgery. Vincent JR, Jones GT, Hill GB, et al. Failure of microvenous valves in small superficial veins is a key to the skin changes of venous insufficiency. *J Vasc Surg.* 2011;54:62S-69S.e3, Copyright 2011, with permission from the Society for Vascular Surgery.)

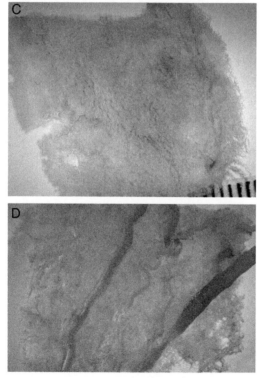

FIGURE 7.—C, D. Tissue excised from venous ulcers (4 cm² regions). C and D, Extensive venous filling in separate ulcer specimens showing the superficial (C) and deep (D) surfaces of the casts. (Reprinted from the Journal of Vascular Surgery. Vincent JR, Jones GT, Hill GB, et al. Failure of microvenous valves in small superficial veins is a key to the skin changes of venous insufficiency. *J Vasc Surg.* 2011;54:62S-69S.e3, Copyright 2011, with permission from the Society for Vascular Surgery.)

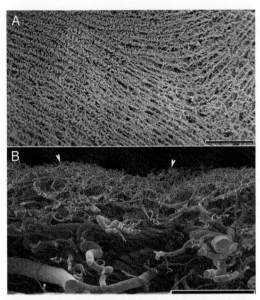

FIGURE 8.—Scanning electron microscopy of extensive superficial venous network filling from a (mixed) ulcer in an 83-year-old male. A, Superficial surface view (scale bar 2 mm), equivalent to that shown in Fig 7, C. B, Lateral view (scale bar 1 mm). Note the extensive filling of the papillary loops (*arrowheads*). (Reprinted from the Journal of Vascular Surgery. Vincent JR, Jones GT, Hill GB, et al. Failure of microvenous valves in small superficial veins is a key to the skin changes of venous insufficiency. *J Vasc Surg.* 2011;54:62S-69S.e3, Copyright 2011, with permission from the Society for Vascular Surgery.)

retrograde phlebography, as used in the clinical demonstration of deep venous and perforator valvular incompetence. The procedure allows the evaluation of progressively smaller vein and microvenous segments and the status of the valves.

Prior to amputation, all limbs underwent duplex color flow ultrasonography to assess the venous system and reflux in the great saphenous vein and its tributaries. In the "normal limbs" and despite competent great saphenous vein, the authors found a system of sequentially smaller generations of tributaries leading to a small venous network, with competent and incompetent microvalves. The regions are divided into 6 generations before reaching the small venous network. In regions where incompetence existed in microvalves out to the third-generation tributary (the boundary), the resin was able to penetrate deeper into the microvenous networks of the dermis (Fig 1D). The majority (94%) of incompetent valves were in the first three generations of the draining venous network (Fig 4), and the majority (65%) of these boundary valves were in the third-generation microvalves of the draining venous network (Fig 6). In limbs with varicose veins and venous ulcers, reflux into the small venous networks and capillary loops was more extensive, with more dense networks and greater tortuosity (Fig 7C,D). There was resin reflux into the venules of the papillary plexus and reaching up into the capillary loops of the skin, as best observed with a scanning electron microscope (Fig 8). Once there is incompetence of the third-generation "boundary" microvalves, reflux can extend into the microvenous networks in the skin. These effects are markedly worse in the presence of great saphenous vein incompetence. In addition to superficial axial saphenous vein insufficiency, microvalve insufficiency also exists, and once it compromises the third-generation set of microvalves, there is a greater risk for development of dermal venous ulceration. In addition, these findings may help explain why some patients with long-standing varicose veins do not develop venous ulcers, since the microvalves may be intact at the third-generation network, preventing clinical deterioration. In addition, these findings may explain why skin changes consistent with venous disease (hyperpigmentation and even small skin ulceration) are seen clinically in patients with normal duplex ultrasound of the superficial, deep, and perforator venous systems.

Future work will need to define the microvenous and microvalve network across the clinical class of the CEAP spectrum, and hopefully it will introduce noninvasive techniques that can measure the microvalve function and identify patients who may be at risk for advancing their disease and offer earlier treatment in an effort to avoid progression of advanced CVD from skin changes and venous ulcers.

J. D. Raffetto, MD

A Systematic Review and Meta-analysis of Randomised Controlled Trials Comparing Endovenous Ablation and Surgical Intervention in Patients with Varicose Vein

Siribumrungwong B, Noorit P, Wilasrusmee C, et al (Mahidol Univ, Rachatevi, Bangkok, Thailand; Chonburi Hosp, Thailand; et al)
Eur J Vasc Endovasc Surg 44:214-223, 2012

Objectives and Design.—A systematic review and meta-analysis was conducted to compare clinical outcomes between endovenous laser ablation (EVLA), radiofrequency ablation (RFA), ultrasound-guided foam sclerotherapy (UGFS) and surgery.

Methods.—We searched MEDLINE and Scopus from 2000 to August 2011 to identify randomised controlled trials (RCTs) comparing EVLA, RFA, UGFS, and surgery or combinations of these for treatment of varicoses. Differences in clinical outcomes were expressed as pooled risk ratio and unstandardised mean difference for dichotomous and continuous outcomes, respectively. Methodological quality was assessed using Cochrane tools.

Results.—Twenty-eight RCTs were included. The primary failure and clinical recurrences were not significantly different between EVLA and RFA versus surgery with the pooled RR of 1.5 (95% CI:0.7, 3.0) and 1.3 (95% CI:0.7, 2.4) respectively for primary failure, and, 0.6 (95% CI:0.3, 1.1) and 0.9 (95% CI:0.6, 1.4) respectively for clinical recurrences. The endovenous techniques had advantages over surgery in lowering wound infections (RR = 0.3 (95% CI:0.1, 0.8) for EVLA), haematoma (RR = 0.5 (95% CI:0.3, 0.8) and 0.4 (95% CI:0.1, 0.8) for EVLA and RFA), and return to normal activities or work (mean differences = −4.9 days (95% CI:−7.1,−2.7) for RFA).

Conclusions.—The primary failure and recurrence in EVLA and RFA were non-significantly different compared with surgery. However, they had lower haematoma, less wound infection, less pain and quicker return to normal activities.

▶ There are multiple therapeutic options for treating symptomatic saphenous vein reflux, including endothermal ablation, ultrasound-guided foam sclerotherapy, and traditional surgical ligation and stripping. This article reviews the outcomes and compares data on all types of interventions via systematic review. This meta-analysis looked at only randomized controlled trials that met appropriate quality indicators for methodological value. This article is a must for any venous surgeon in order to have the latest high-quality comparative data from well-constructed trials. As would be expected, the minimally invasive techniques of radiofrequency and laser ablation have similar outcomes and recurrence rates when compared with surgical intervention, but with better short-term profiles in terms of patient comfort and return to normal activities including work. Ultrasound-guided foam sclerotherapy, while effective, does not perform as well when compared to surgical intervention.

In this day and age of health care finance scrutiny and tightening of hospital budgets, one may perceive that surgical intervention is a less-expensive modality compared with endothermal techniques because of the lack of capital outlay and lower supply expenses. This, however, has to be weighed against the benefits of an outpatient procedure, patient satisfaction, and a faster return to the workplace. In informing hospitals and their finance personnel as well as third-party payers, the social costs should be considered along with the bottom line. In addition, one can also extrapolate that patients having endothermal ablation had fewer postprocedure clinic visits, made fewer phone calls to providers and their staff, and, possibly, were more likely to make positive recommendations based on their experiences. This article provides both information and such inferences in a well-written format with appropriate statistical analysis.

R. L. Bush, MD, MPH

15 Technical Notes

A New Unibody Branched Stent-graft for Reconstruction of the Canine Aortic Arch

Li W, Xu K, Zhong H, et al (The First Affiliated Hosp of China Med Univ, Shenyang, Liaoning, PR China)

Eur J Vasc Endovasc Surg 44:139-144, 2012

Objectives.—To evaluate the feasibility and safety of a new unibody branched stent-graft for reconstruction of the canine aortic arch.

Materials and Methods.—Twenty adult hybrid dogs were used for the experiments. Ten dogs were implanted with single-branched stent-grafts; the other ten dogs were implanted with double-branched stent-grafts. The stent-grafts were implanted transluminally via the abdominal aorta. The branched limbs were caught and pulled into supra-aortic vessels using gooseneck snare wires introduced via the axillary arteries. The animals were euthanized 4 months after implantation.

Results.—One of the ten dogs implanted with a single-branched stent-graft died from failure of the implantation procedure, and two of the ten dogs implanted with double-branched stent-grafts died from failure of the procedure and excessive blood loss. After month 4, the remaining unibody branched stent-grafts were patent and did not migrate.

Conclusions.—This new unibody branched stent-graft could be used to reconstruct the aortic arch. This is a total endovascular technique, and compared to other branched stent-grafts appears to be safer and easier to implant (Figs 1 and 3-5).

▶ This report describes an elegant concept for a branched aortic arch device utilizing detachable sleeves, snares, and traction wires. Essentially, the procedure was carried out in dogs as follows: The device was handmade for each dog and loaded into a delivery sheath utilizing a detachable sleeve anchored over the branch (either single or dual branches; Figs 4, 1, and then 3).

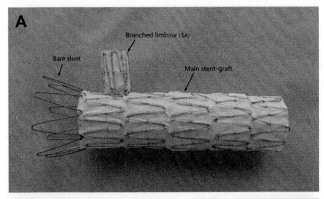

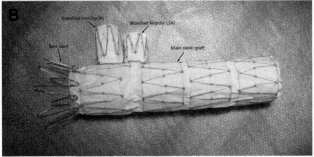

FIGURE 1.—The unibody branched stent-graft. (A) The single-branched stent-graft consists of a branched limb for the left subclavian artery (LSA) and the main stentgraft. The first Z segment of the main stent-graft is bare. (B) The double-branched stent-graft consists of two branched limbs and the main stent-graft. The first limb is for the innominate artery (IA) and the second limb is for the LSA. The first Z segment of the main stent-graft is bare. (Reprinted from European Journal of Vascular and Endovascular Surgery. Li W, Xu K, Zhong H, et al. A new unibody branched stent-graft for reconstruction of the canine aortic arch. *Eur J Vasc Endovasc Surg.* 2012;44:139-144, Copyright 2012, with permission from European Society for Vascular Surgery.)

The device was then implanted into the aorta, and a snare from the left brachial artery was advanced to capture the detachable sleeve. A traction wire in the cavity of the detachable sleeve ensures that the detachable sleeve cannot be accidentally detached (Fig 5).

This simple and elegant design may prove helpful for future device designs incorporating the arch vessels of humans.

B. W. Starnes, MD

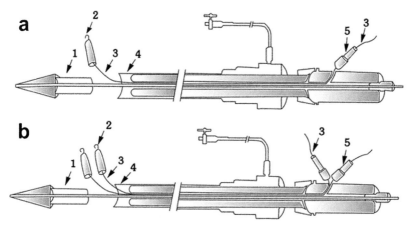

1.Top–cap: 2.Hook: 3.Traction wire: 4.Outer sheath: 5.Fixing device

FIGURE 3.—Line drawings of the vertical section of the delivery system. (a) The delivery system of the single-branched stent-graft consists of a top-cap opening backward, an outer sheath, and a detachable sleeve. The traction wire of the detachable sleeve passes through the delivery system, and its end is fixed outside the handle of the delivery system using the fixing device. (b) The delivery system of the double-branched stent-graft, with two detachable sleeves, is similar to the single-branched stent-graft. (Reprinted from European Journal of Vascular and Endovascular Surgery. Li W, Xu K, Zhong H, et al. A new unibody branched stent-graft for reconstruction of the canine aortic arch. *Eur J Vasc Endovasc Surg.* 2012;44:139-144, Copyright 2012, with permission from European Society for Vascular Surgery.)

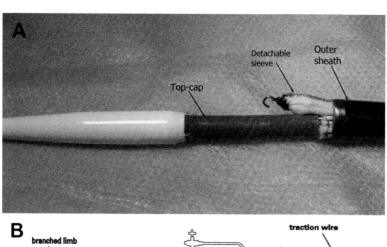

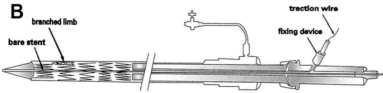

FIGURE 4.—Assembly of the stent-graft system. (A) The top-cap folds the bare segment of the main stent-graft, the detachable sleeve folds the branched limb, and the outer sheath constrains the whole branched stent-graft. (B) Line drawing of the assembled stent-graft system. The bare Z segment of the main stent-graft is constrained into the top-cap, the branched limb is folded into the detachable sleeve, and the whole stentgraft is folded into the outer sheath. (Reprinted from European Journal of Vascular and Endovascular Surgery. Li W, Xu K, Zhong H, et al. A new unibody branched stent-graft for reconstruction of the canine aortic arch. *Eur J Vasc Endovasc Surg.* 2012;44:139-144, Copyright 2012, with permission from European Society for Vascular Surgery.)

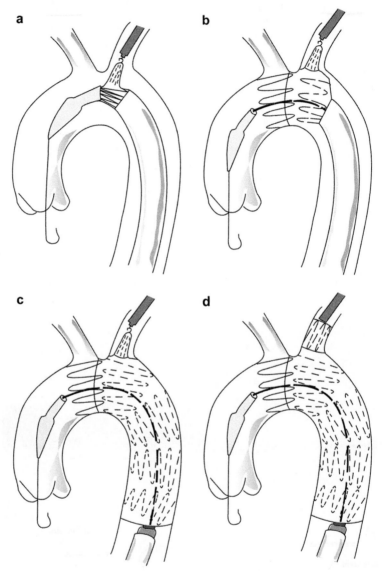

FIGURE 5.—Line drawing of implantation procedure for the single-branched stent-graft. (a) The hook is caught and pulled into the LSA using the gooseneck snare wire introduced from the left axillary artery. (b) The bare segment of the main stent-graft is released from the top-cap by pushing the central core of the delivery system forward. (c) The main stent-graft is released by retracting the outer sheath. (d) The branched limb is released by pulling the detachable sleeve out through the long sheath. (Reprinted from European Journal of Vascular and Endovascular Surgery. Li W, Xu K, Zhong H, et al. A new unibody branched stent-graft for reconstruction of the canine aortic arch. *Eur J Vasc Endovasc Surg.* 2012;44:139-144, Copyright 2012, with permission from European Society for Vascular Surgery.)

Bidirectional endovascular treatment for chronic total occlusive lesions of the femoropopliteal arterial segment using a hand-carried ultrasound device and a retrograde microcatheter

Nishino M, Taniike M, Makino N, et al (Osaka Rosai Hosp, Sakai-City, Japan)
J Vasc Surg 56:113-117, 2012

Background.—Although endovascular therapy for complex lesions in the lower limbs has frequently achieved successful recanalization by improvement of techniques and devices, chronic total occlusion in the femoropopliteal arterial segment still remains a challenge for treatment by endovascular therapy. We investigated the efficacy and safety of endovascular therapy for chronic total occlusion in the femoropopliteal arterial segment guided by a hand-carried ultrasound (HCUS) device and supported by a retrograde microcatheter.

Methods.—We attempted endovascular therapy for chronic total occlusion lesions in the femoropopliteal arterial segment using a protocol involving a dual-access procedure using the HCUS device and a retrograde 2.7F microcatheter from January 2008 to June 2010. We evaluated the success rate, complications, and clinical outcomes, including the ankle-brachial index (ABI) and primary and secondary patency.

Results.—Success was achieved in 18 of 19 patients (95%), without major complications (only two small hematomas). The HCUS device was useful in reducing the personnel and space requirements, radiation exposure, and the required amount of contrast agent. The retrograde flexible 2.7F microcatheter was also useful in achieving successful recanalization and contributed to reducing puncture-related complications. The ABI was significantly improved, from 0.56 ± 0.12 to 0.81 ± 0.11 at 1 year

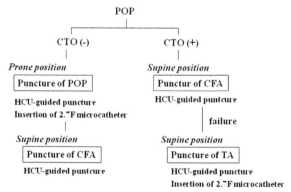

FIGURE 1.—Flow chart shows puncture position and location for endovascular therapy. *CFA,* Common femoral artery; *CTO,* chronic total occlusion; *HCU,* hand-carried ultrasound device; *POP,* popliteal artery; *TA,* anterior or posterior tibial artery. (Reprinted from the Journal of Vascular Surgery. Nishino M, Taniike M, Makino N, et al. Bidirectional endovascular treatment for chronic total occlusive lesions of the femoropopliteal arterial segment using a hand-carried ultrasound device and a retrograde microcatheter. *J Vasc Surg.* 2012;56:113-117, Copyright 2012, with permission from The Society for Vascular Surgery.)

(P < .01) and this effect remained stable. Primary and secondary patency was 63% and 89%, respectively, at 3 years.

Conclusions.—HCUS-guided and retrograde 2.7F microcatheter-supported endovascular therapy for chronic total occlusion lesions of the femoropopliteal arterial segment can achieve a favorable clinical outcome without major complications (Fig 1).

▶ The 95% rate of technical success with the bidirectional technique in this small series is comparable with results reported with other devices available for endovascular management of chronic total occlusions (CTO). Although other techniques for CTO management do not routinely require a second arterial access site distal to the lesion, the described technique has the advantage of avoiding highly specialized disposable devices that can contribute significant costs to endovascular treatment. Although the authors assert that spot ultrasound scan is useful to reduce both radiation exposure and contrast administration associated with endovascular treatment, neither of these were included as endpoints in the study, and all patients underwent diagnostic angiography as a separate procedure before attempted revascularization. The proposed algorithm for access in patients without a popliteal CTO (Fig 1) involves establishment of popliteal artery access with the patient in the prone position before attempting lesion crossing from a femoral approach with the patient repositioned supine. This approach would, therefore, presumably lead to an unnecessary popliteal access (and associated increases in procedure duration and complications) when lesion crossing is successful from the femoral access alone. By comparison, use of a tibial artery approach permits selective utilization of distal access and, therefore, seems more practical.

M. A. Corriere, MD, MS

16 Miscellaneous

How can good randomized controlled trials in leading journals be so misinterpreted?
Veith FJ (New York Univ Med Ctr)
J Vasc Surg 57:3S-7S, 2013

The results of good randomized controlled trials (RCTs) published in leading peer-reviewed journals have been deemed the best possible basis for good medical practice. However, several limitations may decrease their value. These include flaws and weaknesses in the design and the timeliness of RCTs. Progress in a treatment method or control arm may invalidate a trial. So too can defects in patient selection, physician competence, randomization, applicability, end points, and the population being studied. Idiosyncratic flaws can also invalidate an RCT. Examples of these flaws and weaknesses are presented. Another problem with articles describing RCTs is the potential for the conclusions of the trial report to be misleading because of error or bias. This plus subsequent misinterpretation of the trial results or conclusions by others can make the effect of the trial misleading with an unintended detrimental result on medical practice. Guidelines based on such errors or bias-based conclusions and misinterpretations can further compound the problem. This article provides examples of misleading conclusions and/or misinterpretations (spinning) of trial results in articles describing RCTs in leading journals. All physicians should recognize these value-limiting processes so that RCTs can be evaluated adequately and fairly. In that way, they can be used along with good physician judgment to optimize the care delivered to individual patients and to society at large (Table 3).

▶ This author has been a formidable influence in vascular surgery for the past 5 plus decades. For anyone who sifts through the medical literature as it relates to the practice of vascular surgery, this article is a must read.

The author presents compelling data on perspectives, flaws, and weaknesses and biased or erroneous conclusions and interpretations of several recent randomized, controlled trials (RTCs) published in our most leading medical journals (Table 3).

The conclusions of this article can be no better stated than by the author himself:

All these RCTs show that unjustified conclusions can sometimes be reached in leading peer-reviewed journals. This occurs because of flaws

TABLE 3.—Other Randomized Controlled Trials that Reached Misleading Conclusions

RCT	Publication Site	Year	Trial Conclusion	Flaws	Appropriate Conclusion
ACAS ACST	JAMA Lancet	1995[3] 2010[4]	CEA decreased SR more than BMT; CEA for ACS reduces 10-year SR from 2% to 1% per year	Obsolete BMT; decreasing SR with ACS	Need RCT in ACS of CAS and CEA vs BMT; need way to identify high-SR patients; BMT best for most ACS patients
SAPPHIRE	NEJM NEJM	2004[5] 2008[14]	No significant difference in outcome of CAS and CEA at 30 days, 1 year, or 3 years	71% asymptomatic CAS patients; ~6% 30-day SR	High-risk ACS patients should be treated with BMT, not by CAS or CEA
EVAR 2	Lancet	2005[11]	In unfit patients, EVAR did not improve survival over no intervention	Half of deaths (9) in EVAR arm were caused by rupture before treatment, average delay = 57 days	Timely EVAR justified in some unfit patients (see text)
EVAR 1	NEJM	2010[17]	EVAR and open repair yielded equivalent long-term mortality with increased graft complications, need for reinterventions, and cost		EVAR prolonged patient survival longer than open repair

ACAS, Asymptomatic Carotid Atherosclerosis Study; *ACST*, Asymptomatic Carotid Surgery Trial; *ACS*, asymptomatic carotid artery stenosis; Trial; *BMT*, best medical therapy; *CAS*, carotid artery stenting; *CEA*, carotid endarterectomy; *CREST*, Carotid Revascularization Endarterectomy Versus Stenting Trial; *EVA-3S*, Endarterectomy Versus Angioplasty in Patients with Symptomatic Severe Carotid Stenosis; *EVAR*, endovascular abdominal aortic aneurysm repair; *EVAR 1 (2)*, Endovascular Abdominal Aortic Aneurysm Repair 1 (2) study; *JAMA*, *Journal of the American Medical Association*; *NEJM*, *New England Journal of Medicine*; *RCT*, randomized controlled trial; *SAPPHIRE*, Stenting and Angioplasty With Protection in Patients at High Risk for Endarterectomy; *SR*, stroke rate.
Editor's Note: Please refer to original journal article for full references.

in the RCTs, unrecognized author bias, or both. More importantly, these unjustified conclusions and the trials on which they are based can be further misinterpreted or spun to reach even more erroneous or unjustified conclusions. Presumably, much of this spinning results from the bias or biases that all of us in medicine have. By being aware of the influence of bias along with the possible flaws that RCTs can have, we should be able to interpret and use RCTs fairly and optimally for the care of patients.

B. W. Starnes, MD

Operator-controlled Imaging Significantly Reduces Radiation Exposure during EVAR

Peach G, Sinha S, Black SA, et al (St George's Healthcare NHS Trust, London, UK)

Eur J Vasc Endovasc Surg 44:395-398, 2012

Introduction.—Adoption of endovascular aneurysm repair (EVAR) has led to significant reductions in the short-term morbidity and mortality associated with abdominal aortic aneurysm (AAA) repair. However, EVAR may expose both patient and interventionalist to potentially harmful levels of radiation, particularly as more complex procedures are undertaken. The aim of this study was to assess whether changing from radiographer-controlled imaging to a system of operator-controlled imaging (OCI) would influence radiation exposure, screening time or contrast dose during EVAR.

Method.—Retrospective analysis identified patients that had undergone elective EVAR for infra-renal AAA before or after the change to operator-controlled imaging. Data were collected for radiation dose (measured as dose area product; DAP), screening time, total delivered contrast volume and operative duration. Data were also collected for maximum aneurysm diameter, patient age, gender and body mass index.

Results.—122 patients underwent EVAR for infra-renal AAA at a single centre between January 2011 and December 2011. 57 of these were prior to installation of OCI and 65 after installation. Median DAP was significantly lower after installation of OCI (4.9 mGy m^2; range 1.25−13.3) than it had been before installation (6.9 mGy m^2; range 1.91−95.0) ($p = 0.005$). Median screening times before and after installation of OCI were 20.0 min and 16.2 min respectively ($p = 0.027$) and median contrast volumes before and after the change to OCI were 100 ml and 90 ml respectively ($p = 0.21$).

Conclusion.—Introduction of operator-controlled imaging can significantly reduce radiation exposure during EVAR, with particular reduction in the number of 'higher-dose' cases (Fig 1, Table 2).

▶ This reputable group from St. George's Vascular Institute in the United Kingdom took a look at the total radiation does (measured as dose area product)

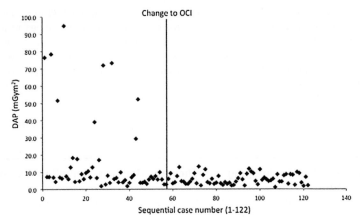

FIGURE 1.—Radiation exposure in cases before/after change to OCI. (Reprinted from European Journal of Vascular and Endovascular Surgery. Peach G, Sinha S, Black SA, et al. Operator-controlled imaging significantly reduces radiation exposure during EVAR. *Eur J Vasc Endovasc Surg.* 2012; 44:395-398, Copyright 2012, with permission from European Society for Vascular Surgery.)

TABLE 2.—Median Values Before and After Change to OCI

	Median Value Before OCI (range)	Median Value With OCI (range)	p Value[b]
Dose area product (mGy m²)	6.9 (1.91−95.0)	4.9 (1.25−13.3)	0.005
Screening time (min)	20.0 (4.8−49.3)	16.2 (3.1−51.1)	0.027
Contrast dose (ml)[a]	100 (60−300)	90 (50−180)	0.21
Operative duration (min)	130 (65−240)	120 (60−205)	0.44

[a]$n = 45$(before)/51(after).
[b]Mann-Whitney U test.

on a cohort of 122 patients treated with endovascular aneurysm repair over 1 year by a single interventionist. During this period, the operators switched from radiographer-controlled imaging to operator-controlled imaging in which 57 patients were treated before this change in technique took place.

To no surprise, operator-controlled imaging was associated with a dramatic decrease in radiation exposure and screening time (we call it *fluoro time*). Also, not surprisingly, the mean contrast volumes did not change significantly (Table 2, Fig 1).

Radiation exposure for both the patient and the operator has become increasingly important, especially with the advent of increasingly complex endovascular repairs such as fenestrated and multibranched graft procedures. With practices such as these, reductions in median emitted radiation dose to as much as 29% can be obtained.

B. W. Starnes, MD

A comparison of 0 + 5 versus 5 + 2 applicants to vascular surgery training programs
Zayed MA, Dalman RL, Lee JT (Stanford Univ Med Ctr, CA)
J Vasc Surg 56:1448-1452, 2012

Objective.—The new integrated 0 + 5 vascular surgery (VS) training paradigm introduced in 2007 required program directors and faculty to reconsider recruiting methods and exposure of medical students to VS. As a means to identify variables important for recruitment of 0 + 5 VS applicants, we sought to analyze national 0 + 5 VS residency application trends and to compare medical school demographics of applicants to both our 0 + 5 residency and 5 + 2 fellowship programs.

Methods.—Electronic Residency Application Service and National Resident Matching Program online public databases were queried to evaluate nationwide trends in the number of applicants to integrated VS residency programs between 2007 and 2010. Demographic data from Electronic Residency Application Service applications submitted to our institution's 0 + 5 and 5 + 2 VS training programs during the same time period were reviewed.

Results.—From 2008 to 2011, there were 190 applicants to our 0 + 5 VS residency program and 161 applicants to our 5 + 2 fellowship program, with 127 (66.8%) and 122 (75.8%) being United States medical graduates, respectively. Annual application volume to our programs over these years remained stable for both training pathways (range, 39-49 for 0 + 5 integrated; range, 39-43 for 5 + 2 traditional). Nationally, applications to 0 + 5 programs increased sixfold over the same time period (52 in 2007 to 340 applicants in 2010; $P < .001$), far exceeding the available training positions. Compared with applicants to the 5 + 2 VS fellowships, medical students applying to the 0 + 5 programs are more likely to be female, be slightly older, have additional postgraduate degrees and publications, have higher United States Medical Licensure Examination test scores, and are more likely to be in the top quartile of their medical school class.

TABLE 1.—Results of 2010 Residency Match into the Most Competitive Surgical Subspecialties Based on Applicant:Position Ratios

| Specialty | Residency Positions | ERAS Applicants | | NRMP Participants | |
		Total Applicants	Applicant: position Ratio	Total Participants	Participant: Position Ratio
Thoracic surgery	10	170	17	74	7.4
Vascular surgery	22	340	15.5	72	3.3
Plastic surgery	69	330	4.8	200	2.9
Neurosurgery	191	565	3.0	309	1.6
Orthopedic surgery	656	1535	2.3	996	1.5
Otolaryngology	280	647	2.3	395	1.4
Urology	268	445	1.7	337	1.3

ERAS, Electronic Residency Application Service; *NRMP*, National Resident Matching Program.

Conclusions.—Nationwide interest in the 0 + 5 vascular surgery residency training paradigm continues to significantly increase. Significant differences exist between the cohorts of 0 + 5 residency and 5 + 2 fellowship program applicants at the completion of medical school, suggesting that 0 + 5 VS residency programs are attracting a different medical student population to the VS specialty. VS program directors should continue to foster interest in this new applicant pool through early exposure, mentorship, and extracurricular research activities (Table 1).

▶ You have to have been asleep for the last 6 years to have missed the dramatic change in vascular residency training with the implementation of the new integrated "straight 5" training pathway.

These authors at Stanford, in 1 of 4 integrated programs in California and 6 on the entire west coast of the United States, examined national statistics regarding the applicant pool for integrated vascular residencies.

Medical students applying for these programs were more likely to be women, slightly older, more likely to have additional postgraduate degrees and publications, and more likely to be in the top quartile of their medical school class. Vascular surgery now ranks slightly second behind thoracic surgery as the most competitive surgical specialty (Table 1).

These facts, along with a 6-fold increase in the number of applications nationally, make vascular surgery one of the hottest surgical specialties in America at the moment. Good mentorship and exposure of the specialty to medical students will be needed to continue this pathway of success and elevate the quality of our specialty.

B. W. Starnes, MD

A Randomized Prospective Multicenter Trial of a Novel Vascular Sealant
Stone WM, Cull DL, Money SR (Mayo Clinic, Scottsdale, AZ; Greenville Memorial Hosp, SC)
Ann Vasc Surg 26:1077-1084, 2012

Background.—Increasing use of anticoagulant medications, particularly antiplatelet therapies, can increase the difficulty in obtaining adequate suture line hemostasis. Multiple vascular sealants have been used as adjuncts to surgical procedures, but none of them have been universally successful. The aim of this study was to evaluate the safety and effectiveness of a new prophylactic vascular sealant in arterial surgery.

Methods.—A randomized prospective multi-institutional trial was undertaken comparing ArterX Vascular Sealant (AVS) with Gelfoam Plus during open arterial reconstruction.

Results.—Three hundred thirty-one anastomotic sites in 217 patients were randomized. One hundred one of 167 (60.5%) anastomotic sites in the AVS group achieved immediate hemostasis compared with 65 of 164 (39.6%) in the control group ($P = 0.001$). In anastomoses with polytetrafluoroethylene grafts, 105 of 167 (62.5%) in the AVS group achieved immediate hemostasis compared with 56 of 164 (34.0%) in the control group ($P < 0.001$). No significant differences were noted in morbidity or mortality. Operative time was significantly less in the AVS group compared with the control group (3.2 vs. 3.8 hours, $P < 0.01$).

Conclusion.—Use of AVS results in superior hemostatic effectiveness compared with Gelfoam Plus, with no difference in safety. Although no cost analysis was performed, cost savings likely resulted from significantly decreased operative time.

▶ Topical hemostatic agents are commonly used in the operating room during vascular (and other) procedures, either selectively or as a matter of routine, and may contribute to equipment costs but also may reduce overall costs by decreasing operating room time. Because there is little clinical evidence to support or guide topical hemostatic use, these agents represent a topic that is ripe for critical evaluation. Although these results suggest an advantage associated with use of ArterX Vascular Sealant relative to Gelfoam Plus, several aspects of this study make it challenging to draw definitive conclusions from the results. Use of anticoagulation medications were not included among the descriptive statistics or accounted for in the randomization scheme, and lack of a standardized protocol for administration or reversal of intraoperative anticoagulation may have introduced bias because of variability in these factors given the nonblinded study design. The definition of a significant bleeding event used by the authors would also potentially include bleeding resulting from technical factors (eg, a gap in an anastomosis), some of which would not be expected to seal with any topical agent. Finally, the results include more than 20 statistical comparisons, but the significance criteria are not adjusted for multiple testing. Despite these limitations, this study suggests that the novel sealant may reduce operating room time through more rapid hemostasis. It may be that the true utility of these agents will ultimately be determined by the relative costs of their administration compared with the savings achieved through reduced procedure duration.

M. A. Corriere, MD, MS

Therapeutic angiogenesis in patients with severe limb ischemia by transplantation of a combination stem cell product
Lasala GP, Silva JA, Minguell JJ (TCA Cellular Therapy, Covington, LA)
J Thorac Cardiovasc Surg 144:377-382, 2012

Objective.—Angiogenesis involves the interplay of endothelial progenitor cells, pericytes, growth factors, and cellular matrix components. The use of mesenchymal stem cells, which are closely related to pericytes and produce diverse angiogenic growth factors and matrix molecules, seems to be a promising therapeutic modality. We postulate that the use of a combination cell product (mesenchymal stem cells in conjunction with a source of endothelial progenitor cells) is safe and efficient and may optimize the clinical results obtained with the use of endothelial progenitor cells alone. This study assessed whether the intramuscular infusion of a combination cell product represents a viable, effective, and lasting therapeutic modality to improve perfusion in severely ischemic limbs.

Methods.—Patients with limb ischemia (n = 26) received an intramuscular (gastrocnemius) infusion of the combination cell product in the most ischemic leg and a placebo product in the (less ischemic) contralateral leg. Clinical follow-up (months 0.5, 1, 2, and 4 postinfusion) included evaluation of pain-free walking time, ankle-brachial index, perfusion scintigraphy, and quality of life survey.

Results.—No adverse events occurred after infusion. Efficacy assessment indicated that after cell infusion there was a significant improvement in walking time and ankle-brachial index. In addition, technetium-99m-tetrofosmin scintigraphy demonstrated a significant increase of perfusion in the treated limbs compared with the respective control legs.

Conclusions.—This phase II clinical trial shows that the use of a combination cell therapy is safe and effective in increasing blood flow in the ischemic legs of patients with limb ischemia.

▶ Angiogenesis, presumably from bone marrow (BM)—derived endothelial progenitor cells (EPC), was originally pursued by Judah Folkman et al when studying childhood vascular malformations in the 1990s. Improvements in cell harvest and identification have led to the emerging efforts at therapeutic angiogenesis in the current era, and the work of Dr Lasala represents some of the first steps in the transition from bench to bedside. Not uncommon in the biological therapy realm, the authors have financial interest in favorable outcomes given their stock investment in the sponsor of the work. The trial design is predicated on BM harvest of mesenchymal stem cells and mononuclear stem cells, the latter a source of EPCs. Harvest to expansion to injection took 24 days on average, and the stem cells were not labeled to determine trafficking before injection. The less-affected extremity was injected with the cell media. The authors appreciated a minimal 0.15 average increase in ankle-brachial index (ABI) and 3-fold walking distance increase on the treated legs. Because the results are predicated on entirely noninvasive metrics, we are left with more questions than the studied answers: Are blood vessels recruited by signals or created by EPC and new mesenchyme? Are the injected cells trafficking to the ischemic area or back to spleen and marrow to deliver signals in a paracrine fashion? How long can neovascularity last? So far, therapeutic angiogenesis has delivered the minimum significant ABI increase to the bedside, perhaps another generation of "back to the bench" will provide a better kick for sore legs.

J. Black, MD

Dynamic contrast-enhanced ultrasound and transient arterial occlusion for quantification of arterial perfusion reserve in peripheral arterial disease

Amarteifio E, Wormsbecher S, Krix M, et al (Univ Hosp of Heidelberg, Germany; et al)
Eur J Radiol 81:3332-3338, 2012

Objective.—To quantify muscular micro-perfusion and arterial perfusion reserve in peripheral arterial disease (PAD) with dynamic contrast-enhanced ultrasound (CEUS) and transient arterial occlusion.

Materials and Methods.—This study had local institutional review board approval and written informed consent was obtained from all subjects. We examined the dominant lower leg of 40 PAD Fontaine stage IIb patients (mean age, 65 years) and 40 healthy volunteers (mean age, 54 years) with CEUS (7 MHz; MI, 0.28) during continuous intravenous infusion of 4.8 mL microbubbles. Transient arterial occlusion at mid-thigh level simulated physical exercise. With time—CEUS—intensity curves obtained from regions of interest within calf muscles, we derived the maximum CEUS signal after occlusion (max) and its time (t_{max}), slope to maximum (m), vascular response after occlusion (AUC_{post}), and analysed accuracy, receiver operating characteristic (ROC) curves, and correlations with ankle-brachial index (ABI) and walking distance.

Results.—All parameters differed in PAD and volunteers $(p < 0.014)$. In PAD, t_{max} was delayed $(31.2 \pm 13.6$ vs. 16.7 ± 8.5 s, $p < 0.0001)$ and negatively correlated with ankle-brachial-index $(r = -0.65)$. m was

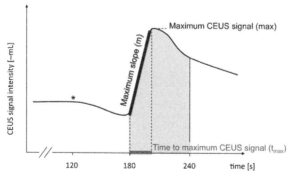

FIGURE 1.—Sketch of a contrast-enhanced ultrasound (CEUS) signal—intensity—time curve. CEUS of the gastrocnemius muscle starts at time 0 s. At 120 s, a steady state level of contrast media is reached. Arterial inflow to the calf is blocked with a conical cuff tied around the thigh after 120 s of continuous intravenous contrast media injection. Consecutively, the CEUS signal decreases (star). After 180 s, the arterial block is released, and the CEUS signal increases due to reactive hyperaemia. The maximum CEUS signal reached is called "max". The time interval from end of arterial block to maximum CEUS signal is called "t_{max}". The maximum slope of the CEUS curve between end of arterial block and maximum reached CEUS signal is called "m". The integral under the curve between end of arterial block (at 180 s) and 240 s is called "AUC_{post}". (Reprinted from the European Journal of Radiology. Amarteifio E, Wormsbecher S, Krix M, et al. Dynamic contrast-enhanced ultrasound and transient arterial occlusion for quantification of arterial perfusion reserve in peripheral arterial disease. *Eur J Radiol.* 2012;81:3332-3338, Copyright 2012, with permission from Elsevier.)

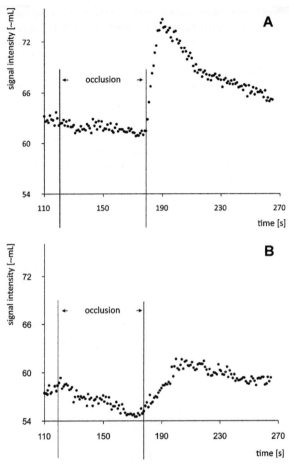

FIGURE 4.—Representative examples of signal—intensity—time curves obtained from dynamic contrast-enhanced ultrasound (CEUS) examinations: a rapid increase in the measured CEUS signal is observed after release of arterial occlusion in a 58-year old healthy male volunteer (A), while the time—intensity curve of a 55-year-old man with peripheral arterial disease (walking distance, 130 m) increases less rapid with a delayed and lower maximum after provocation (B). (Reprinted from the European Journal of Radiology. Amarteifio E, Wormsbecher S, Krix M, et al. Dynamic contrast-enhanced ultrasound and transient arterial occlusion for quantification of arterial perfusion reserve in peripheral arterial disease. *Eur J Radiol.* 2012;81:3332-3338, Copyright 2012, with permission from Elsevier.)

decreased in PAD (4.3 ± 4.6 mL/s vs. 13.1 ± 8.4 mL/s, $p < 0.0001$) and had highest diagnostic accuracy (sensitivity/specificity, 75%/93%) for detection of diminished muscular micro-perfusion in PAD (cut-off value, $m < 5 \sim$ mL/s). Discriminant analysis and ROC curves revealed m, and AUC_{post} as optimal parameter combination for diagnosing PAD and therefore impaired arterial perfusion reserve.

Conclusions.—Dynamic CEUS with transient arterial occlusion quantifies muscular micro-perfusion and arterial perfusion reserve. The technique is accurate to diagnose PAD (Figs 1 and 4).

▶ This exploratory study quantifies muscular perfusion at the level of the microcirculation using dynamic contrast-enhanced ultrasound (CEUS) with transient arterial occlusion. The signal-intensity time curve (Fig 1), evaluating increases related to reactive hyperemia, generated several parameters useful in discriminating between individuals with peripheral arterial disease and healthy volunteers (Fig 4). The authors demonstrate proof of concept for assessment of muscular perfusion with this technique in the hands of expert operators with very specialized skills and experience. Although the authors focus on muscle perfusion in patients with intermittent claudication in this study, the technique does not localize occlusive lesions and seems more cumbersome than conventional pulse volume recordings; it is, therefore, unclear what CEUS would add to routine care of claudicants. Conversely, one could envision applications of CEUS for intra- or postoperative assessment of muscle flap reconstructions, compartment syndrome, or critical limb ischemia. It will be interesting to see what clinical niche this imaging modality occupies as it is further developed and standardized.

M. A. Corriere, MD, MS

Evolving Patterns of Vascular Surgery Care in the United States: A Report from the American Board of Surgery

Valentine RJ, Members of the Vascular Surgery Board of the American Board of Surgery (Univ of Texas Southwestern Med Ctr, Dallas; et al)
J Am Coll Surg 216:886-893, 2013

Background.—The purpose of this study was to analyze the distribution of major vascular procedures among general and vascular surgeons and to compare the evolution of vascular surgical practice of general and vascular surgeons at specific points in their careers.

Study Design.—Case logs of surgeons seeking recertification in surgery from 2007 to 2009 were reviewed. Data from 3,362 physicians certified only in surgery (GS) were compared with 363 additionally certified in vascular surgery (VS). Independent variables were compared using factorial ANOVA.

Results.—The mean numbers of major vascular procedures ($\pm$SD) were 10 $\pm$ 51 for GS and 192 $\pm$ 209 for VS ($p < 0.001$). Thirty-three percent of the total vascular procedures reported were performed by GS. Compared with VS, GS performed significantly fewer vascular procedures in all major procedure categories, and GS certifying at 10 years performed fewer vascular procedures (6.7 $\pm$ 47) than those recertifying at 20 years (11.5 $\pm$ 48) and 30 years (13.6 $\pm$ 59) ($p < 0.01$). In contrast, VS certifying at 10 years performed more vascular procedures (235 $\pm$ 237) compared with those recertifying at 20 years (157 $\pm$ 173) and 30 years (104 $\pm$ 115). The mean number of vascular procedures was not different for sex, geographic location, or practice type, after controlling for other variables in the study.

Conclusions.—The majority of GS currently do not perform any major vascular procedures, and younger GS are performing fewer such procedures than their older counterparts. The opposite is true for VS. These opposing trends indicate that vascular procedures are shifting from GS to VS in modern surgical practice, and this may have important implications for patient access to vascular surgery care, considering the limited capacity for VS to assume the excess case load.

▶ It is clear that there is an increasing chasm growing between vascular surgeons and general surgeons. The shift in techniques from open to endovascular has propelled our specialty into the stratosphere. The scope of work for all vascular surgeons has seen a coinciding increase. As a result, general surgery residents are getting less exposure to our specialty and feeling less competent in the care of vascular patients because of a lack of experience with endovascular skills. This very timely article by Valentine et al analyzes these evolving trends in vascular surgery care in the United States. Over the study period from 2007 to 2009, general surgeons performed only 33% of vascular surgery procedures compared with vascular surgeons (67%). The authors use self-reported case volumes from surgeons seeking American Board of Surgery recertification in surgery. This analysis shows that general surgeons' vascular surgery case volumes have greatly decreased over the last 30 years. In fact, they are seeing continuing declines in vascular surgery volumes by general surgeons 10 years out of practice compared with those 20 and 30 years out. In direct contrast, the authors found that the vascular surgery volumes of younger vascular surgeons are higher than those out of practice for longer periods. These results give the authors concern that there is likely to be a shortage of vascular surgeons over the next several years as the baby boomer generation ages. In addition, the care of the vascular patient in the rural setting will definitely be a challenge. The authors give no solutions but highlight that these findings will have important implications on the future care of the vascular patient.

D. L. Gillespie, MD, RVT, FACS

Inhibition of experimental neointimal hyperplasia and neoatherosclerosis by local, stent-mediated delivery of everolimus

Zhao HQ, Nikanorov A, Virmani R, et al (Abbott Laboratories, Abbott Park, IL; CVPath Inst, Inc, Gaithersburg, MD)
J Vasc Surg 56:1680-1688, 2012

Introduction.—A novel self-expanding, drug-eluting stent (DES) was designed to slowly release everolimus in order to prevent restenosis after percutaneous peripheral intervention. The purpose of this experimental animal study was to test the hypothesis that long-term local, stent-mediated delivery of everolimus would reduce neointimal hyperplasia in porcine iliac arteries.

Methods.—The iliac arteries of 24 Yucatan mini-swine were percutaneously treated with overlapping 8- × 28-mm self-expanding nitinol stents loaded with everolimus (225 µg/cm^2 stent surface area) formulated in a poly(ethylene-co-vinyl alcohol) copolymer intended to deliver the drug in a sustained fashion over about 6 months (DES). Bare nitinol self-expanding stents (bare metal stent [BMS]) were implanted in an identical fashion on the contralateral side to serve as controls. After 3, 6, or 12 months, the animals were sacrificed and the stented arteries perfusion-fixed for histomorphometric analysis.

Results.—The chronic presence of everolimus in arterial tissue reduced stent-induced inflammation after 3 months (inflammation score: BMS 2.29 ± 0.44 vs DES 0.17 ± 0.17; $P = .001$) and 6 months (BMS 2.06 ± 0.43 vs DES 0.50 ± 0.5; $P = .007$), although some late inflammation was observed after drug exhaustion (BMS 1.00 ± 0.25 vs DES 2.56 ± 0.62 after 12 months; $P = $ not significant [NS]). Treatment with locally delivered everolimus significantly reduced neointimal hyperplasia after 3 months (neointimal thickness: BMS 0.79 ± 0.20 vs DES 0.37 ± 0.04 mm; $P = .03$) and 6 months (BMS 0.73 ± 0.14 vs DES 0.41 ± 0.08 mm; $P = .05$), although the effect had dissipated after 12 months (BMS 0.68 ± 0.11 vs DES 0.67 ± 0.11 mm; $P = $ NS). Remarkably, stent-induced neoatherosclerosis, characterized by the histologic presence of foamy macrophages and cholesterol clefts, was significantly attenuated by treatment with everolimus (atherogenic change scores at 3 months: BMS 0.56 ± 0.15 vs DES 0.04 ± 0.04; $P = .003$; 6 months: BMS 0.84 ± 0.23 vs DES 0.00 ± 0.00; $P = .004$; and 12 months: BMS 0.09 ± 0.10 vs DES 0.19 ± 0.19; $P = $ NS).

Conclusions.—In this experimental animal model, local arterial stent-mediated delivery of everolimus inhibited the formation of neointimal hyperplasia and neoatherosclerosis during the first 6 months. The effect was transient, however, as arterial morphology and histology appeared similar to control stented arteries after 12 months.

▶ Percutaneous coronary intervention with stenting is the most common procedure for the treatment of symptomatic coronary and peripheral artery disease; however, 30% to 50% of stent-based coronary and peripheral interventions will fail during the first year because of the development of neointimal hyperplasia and restenosis. The introduction of drug-eluting stents (DES) has contributed a major breakthrough to medical technology in relation to coronary artery disease, but they have yet to be shown to be truly effective in the treatment of all peripheral artery disease. The purpose of this experimental study was to test the hypothesis that a peripheral DES with a relatively high drug dose and prolonged elution profile would inhibit neointimal hyperplasia in a long-term porcine model of percutaneous peripheral intervention. The results were extremely promising during the first 6 months after stenting, which showed that neointimal hyperplasia and neoatherosclerosis were reduced in the presence of everolimus, an antiproliferative drug. However, 12 months after stenting, there was no difference when the coated stents were compared with the bare metal stents. Despite the absence of an effect at 12 months, these results still show great initial promise to prevent stent failure in the treatment of peripheral artery disease. As the authors discuss, the development of DES for the peripheral is more challenging than for the coronary arteries, and the efficacy of these devices may improve with better drug delivery and elution profiles.

J. Cullen, PhD

Description and outcomes of a simple surgical technique to treat thrombosed autogenous accesses
Cull DL, Washer JD, Carsten CG, et al (Univ of South Carolina School of Medicine-Greenville)
J Vasc Surg 56:861-865, 2012

Objective.—Owing to the difficulty of removing acute and chronic thrombus from autogenous accesses (AA) by standard surgical and endovascular techniques, many surgeons consider efforts to salvage a thrombosed AA as being futile. We describe a simple technique to extract acute and chronic thrombus from a failed AA. This technique involves making an incision adjacent to the anastomosis, directly extracting the arterial plug, and manually milking thrombus from the access. This report details the outcomes of a series of thrombosed AAs treated by surgical thrombectomy/intervention using this technique for manual clot extraction.

Methods.—A total of 146 surgical thrombectomies/interventions were performed in 102 patients to salvage a thrombosed AA. Mean follow-up was 15.6 months. Office, hospital, and dialysis unit records were reviewed to identify patient demographics, define procedure type, and determine functional patency rates. Kaplan-Meier survival analysis was used to estimate primary and secondary functional patency rates.

Results.—Complete extraction of thrombus from the AA was achieved in 140 of 146 cases (95%). The studied procedure itself was technically successful in 127 cases (87%). Reasons for failure were the inability to completely extract thrombus from the AA in six, failed angioplasty due to long segment vein stenosis or sclerosis in seven or vein rupture in two, and central vein occlusion in one. Three failures occurred for unknown causes ≤ 3 days of successful thrombectomy. No single factor analyzed (age, sex, race, diabetes status, access type or location) was associated with technical failure. The estimated primary and secondary functional patency rates were 27% ± 5% and 61% ± 6% at 12 months.

Conclusions.—The manual clot extraction technique described in this report effectively removed acute and chronic thrombus from failed AAs. Its use, combined with an intervention to treat the underlying cause for AA failure, significantly extended access durability.

▶ Many of us were trained NOT to intervene in attempts to salvage thrombosed autogenous hemodialysis access sites. The standard consensus has always been that such attempts would be unsuccessful even in the short term and to proceed with creating a completely new access site. Providing an autogenous hemodialysis access is the ultimate goal with a target of 66% set by the Fistula First Breakthrough Initiative. Thus a new yet simple technique for fistula salvage should be welcomed with enthusiasm by those of us who perform access procedures.

The group from Greenville, SC, has written and presented extensively on creation, maintenance, and salvage of autogenous access sites. They have excellent outcomes and meticulously refine their techniques as needed in continual quality improvement. Their work should be read and incorporated into a vascular access practice in salvaging both acute and chronically thrombosed autogenous fistulae. Rather than incorporating newer percutaneous techniques, this group uses standard open thrombectomy and manual clot extraction to clear the fistula. They follow up with a completion fistulogram to identify and treat any stenoses that may be present and contributing to fistula failure. Even chronically thrombosed and aneurysmal fistulae can be salvaged with their technique, which is especially successful if occluded for less than 2 weeks. Over this time, they do not recommend intervention because of very low success rates.

I commend the group for going against conventional thinking concerning the futility of thrombectomy of autogenous access and demonstrating successful salvage and improved utilization of native arteriovenous fistula.

R. L. Bush, MD, MPH

The influence of metabolic syndrome on hemodialysis access patency
Protack CD, Jain A, Vasilas P, et al (Yale Univ School of Medicine, New Haven, CT; VA Connecticut Healthcare System, West Haven, CT)
J Vasc Surg 56:1656-1662, 2012

Objective.—The natural history of patients with metabolic syndrome (MetS) undergoing hemodialysis access placement is unknown. MetS has previously been found as a risk factor for poor outcomes for vascular surgery patients undergoing other interventions. The aim of this is study is to describe the outcomes of MetS patients undergoing primary hemodialysis access placement.

Methods.—The medical records of the 187 patients who underwent hemodialysis access placement between 1999 and 2009 at the Veterans Administration Connecticut Healthcare System were reviewed. Survival, primary patency, and secondary patency were evaluated using the Gehan-Breslow test for survival. MetS was defined as the presence of three or more of the following: blood pressure $< 130/90$ mm Hg; triglycerides < 150 mg/dL; high-density lipoprotein ≤ 50 mg/dL for women and ≤ 40 mg/dL for men; body mass index < 30 kg/m^2; or fasting blood glucose < 110 mg/dL.

Results.—Of the 187 patients who underwent hemodialysis access placement, 115 (61%) were identified to have MetS. The distribution of MetS factors among all patients was hypertension in 98%, diabetes in 58%, elevated triclyceride in 39%, decreased high-density lipoprotein in 60%, elevated body mass index in 36%, and 39% were currently receiving hemodialysis. Patients were a mean age of 66 years. The median length of follow-up was 4.2 years. The forearm was site of fistula placement in 53%; no difference existed between groups (MetS, 57%; no MetS, 50%; $P=.388$). The median time to primary failure was 0.46 years for all patients (MetS, 0.555 years; no MetS, 0.436 years; $P=.255$). Secondary patency was 50% at 1.18 years for all patients (no MetS, 1.94 years; MetS, 0.72 years; $P=.024$). Median survival duration for all patients was 4.15 years (no MetS, 5.07 years; MetS, 3.63 years; $P=.019$).

Conclusions.—MetS is prevalent among patients undergoing hemodialysis access placement. Patients with MetS have equivalent primary patency rates; however, their survival and cumulative patency rates are significantly lower than in patients without MetS. Patients with MetS form a high-risk group that needs intensive surveillance protocols.

▶ Many of us who perform surgical procedures to establish access for hemodialysis do not pay much attention to the overall general health of our patients beyond what is necessary for safe anesthesia. This article is a must-read to point out that we should indeed consider the effects of metabolic syndrome on our outcomes in patients with renal dysfunction. Patients with renal dysfunction are highly likely to have metabolic syndrome with its associated prothrombotic and proinflammatory states. Abnormalities in lipid levels and diabetes mellitus are known risk factors for access failure. The presence of metabolic syndrome (MetS) will only compound these factors, leading to unfavorable outcomes after hemodialysis access procedures. Perhaps the surgeon should consider either delaying an elective access procedure until the patient is medically optimized or instituting a more intensive surveillance protocol.

These authors found 61% of their patients who had access procedures to have MetS. Although maturation and primary patency rates were equivalent, the secondary patency rate was much lower in the MetS group. This led the authors to the appropriate conclusion: Although we may not be able to influence the physiologic impact of MetS, this high-risk group should have frequent surveillance of their access site to identify needs for early intervention or revision. I would also encourage early referrals for fistula creation in those patients for whom dialysis is imminent but not immediate. In our practice, the nephrologists refer patients with chronic kidney disease very early, sometimes 6 to 12 months before the need for dialysis is predicted. This allows time for medical and surgical planning, the unfortunate but expected access failures, and lack of fistula maturation.

R. L. Bush, MD, MPH

Frequency of Coronary Artery Disease in Patients Undergoing Peripheral Artery Disease Surgery

Hur DJ, Kizilgul M, Aung WW, et al (Univ of Virginia, Charlottesville)
Am J Cardiol 110:736-740, 2012

The prevalence of coronary artery disease (CAD) in patients with peripheral arterial disease (PAD) varies widely in published reports. This is likely due at least in part to significant differences in how PAD and CAD were both defined and diagnosed. In this report, the investigators describe 78 patients with PAD who underwent preoperative coronary angiography before elective peripheral revascularization and provide a review of published case series. Among the patients included, the number with concomitant CAD varied from 55% in those with lower-extremity stenoses to as high as 80% in those with carotid artery disease. The number of coronary arteries narrowed by $\geq 50\%$ was 1 in 28%, 2 in 24%, and 3 in 19%; 28% did not have any angiographic evidence of CAD. The review of published research resulted in the identification of 19 case series in which a total of 3,969 patients underwent preoperative coronary angiography before elective PAD surgery; in the 2,687 who were described according to the location of the PAD, 55% had ≥ 1 epicardial coronary artery with $\geq 70\%$ diameter narrowing. The highest prevalence of concomitant CAD was in patients with severe carotid artery disease (64%). In conclusion, despite sharing similar risk factors, the prevalence of obstructive CAD in patients with PAD ranges widely and appears to differ across PAD locations. Thus, the decision to perform coronary angiography should be based on indications independent of the planned PAD surgery.

▶ Preoperative stratification of cardiovascular risk before vascular surgery has taken a truly nihilistic turn since the publication of the CARP (Coronary Artery Revascularization Prophylaxis) trial demonstrated no improvement in myocardial infarction and cardiovascular death whether or not a strategy of preoperative coronary vascularization was used. These authors actually support the CARP contention because they discovered only 19% of the patients had 3-vessel coronary disease. But the import of this study fuels the flame of a last unanswered issue in vascular surgery—the utility of carotid revascularization with coronary bypass surgery. The authors thoroughly review the extant data and series, and the novelty of their study emerges in that the highest incidence of concomitant coronary disease is appreciated in the carotid disease patients (72%). Interestingly, the "other" category had a slightly higher risk, but it was limited by the multiple territories included. I do not suspect the impact of this series to echo very far, yet if one were to contemplate use of combined carotid endarterectomy with coronary artery bypass graft, this article suggests a benefit lies therein.

J. Black, MD

Diagnostic criteria for renovascular disease: where are we now?
Herrmann SMS, Textor SC (Mayo Clinic, Rochester, MI)
Nephrol Dial Transplant 27:2657-2663, 2012

Renovascular disease, especially atherosclerotic renal artery stenosis (ARAS) in older subjects, is commonly encountered in clinical practice. This is at least in part due to the major advances in non-invasive imaging techniques that allow greater diagnostic sensitivity and accuracy than ever before. Despite increased awareness of ARAS, renal revascularization is less commonly performed, likely as a result of several prospective, randomized, clinical trials which fail to demonstrate major benefits of renal revascularization beyond medical therapy alone. Primary care physicians are less likely to investigate renovascular disease and nephrologists likely see more patients after a period of unsuccessful medical therapy with more advanced ARAS. The goal of this review is to revisit current diagnostic and therapeutic paradigms in order to characterize more clearly which patients will likely benefit from further evaluation and intensive treatment of renal artery stenosis.

▶ There definitely has been a decrease among vascular interventionalists in regard to percutaneous renal artery angioplasty and stenting over the past several years. This is mainly because of several excellent studies that failed to demonstrate any advantage over intervention in most patients compared with best medical therapy alone. Importantly, data and details are needed to specifically define which patients would actually benefit from intervention before they are at an advanced stage of chronic renal insufficiency or refractory renovascular hypertension. At this point, intervention may be performed but may not impact positively on renal function if done too late. This article addresses specifically how to determine which patients are failing medical therapy with moderate to severe renal artery stenosis and how to establish that renal artery stenosis is indeed present and treatable.

This article provides good overviews of both clinical and diagnostic imaging criteria for pursuing the diagnosis of renovascular hypertension. This is often-tested information on the vascular surgery in-training and certification/recertification examinations and because it is not a common clinical entity seen in practice, this is a must-read for trainees and attendings alike. Details of the Duplex imaging criteria as well as technical tips for technicians are given. The authors also review when to consider intervention on persons failing medical therapy or with progressive deterioration of renal function should raise a level of suspicion for correctable renovascular disease. Of course, the shorter the duration of medical management failure, the better the outcome will be following vascular intervention. Staying in touch with your nephrologists will ensure timely identification of patients who will be the most beneficial.

R. L. Bush, MD, MPH

Article Index

Chapter 1: Basic Considerations

Chapter 2: Epidemiology

Chapter 3: Vascular Laboratory and Imaging

Chapter 4: Perioperative Considerations

Chapter 5: Grafts and Graft Complications

Chapter 6: Aortic Aneurysm

Chapter 7: Abdominal Aortic Endografting

Chapter 8: Thoracic Aorta

Chapter 9: Aortoiliac Disease and Leg Ischemia

Chapter 10: Upper Extremity Ischemia/Dialysis Access

Chapter 11: Carotid and Cerebrovascular Disease

Chapter 12: Vascular Trauma

Chapter 13: Venous Thrombosis and Pulmonary Embolism

Chapter 14: Chronic Venous and Lymphatic Disease

Chapter 15: Technical Notes

Chapter 16: Miscellaneous

Author Index

Printed and bound by CPI Group (UK) Ltd, Croydon, CR0 4YY

08/05/2025

01864755-0008